Gary Null's Guide to a

Joyful, Healthy

Life

Also by Gary Null

Complete Guide to Sensible Eating
Complete Guide to Health and Nutrition
Alcohol and Nutrition
Man and His Whole Earth
Why Your Stomach Hurts
The Joy of Juicing
The Egg Project
Good Food, Good Mood
Healing Your Body Naturally
Healing with Magnets
No More Allergies
Reverse the Aging Process Naturally
Nutrition and the Mind
Supercharge Your Health
Ultimate Training
How to Rid Your Body of Poisons
Gary Null's International Vegetarian Cookbook
Gary Null's Ultimate Aging Program
Change Your Life Now
The '90s Healthy Body Book
The Women's Encyclopedia of Natural Healing
The Clinician's Handbook of Natural Healing
The Complete Encyclopedia of Natural Healing
Vegetarian Handbook
Secrets of the Sacred White Buffalo
Get Healthy Now

Gary Null's Guide to a

Joyful, Healthy
Life

Gary Null, Ph.D.

CARROLL & GRAF PUBLISHERS
NEW YORK

GARY NULL'S GUIDE TO A JOYFUL, HEALTHY LIFE

Carroll & Graf Publishers
An Imprint of Avalon Publishing Group Incorporated
161 William Street, 16th Floor
New York, NY 10038

Copyright © 2000 by Gary Null, Ph.D.

First Carroll & Graf cloth edition 2000
First Carroll & Graf trade paperback edition 2002

Library of Congress Cataloging-in-Publication Data is available.

ISBN: 0-7867-0994-4

Printed in the United States of America
Distributed by Publishers Group West

The author would like to thank the following people:
Vicki Riba Koestler, Bob Marty, and Mitchell Waters.

Contents

*Co-authored with Vickie Riba Koestler

Preface

The three books included together in this volume provide all the guideposts required in your life journey to personal enrichment and spiritual happiness.

While all three books were written with the same objective—to enable readers to achieve a wholeness and wellness of being—only in the time since their publication has their relationship to one another become fully and organically apparent. Each book, in fact, comprises a guide to your completion of an essential phase in the total and always ongoing process of self-realization. Requisite to this process is the creative use of your life energy. Energy enables and empowers.

Energy is also commonly obstructed, generally with negative effects, and usually by the very selves we optimistically set out to improve. To discover and free your energy, then to channel it creatively, often demands radical measures. Old habits of mind die hard. Consider the thousands upon thousands of people—you may be one of them—who conscientiously pursue self-improvement. They go on a weekend retreat, attending the inspirational words of a charismatic teacher, seeking psychic peace and mental happiness. With renewed spirit and new resolve, they return home to their everyday lives. And too soon their fresh perspective and vigorous resolution dissolve in the face of old problems. They can't effectively adopt and implement new constructs for being because they are still trapped in their old ones. A weekend of self-examination and self-exploration cannot undo a lifetime of conditioning.

Patterns, though, can be broken, and mindsets can be altered. Personal behavior does not have to be limited by such negative components as overdeveloped feelings of inadequacy or over-imagined guilts and fears. Nor should it be. The past may have molded us but it should not imprison us. It should be examined, and challenged, so that the ghosts that haunt and inhibit our evolvement into secure, happily adjusted human beings can be banished.

Easier said than done, you may say. But, as the books in this comprehensive guide demonstrate, the pathway to mental, physical, and spiritual well-being can be simply traveled.

The journey takes you first to the center of yourself, to realize the natural life energy that defines yourself, and then enables you to use that energy not only to empower yourself but also to embrace joyfully the world beyond yourself. Your answer to the question that titles the first book in the volume— *Who Are You, Really?*—will clarify the specific nature of your life energy and discuss the particular ways it can be effectively implemented, whether you design airplanes, file court records, wash dishes, sing opera, teach kindergarten, repair watches, sell real estate, or make movies. The second book, with its encouraging title *Be Kind to Yourself*, proceeds from self-discovery to self-exploration as it offers practical strategies for self-empowerment. Step by simple step, it shows you how to deal efficiently with such issues as eliminating self-defeating habits, developing autonomy, letting go of internalized pain, and making healthy new beginnings. The third book, *Choosing Joy*, makes manifest the possibilities of emotional fulfillment, intellectual stimulation, physical fitness, and spiritual solace that lie in the nurture and growth of a new, positively realized self.

In all, this volume maps the journey to a happy, healthy future. Use it to build your bridge to personal well-being in the twenty-first century.

How To Use This Book

Most of us know that life is a journey, but at any given stage of life, we may not have a clear perspective on where we are on the road to personal growth—emotionally, spiritually, intellectually and physically. *Gary Null's Guide to a Joyful, Healthy Life* is designed to help you determine where you are today and what you need to do to achieve personal fulfillment.

As you read through each section, you will be asked to consider a wide variety of questions about your life. The objective is to delve into your personal experiences, identify your true needs and discover what is meaningful to you. This process will require you to think through many of your life experiences, both negative and joyful. It will encourage you to see who you really are so that you can express that self to the world.

Keep a pen and a notebook with you as you use this book, and take the time to make written notes of your answers to the questions. There is room to jot down notes and lists on the margins of the pages. For more detailed answers, keep a journal. You will find that the questions which are most meaningful to you will stimulate you to write your ideas at length.

I believe that writing about yourself is indispensable to personal development. By making the time to keep a journal, and thinking through what you plan to write, you will stimulate the process of growth and change. With every question you consider, you set into motion a dialogue with your inner self. It is a purely introspective process—one that honestly reflects your feelings without the interference of outside influences.

This is not to say that other approaches to self-expression, such as talking to a counselor or a friend, are not viable as well. However, I truly believe that the first step toward personal development is to get in touch with your own feelings. After all, no one knows you as well as you know yourself.

Throughout this book I ask you to assess both your positive and negative qualities. To benefit from the process, you must be honest with yourself. Only then will you be able to eliminate negative behavior and identify the positive attributes that deserve more of your time and energy. This process, in turn, will allow you to steer your life in a more constructive direction.

The process of personal growth is certainly not easy. What's easy is to lose sight of your real needs, stagnate in your growth, and experience more of the same each day. It takes courage, resolve and a commitment of time and energy to make positive changes in your life and stimulate your growth. It is hard but ultimately rewarding work, and I welcome you to the challenge.

Who Are You, Really?

Understanding Your Life's Energy

Here, Gary Null shares his insights into the power of our natural life energy (NLE), that accompanied his spiritual reawakening one star-studded night in the Arizona desert. Redefining human behavior patterns in terms of the NLE that characterizes and motivates all of us, he presents a spectrum of seven distinct personality types that ranges from the Dynamic Aggressives (The Ultimate Go-Getters) to the Adaptive Supportives (Most of the People You'll Ever Meet). In the terms of this spectrum, readers can not only identify the attributes that constitute their essential selves, but also clarify their relationships with other types, thus bringing harmony into their own, and others', lives.

Contents

Introduction

Several years ago, when I least expected it, life did an about-face, and I found myself needing to make a radical shift in my whole way of thinking and living. Within a few days, everything I had worked for and, more dismayingly, everything I had thought I was, were called into question. It started one evening, at the end of a weekly class on nutrition I taught to a large group of students in Manhattan. My brother and I were discussing the class after everyone else had left.

"They're not getting it, Gary," my brother observed as we walked to the car. "The same people show up week after week, year after year, but nothing changes. The fat people haven't lost weight, the hyper ones haven't calmed down, the stress cases haven't relaxed. I don't think they're changing their diets at all. In fact, some of them head straight for McDonald's when your talk is over and load up on junk."

I stopped in my tracks, dumbfounded. It wasn't that all this was new to me—I'd basically known it subconsciously because

I'd been seeing it—but this was the first time the whole picture had crystallized, perhaps because someone had verbalized it. Here I had dedicated my entire working life to helping people change their lives for the better, and my brother could see the terrible truth that I had failed to consciously grasp: I wasn't making a difference—not even for those who personally attended those weekly sessions. It was shocking. How could I have missed it?

I was, by then, twenty years into my career as a health educator and had become very well known. My daily afternoon show enjoyed the largest radio audience in America in my time slot; my books on nutrition and health had been on the bestseller lists; I was much sought after as a lecturer. And all along, the idea that I had been making a difference had been the great motivating factor that had kept me working very hard. I had always operated under the assumption that I had a real mission in life—to find out the truth about health and stay healthy. I took great satisfaction from fulfilling what I considered my important, worthwhile function in society.

Now it seemed that my bright dream lay shattered at my feet under the dim light of the corner streetlamp. I didn't know which way to turn—an unfamiliar, highly disturbing feeling for me, who had always been so sure of things.

Maybe I didn't belong in the health field. Perhaps I should change careers, follow other interests. I blamed myself for not seeing the obvious. Maybe I was just too idealistic; maybe I should be satisfied to be like other nutritionists I knew who dispensed advice for years while indulging all the while in unhealthful habits such as smoking and drinking. No, I had too much integrity for that—I'd always put into practice in my own life the health rules I'd advocated. As the shock began to subside, I started to wonder about my audience. It just didn't make sense. I knew that they were intelligent. So why had they failed to take all the information they had received and apply it to making positive changes in their lives? What is there about people that keeps them from acting in their own best interests—even when they show up week after week to learn what to do? There didn't seem to be an answer.

I'd made a deep study of psychology and had delved into more arcane systems for understanding personality, character, and human behavior, but I was still at a loss to explain what was going on with my students, and I felt anxious and confused. The next morning I was up at the crack of dawn, knowing that I had to get away, to think, to be alone for a few days. It didn't matter where I went; I'd just take the first plane I could to get out of New York after my midday broadcast.

Luckily, the first plane with an empty seat was headed for Arizona, and the desert has always been a special place for me. On the cross-country flight I kept puzzling about those students of natural health who ran around the corner for fast food the minute class was out. Some of them had been coming for years and could easily have passed a master's-level test in nutrition.

As the plane flew westward my mind was working full-time, flooded with memories of other incidents when people's behavior had surprised me. On one occasion I'd invited several friends to my farm in upstate New York for a weekend. Because I was busy in the city until late on Friday, I couldn't arrive ahead of the guests to take care of preparations. I didn't worry about it, though. There were just everyday things to do—putting away the groceries that had been ordered, making dinner, bedding down the animals in the barn. The caretaker always left early on Fridays, but my friends would figure it out. The group of friends I'd invited up the previous month had taken care of everything without being told. They'd started a roaring fire in the fireplace, made a great dinner, taken the goats into the barn, and had the bedrooms ready to sleep in. They'd even chipped in to pay for the groceries, presenting me with a bowlful of tens and twenties when I arrived. We'd had a great time. I was looking forward to another pleasant weekend with this new group.

But when finally I arrived, at about ten o'clock, I found utter chaos. The boxes of food the organic food co-op had delivered were still on the porch; no one had put anything away. Fresh linens were available in neat piles in the laundry room, but no one had made a bed. The animals were loose in the yard, running around hungry, but the guests hadn't even made dinner for themselves, much less fed the animals. How could they just sit there when there were so many simple, obvious things that needed attention? Why hadn't someone taken charge? I had no answers to that puzzle either.

No use dwelling on the problems, I reminded myself as the plane started its descent. I knew that the time had come to stop trying to figure things out. I've always believed that if you send your questions out to the universe, your answer will come. Sometimes it comes in an unexpected form before you even formulate your questions. I needed the stillness the desert would provide. I settled back in my seat, feeling confident now that I was on the right track. Sooner or later, the answers would come.

By the time we'd landed and I'd rented a car, the sun was beginning to set, and the heat of the day was subsiding. I drove out of town, toward some distant mountains, enjoying the sight of the desert changing color as the golden light gave way to dusky shadows. As night fell, I pulled to a stop, parked the car, and climbed to the top of a mesa. I was surrounded by stars, above me and on every side. It was mesmerizing.

I sat in the desert all night, in what might be called an altered state of consciousness, oblivious to everything around me. I gave no thought to tarantulas or fire ants or scorpions or rattlesnakes or any of the other dangers I'd learned about as a Boy Scout. There were millions of stars, and I felt safe there, peaceful and at one with the universe. I know that many people have had similar moments on clear nights when they experienced timelessness—they could have been at any point in history, a hundred, a thousand, or ten thousand years back, looking at the same panorama, having the same feelings. My anxiety left and I stayed there all night, enjoying a sense of unity with nature.

As the night wore on, I became more and more absorbed in

the totality of the universe. I lost track of my problems and why I had come. I simply gave up my ego and listened to the silence, and as I did, I became increasingly aware of the magnificent overriding harmony of life. I felt that I was having a spiritual reawakening.

Insights began to arise within me, about the nature of human beings and our special, individual places in the universe. I understood how interrelated we are with one another, how each of us has a certain natural energy that is there for the good of the whole. Some people's energy impels them to change—to change their own circumstances and lifestyles, to change their communities, even to change the world. Some people's energy, by contrast, is channeled into adapting to what exists, and even nurturing it. Some people can naturally, and with ease, assert what they believe in, some to the point that they become leaders of others. Some people never lead; they just don't have that energy within them. But they can do the valuable work of supporting other people and enterprises, and the quality of their support can be extraordinary, of a caliber that the leaders would not be capable of.

So was one type of natural life energy better than another? Well, perhaps from my point of view when I had arrived at the farm that night and found the place in disarray, a guest or two with the dynamic, take-charge kind of energy would have been nice. But wasn't that idea really shortsighted, even selfish? After all, think of all the vital parts of society that are kept running day to day by the adaptive, supportive energies of nonleaders: farms, hospitals, stores, banks, factories. . . .

As I became immersed in that state of receptivity that allows inspiration to flow, I sensed that it was time to broaden my perspective on human behavior. People's natural life energies were too diverse to expect anyone to behave in any particular way. Perhaps the important thing was whether a person was living up to the highest potential for her or his type of energy.

At the first light of dawn, I looked around, and not too far from me was a woman, sitting very still, facing the lightest part of the sky, where the sun would soon rise. I got up and walked over to her slowly, and as I approached I realized she was an Indian, quite old, though how old I couldn't say. The deep lines etched in her face by the sun made her look ninety, although she might have been only sixty. She had the timeless quality of the stars above, still in evidence in the early light of dawn.

Thinking I might be on her land, I started to say I was sorry to have imposed, but my words seemed not to matter. She looked at me kindly and asked, "Have you found what you came for?"

"Yes, more than I could ever have hoped for," I responded. "This has been a very short journey for me, but perhaps the most significant I have ever taken."

She gestured with her hand out over the landscape where there was nothing but empty mountains and desert. "When you have nothing to lose, then everything is yours to enjoy."

I didn't know in what context she meant that, so I said, "I've made my life about acquiring knowledge and sharing that knowledge."

The woman looked at me again and said something that startled me and enabled me to see my life from a whole new perspective. "Knowledge is the most important gift you must learn to let go of."

I understood immediately. I had thought that as long as I brought people knowledge, they would use it—facts and blueprints for change that they said they wanted for their ailments—their arthritis, depression, cancer, insomnia. I really believed in the hundredth-monkey syndrome—that when enough people believe in something new and better and do something to actualize it, there's a general shift in the consciousness of the populace at large. Marilyn Ferguson had said it in *The Aquarian Conspiracy*; Herman Kahn said it in a slightly different way: When the critical mass shifts, the paradigm shifts. Believing in these notions, I had thought I could help change things by educating people to adopt a healthier, more spiritual life.

Now, as this Indian woman's simple words sank in— "Knowledge is the most important gift you must learn to let go of"—I realized that there had been no paradigm shift, there had never been a quantitative spiritual change in the consciousness of most Americans. I had been operating on a false premise, thinking I could transmit data and change some destructive habits in the world. I knew in a second that I had to give up all my knowledge, release everything that I'd felt offered me intellectual certainty, and become a student again. The difference between the facts and the truth became very clear to me. The facts, which I had been dispensing right and left, were not the answer. I felt humble, intellectually naked. I was very thankful to the universe for all the insights into human nature it had inspired in me, and grateful to the Indian woman with her deep, intuitive wisdom. I knew I must begin again, on a new and different path. There was a lot of work ahead, many changes to be made. But I had a clear vision now of the dynamic workings of human nature, and knew what I must do to fulfill my highest potential in the great scheme of things. I couldn't just think my thoughts anymore; I had to live them. And that meant I had to change.

My first day back in the studio I made some radical changes in my program and in the way I dealt with my audience. I went on the air and really got honest. I told my audience that I couldn't help them anymore. They had been calling in because they wanted instantaneous cures for their sicknesses. But I knew that they were not using the information I was providing—some of them might have called in fifty times with questions about their arthritis, but they still had it. So I refused to give another sixty-or ninety-second answer to a question. I just couldn't dispense another fact or figure. Then I told the audience that I was turning the tables on them—instead of my getting a rating as a broadcaster, I was rating them as an audience, and they rated a zero. They were just not living up to their potential. I had been honoring them as if they were trying to be healthy, but they were working very hard at being sick.

The station manager and program director were frantically gesturing from the control room. They thought I had really gone over the edge. Of course, they decided to fire me. That would take several months, because I had a full roster of sponsors, so my program stayed on the air in the meantime. My ratings plummeted into oblivion. Before, I had received as many as twenty-five thousand phone calls during a one-hour show, which is a phenomenal number of calls. Once the telephone company circuits had actually blown out with all the busy signals they had to give. But now I was getting only three or four calls per hour, which was just as well, because I had decided that what I needed to do was put every question and answer into a context. I would provide as deep and integrated a view to my listeners as I possibly could.

If someone called in and asked about fat in a hamburger, my answer had to do with everything that was connected to the fat. I felt that I wasn't living up to my potential, living at the high end of my life energy, if I didn't put things into context for people, take the time to tell them, in depth, everything they needed to make intelligent choices for themselves. So instead of reciting the data about cholesterol counts, I told the whole story of the destruction of the rain forests to plant grass for cattle on a pasture that was only a temporary pasture because the topsoil was so thin it would not support a second growth. They heard about the decline in rainfall on the planet because of destruction of South American rain forests, about destruction of species of plants and animals, about eradication of indigenous cultures so a restaurant chain could buy cheap hamburger meat that is high in fat, high in sodium, high in animal protein, high in disease-producing microorganisms— none of which we need. When I was finished, they would have enough of a feel for the process to make intelligent choices for themselves about being part of the whole destructive cycle.

I had stopped living by the headlines of life, and as I changed the way I shared my knowledge with people, my life grew richer and deeper. Over the course of the following six months, while the station was looking for my replacement, the next rating book came out, and I had more than doubled my number of listeners and ended up with the largest afternoon radio audience in the United States. No one had known that this audience wanting health and wholeness was there.

Developing the Life Energies System

After I made the necessary changes in my own life, I turned my attention to the amazing insights I had had about natural life energies. The theory of natural patterns of energy of human beings was, in one sense, easy to put together. So much had been given to me that starry night in the desert—a complete gestalt, a holistic view of the human race, with people naturally fitting into the total picture.

While I knew intuitively that my concepts were right on target, I realized that they needed to be expanded. Also, to convince other people of the concepts' validity, I would have to take a scientific approach to testing my hypotheses. The rule in scientific research is that you must try to disprove your own theory. If you can't, then it may have merit.

I set up some studies and enlisted the aid of several psychologists, psychiatrists, and behaviorists to see if the model worked for them. They came from different schools of psychoanalytic thought and employed different psychotherapeutic models—Freudians, Jungians, Gestaltists. I had received a Ph.D. in psychology myself, and though I was not in clinical practice, I had the opportunity, through my work, to meet and interview people from all walks of life.

I saw that there are different qualities in each energy that make each one uniquely valuable. I developed a range of possibilities for each energy and checked to see which kinds of people had it in them to go to certain extremes.

We tested the natural life energy theory with thousands of people, and I taught it to thousands more over the course of eight years. Those who have learned it, whether or not they are professional therapists, have found it a powerful tool for understanding themselves and others.

One thing I've found is that the natural life energy model can be really helpful in conjunction with selecting the right person for a job. For example, if you were hiring a secretary, you would want to get someone who was an energy match in the supportive role. If you were hiring a salesperson, you'd probably look for a candidate displaying aggressive energy. Also, if you were looking for a job for yourself, or starting a career, it would be particularly important that your efforts suited your energy. If you had been told all your life that you should be a lawyer, for example, but your life energy was predominantly creative, you'd do best to follow your creativity, or all your life you would be a square peg in a round hole. You'd be unhappy—and probably not a very good lawyer.

I tested the theory in my own office and found that I had someone in an important supportive position who did not have the highest level of supportive energy. I replaced that person with someone for whom reliability and dependability were second nature. She was not willing to take risks, but she was practical and efficient, and within two weeks the office started humming along. The atmosphere was harmonious, and it was easy to be there. Her life energy category was absolutely on target. I have never failed when I've set up an enterprise according to people's life energies.

In the area of personal relationships, too, looking at things from the perspective of natural life energies can be enlightening. In my own life, I reflected, I seemed to be attracted to a certain type of woman over and over again. Though the initial attraction was always compelling, this was never the kind of person I could be with for any length of time without conflict. When I applied the life energy principles to this area, they worked beautifully to help me identify that particular energy. I am still attracted to and like that particular type of woman, but I don't pursue a relationship. No matter how exciting it might be at the outset, there's no point in wasting our time and setting ourselves up for stress and anguish.

This book is the result of more than eight years of research into the natural life energies concept that began to evolve for me that night in the desert. I hope you find it valuable and easy to apply to yourself, your family, and your friends, and that you come to benefit from it as much as I have in terms of discovering a higher, more balanced use of your own energy and, through that discovery, a more satisfying life.

I extend my deep thanks and appreciation to all of the thousands of people who have contributed to our understanding, and to the powerful forces of the universe that always provide more than you'd hoped for when you take the time to quiet your mind, ask, and listen for the answer.

—Gary Null, New York
March, 1996

Who Are You, Really?

Life Energy and
How it Works

❖

Each person comes into the world with an essence, a unique constellation of attributes that make him or her different and special. We have certain capacities for physical growth, strength, and intellectual development programmed into our DNA, right along with the genes that make our eyes blue and our hair brown.

One of these original attributes of the self is a unique spiritual energy that is manifested as charisma, or magnetism, a dynamic quality that gives a person the ability to attract or influence other people—and maybe even the ability to attract and influence events. At one end of the spectrum of this dynamic energy are those supercharged few who have what we call "star quality," which we see played out not just on the stage but also in all of life's arenas—business, sports, religion, academia, medicine, the military, and so on.

At the other end of this energy spectrum are people who have no need to stand out in any way. No matter how physically strong they may be or how high their IQ, the energy of their spirit is adaptive rather than dynamic. Their joy is more low-key, and their gift is the ability to adapt to their circumstances and make life work no matter what.

This special life energy is separate and distinct from all other essential qualities of the self. It is impossible to measure, and yet it is, I believe, the determining factor in how a person addresses life. This property of the self is what I refer to in this book as natural life energy (NLE).

When I had these insights, I was quite sure that we are all interconnected in a web of energy. No one has too much, no one has too little to fulfill his or her place in the universe. Each individual energy has its own resonance, its own note to play in this harmonious symphony called life. In a way that is truly ecological, each human being has value for and a connection to every other.

The Main Energy Types

As I see it, the two main types of people in terms of natural life energy are the Dynamics and the Adaptives. The basic difference between them is that charismatic quality, a personal magnetism that enables individuals to inspire and lead others. The Dynamics are the ones who have charisma, as well as an affinity for change and often a strong sense of ego. Adaptives are not charismatic, nor are they looking to change things; their sense of ego tends to be less than that of the Dynamics. There is a third type—the Creative. Creatives have a different kind of personal rhythm, awareness, and sensitivity, which allows them—and even makes it necessary for them—to bring their creations into the world. Of course, adaptive people can be creative, dynamic people can adapt to certain things, and creative people may be dynamic or adaptive, too. What we are pinpointing when we refer to a person's natural life energy is that person's *predominant* energy type.

Refining the Focus:
The Secondary Qualities

Within the three broad types there are further divisions. Some people are characteristically Aggressives, some are Assertives, and some are Supportives.

Aggressives

Aggressives have a driving, forceful energy, and tend to lead or want to dominate others. They like to take charge of whatever they're engaged in, whether it's a business, a family, or the PTA. If you've ever been involved in an informal, unstructured meeting of several people, you've seen how the group takes on its own structure after a while, as Aggressives come to the fore and assume leadership roles. There are Dynamic Aggressives and Adaptive Aggressives.

Assertives

Assertives put forth their own point of view with confidence. While they are willing to take an aggressive responsibility for their own actions and deeds, they have no particular need to lead others. In a group, Assertives would be the ones who are comfortable expressing their views but who are not particularly driven to take charge. There are Dynamic Assertives and Adaptive Assertives, and virtually all of the Creative group consists of Creative Assertives.

Supportives

There are both Dynamic and Adaptive people who are at their best in a supportive role. Qualitatively, they are basically nurturing, happy to help, and are truly concerned about other people's welfare. In a group, Supportives are not the natural leaders, and they're usually not the most eloquent speakers. But they are ultimately the people who make things happen.

Putting It All Together:
The Seven Energy Types

The three basic spiritual energies and the three basic qualities are like strands that form the warp and woof of personality. They weave together in certain patterns that produce the rich tapestry of the seven NLE types. Of course, there is no end to the variations that nature produces, and each person is born completely unique. And yet, at the same time, everyone will tend to fall into one of the following seven categories, based on their predominant energy type:

Dynamic Aggressives

These people are the charismatic natural leaders of society. Think of presidents, prime ministers, generals, corporate CEOs, authority figures—they're all Dynamic Aggressives. For these self-made men and women, being goal-oriented and entrepreneurial, as well as controlling others, come naturally. You can just about feel their drive to direct things.

Dynamic Assertives

Charismatic, nonconformists, creators of social change: Dynamic Assertives, while they may be trendsetters and revolutionaries, are basically looking to control only their own lives, not others'. They know what they believe in and why, and what they don't believe in and why, because these are the types of things they think about. They are conceptually creative and process-oriented.

Dynamic Supportives

Charismatic, warmhearted, sincere, reliable, humorous, compassionate, strong yet gentle—all these words describe Dynamic Supportives. The Dynamic Supportive energy is typified in therapists, doctors, conciliators, clergy, teachers, and communicators. Dynamic Supportives are independent, intuitive, and good at bringing people together, sometimes serving as bridges between Dynamics and Adaptives.

Adaptive Aggressives

While Adaptive Aggressives are not charismatic themselves, they are drawn to powerful people and have the resourcefulness to work with them. They are socially aware, goal-oriented, survivor types, expert at finding their niche within the power structure and using it. Successful sales and public relations people, as well as behind-the-scenes "operators," are often Adaptive Aggressives. Many actors are, too.

Adaptive Assertives

Adaptive Assertives are not charismatic, but they do have the kind of practical leadership skills that make them good foremen, supervisors, office managers, and teachers. They're solid and dependable hard workers, and highly responsible.

Adaptive Supportives

This group comprises the great majority of the population. They are the nonglamorous supporters of the status quo, and society runs because of them. This group, which has the gift of helping others, includes blue-collar workers, administrative assistants, "support staff," "the troops." Sometimes security-seeking, they're often good citizens: compassionate, charitable, even selfless.

Creative Assertives

Creatives seem to manifest only as Creative Assertives. They often display heightened sensitivity and perceptual ability. They're absorbed in their work, reflective, self-sufficient, sometimes volatile, and visionary; they question life and themselves. They're designers, artists, novelists, dancers, and musicians.

High Side, Low Side

The qualities just listed for each type of energy are generally positive ones, and in describing people this way I've been purposely upbeat. In truth, each NLE has a high side and a low side, an up side and a down side. When we are living in harmony with our NLE, we feel comfortable with ourselves and are able to live a balanced, healthy life on the high side of our energy. We are fulfilled and able to do our best to make our special contribution to the world, whether we are Dynamics, Adaptives, or Creatives. We don't have to be champions in a competition; we just need to be the best of who we are to fulfill our life's purpose.

In actuality, though, very few people are truly living up to the potential of their NLE. Perhaps this is an unrealistic expectation—to do so you would have to be like an athlete playing on top of his or her game every day. Yes, there is always a champion, like Arnold Palmer, who comes close to shooting four under par every time he goes out to play golf. Arnie plays on the high side of his golf game virtually all the time. But for every Arnold Palmer, there are millions of golfers on the course with less natural talent, interest, and determination.

On the negative end of the living-up-to-one's-potential spectrum, when we are not in touch with our innate energy at all, we may waste a great deal of time and effort trying to be what we are not. We become fragmented, unbalanced, and diseased in the process. Then we are living on the low end of our NLE, and we are unhappy and frustrated, or perhaps even dangerous to ourselves and others.

I believe that if everyone on the planet was living on the high side of his or her energy, the world would be a peaceful, joyous place. But when you look at the reality of our world today, with all its strife, pollution, crime, and political unrest, and with millions of people living dysfunctional, self-destructive lives, you can see that society is far from the harmonious whole that nature intended. A staggering number of people are living on the low side of their energies, and there doesn't seem to be a remedy in sight. Why are we so far from our natural spiritual birthright? What happens that creates misery where there should be happiness, war instead of peace?

Conditioning

What happens is that our conditioning often stunts or distorts our true nature. From the minute we are born, our essential being is shaped by the circumstances of our lives, and our natural life energy is influenced by these conditions. We learn from and are influenced by our families, our physical surroundings, our culture, and many other factors. We must fit in with, and meet the expectations of, other people. As we become acculturated, many layers of conditioning are superimposed over our natural selves. Much of it is useful and appropriate—we need to know how to behave in the world; we have to learn those kindergarten-level lessons about manners and traffic and consideration for others.

The problem comes when your conditioning diverts the development of your potential in a major way. Your true energy may be so blocked that you can't feel it, and as a result you may lose touch with the real you.

By the time we reach adulthood, we are an amalgam of our natural life energy, circumstances, and conditioning. If we have had positive conditioning, appropriate to our particular energy, then chances are we are ready to live a satisfying, fulfilling life. But if, instead of having had our special gifts nurtured, we have been bent to fit into a framework that is foreign to our nature, we may grin and bear it and settle for a forced kind of existence, not even acknowledging our unhappiness. We may end up spending a great deal of time and money going to groups, reading self-help books, or going to counselors and therapists to learn what makes us tick, or to find out why we're not satisfied or happy with our lives.

Here's an example of the negative effects of conditioning. A young boy is conditioned to be competitive, aggressive, ambitious, and highly driven, as boys often are; it's all intended to help him be successful, to win at any cost. So that's what he does. He fights for power and control, working hard to win recognition and enhance his self-esteem through every possible avenue. He pushes himself to get degrees, make money, achieve social standing. It looks good from the outside. But on the inside, he's living in an arid emotional desert because his real self wanted to be an artist— someone who had a cooperative rather than a competitive approach to life. He doesn't like to make other people lose so he can win; it just doesn't resonate with his spirit. But because of his relentless conditioning, he goes ahead and gives his all to the "proper" life his family and culture have ordained for him. In doing so, he denies any connection to his natural life energy. In short, he's made an outward success of a journey down the wrong road. Only in the innermost reaches of his heart, a place where he rarely feels comfortable, does he know that the trappings of success cannot compensate for the loss of his true self.

If this individual had become an alcoholic or drug addict, or had failed at every business he'd started, it would take some doing to get through his dysfunction, but he might. Perhaps he'd go back to school as an adult, or go to support groups, to give himself a new beginning. Many people take those steps as they recover from addictions and other dysfunctional behavior. But it's a curious paradox that if this person makes a success of his career and never has glaring disasters in life, he earns so much approval from others that it becomes very hard for him to consider that he's been riding down a road through the wrong forest. In fact, he'll find it almost impossible to separate from his artificial self, renew his acquaintance with his real self, and start over. In those "wee, small hours of the morning," when his mind is quiet, the yearning will be there, but he may not even know what he longs for.

Well-meaning parents and society teach children what they think they need to know for survival: how to adapt, earn a steady wage, and become integrated into society. If there's some other urge inside a child, an energy that wants to manifest itself, it can be submerged very easily at an early age by adults who think they're doing the child a favor by teaching him that doing well and fitting in are the most important tasks in life.

In some families, parents don't agree with each other about what conditioning to give the child, and they work at cross-purposes. The mother may be influencing the youngster to be a Creative Assertive, the father may be instilling the values of a Dynamic Aggressive, and the church may be trying to force the child into being an Adaptive Supportive. The child's natural life energy might ultimately be something different from all of these. The result can be a person who will try to manifest all of these energies, superimposed over one another, and who will consequently have trouble being himself. The person will always be confused, and rarely happy.

This is not to say that each baby born is of a particular life energy type, and that it is up to the parent to figure out, as soon as possible, what type that is and then bring the child up accordingly. Being predominantly one type is something that will come much later. Young children are more amorphous than that; even though each individual has an underlying energy, as developing creatures children experiment with different energies and grow from living awhile with each (and note—in the case of very young children, "awhile" can mean a few minutes!) It's sort of like trying on different pairs of shoes— the child sees which ones fit, which ones feel even better, and which, ultimately, are the most comfortable to walk in, and give him the most joy. And just as children are periodically in need of new shoes, they periodically have to live with new energies. They try them all on for size. That's how they learn who they are.

So a parent's job is not to find a slot and then place the child into it, but rather to encourage whatever potential the child is developing at the moment. If at a particular time you as a parent find that your child's life energy seems to coincide with your own, that's fine. Your child will learn easily by example, because you are his (or her) best teacher. The challenge comes when your child's tendencies and your own are disparate. Then you have to let go of your preconceived notions and fear of a nature that may seem foreign to yours. People joke about not understanding their kids, but it happens all the time, and it's normal. The key is supporting your children as they metamorphose through their lives *without* your understanding them fully. You simply have to respect them.

The idea of respecting the child is fairly new in many segments of society, but now some enlightened parents and teachers are taking time to listen to children to find out what they feel ready to do. When they really know the child's inner landscape, they have a better chance of providing appropriate activities and exposing the child to things of interest. The father who wants his musically inclined son to be a quarterback, for example, might take him to concerts instead of football games instead, at least some of the time, to further his musical interests.

Inappropriate Conditioning: The Price We Pay

Conditioning can subvert our natural energy in many ways that lead to disharmony and disease. If a Dynamic Assertive woman has been taught at every turn to be subservient to the men in her life—from her father to her husband to authority in general—she will have to deny her dominant energy and learn not to let her charisma show. She may pay a very high price for that: cancer, heart disease, ulcers. Ultimately, one cannot live happily with such conflict, and yet people try anyway. They end up with psychic pain that manifests itself as disease.

The ideal, of course, is when a person's conditioning is attuned to her underlying nature. Generally, when I see conflict in a person, this hasn't been the case. And there are so many ways in which inappropriate conditioning occurs. The examples already given—of a boy pushed to be a Dynamic Aggressive when he was really, by nature, a Creative, and of a Dynamic Assertive girl conditioned to be an Adaptive Supportive, illustrate very common situations, but they are by no means the only ones. There are myriad variations on thoughtless conditioning, but what they all have in common is that they result in psychic pain on some level, as well as in waste.

That waste can be enormous. Some people go through their entire lives never really experiencing even the feeling of who they really are, because the moment they start to get to that feeling, they deny it. That's what they were taught to do.

I've seen it all. I've seen so many Dynamics who had to live as Adaptives. Why? Because they were conditioned to fear being their true selves. This is how it happened:

As youths, they would periodically get new ideas and attempt to act on them.

"Stay in your place," their parents said.

"I feel—"

"Don't."

"But I think—"

"Don't."

After a while, they didn't. The only problem is, they are now trapped, and on some level, they know it. Perhaps they sense that that's why their adult lives are beset by frustration and anger.

I've also seen Adaptives try to live as Dynamics, because they were conditioned to be dynamic. It didn't work, though. They were just pushy.

Sometimes a child does grow up to follow the path dictated by his or her own natural life energy, and the parents can't understand it. They view their grown child as a failure, and the irony is that the child is living a happy life, one that's right in sync with his or her essential self.

Think of two Creative Assertive types who are highly involved in the arts and who have always just assumed that their son would follow in their footsteps and become a writer or a poet or a painter or a musician. Despite years of the best schooling and special lessons, though, nothing "takes," and the son grows up and goes on to a career in an area with less glamour than those the parents have been involved in. Nor does the son have any desire to move in the same circles his parents have enjoyed. He works as a manager in a hardware store, and thus seems to have rejected everything his parents have lived by. They view him as a disappointment. It's not a monetary thing particularly, but a cultural one. Their son seems to have turned his back on their whole world.

The problem here? There is none, except in the parents' minds. Maybe the son is simply not a Creative Assertive. Maybe he's an Adaptive Assertive. Maybe if his parents had thought in terms of natural life energies, and the possibility of people within families having different ones, their conditioning of their son would have been less one-sided. They would have been more open to life's possibilities—from their son's perspective. They would have encouraged him to enroll in business courses instead of art school when he'd shown a leaning in that direction. With a broader, life-energy-based view, they would have had no trouble seeing their child not as a failure, but as a success, because they would have seen immediately that he's happy doing what he's doing. They would have understood that in his quiet mind, he is at peace when he thinks about his life. There is no dissonance between how he is living and what he is all about.

Listening to the Quiet Mind

Your natural life energy is the mode of living you acknowledge as your own when you give yourself a quiet mind. It's the mode you're operating in when you're in your happiest, most comfortable, and most relaxed state. It is not the mode you're operating in—no matter how "successfully"—under pressure, be it financial or status pressure, or the pressure of conditioning.

Here's a way to visualize it. Let's say you were in a roomful of randomly selected people and you were all given art lessons. Everyone in the room would end up painting something. For some of the people in the room, the act of creating a painting would be natural. If you were part of this group, that natural feeling would show in your work, and you would have experienced a comfortable flow while working. But for others in the room, painting would be a very uncomfortable process. If you were part of this group, you wouldn't be happy with what you did, and you wouldn't have felt particularly happy doing it.

But what if you had been conditioned to always be a creative person? You could fake it; you could force it; technically, you could do it; and if you had the right connections and knew how to "talk the talk," you might even be able to base your whole life around painting. But your life wouldn't be real. And if you went on to live as a Creative Assertive when in fact your energy was a different one, you would feel terrible when you gave yourself a quiet mind.

People can sometimes live lives dramatically split between their true life energies and those they were conditioned to display. There was a very well known man who, at work, was a champion of industry and a major American force both in economics and in politics. But in his personal life—I was in his home many times—his wife was an absolute Dynamic Aggressive and he was an Adaptive Supportive. That's how extreme the differences can be. I talked with him on a personal level, asking him, "Where do you feel happiest?" Because, again, that's the key: Where do you feel most satisfied, comfortable, and happy?

He said, "At home."

I said, "Even, you know, with the family—"

He said, "I love it. I feel so relaxed and at ease. I feel it's like me."

"So how do you feel being this great icon of industry?"

He said he feels very uncomfortable. He said, "I have to force myself. I know I've got enemies and people think I'm this crude and harsh bastard. But look, I was told that if you want to get on in business, this is what you have to do."

His parents had both been Dynamics, and they had pushed him and pushed him and pushed him. And so he grew up believing that that's how you should be, that's how you got ahead. His conditioning was so pervasive that he accepted it. But it wasn't his real nature.

I also know a few very lucky people whose parents and schooling encouraged them to grow in the direction of their own naturally developing energies. These people tend to be more balanced and happier than those whose lives are split between an inborn and a conditioned mode of living, or those whose natural life energies have been suppressed completely.

You're Not a Prisoner of Conditioning

While conditioning is a powerful factor, it's not an insurmountable one. People can overcome it, and some people's natural life energy is so strong that they just *have* to transcend it. We can probably all think of the kid who we always knew was going to turn out a particular way because the energy was there. The conditioning didn't matter: that's how strong the energy was.

Also, it's sometimes possible to change course after living a certain way for a long period. I saw that a few years ago, after my high school reunion.

At the reunion, I was disappointed to find that one of my best friends through high school and college was not there, and that no one had heard anything as to his recent whereabouts. We knew he'd had problems—he'd been an alcoholic, he'd been on drugs, he'd had businesses that had come and gone. We were all concerned about him.

I remembered Bob as a fun guy but very aggressive. He was definitely an Adaptive Aggressive to the max—often living at the low end of that energy. I can remember in high school that even in an intramural game, if he didn't win he'd get really angry and throw the basketball at someone. He was an exaggerator; he liked to be the center of attention; he bragged. It wasn't that he'd had a bad upbringing; he'd had a good upbringing with loving parents, but they had tried to condition him to be an Adaptive Supportive in that they expected him to grow into the kind of person who lives quietly and works in a factory without calling attention to himself—and that could never be Bob. So he seemed to me to be acting out in his sometimes obnoxious way as a kind of reaction to these expectations.

Anyway, his not being heard from by any of his former classmates was disturbing, so we searched for him, calling all over the United States. But nobody knew where he was. And I mean nobody—his biological father didn't know, his stepfather didn't know, his stepmother didn't know—*no one* had seen him in four years. I tried tracking him down in Los Angeles but couldn't find him. And then, some time later, I called my older brother, Howard, just to see how he and his family were at Thanksgiving time. And I happened to say, "Just as a point of curiosity, whatever happened to Bob? Remember Bob?"

And to my surprise, my brother said, "Sure I do; I just saw him."

"You just saw Bob?—Where?"

"He dropped in here," Howard said.

"You're kidding!"

But he wasn't kidding. It turned out that Bob was trying to keep a low profile at the moment. My brother explained the he hadn't seen Bob in ages either—in about a decade, in fact—but that recently there had been a knock at the door. Howard had gone to open it, and there was Bob, just standing there.

"He was dressed in old clothes," Howard reported. "He kind of looked like he'd been wearing these same clothes for a long period of time, and he said he'd lost everything. But then Bob said that he had given up on drugs, and on alcohol, too. He told me that he was in the process of changing his entire life radically, and that he didn't want the whole world to know about it just yet."

Howard went on to tell me that Bob was going back to school, studying soil science and landscaping. He was simply starting over, because he realized that where he had started the first time was on the wrong track.

As Howard explained more about our old friend's troubles, and about his new plans, I marveled at the human potential for self-understanding and transformation. Sometimes the realization of this potential can be quite dramatic, as it was in Bob's case. It seemed that Bob had been living for years through an artificially constructed winning-is-everything self. When Bob began to experience the inevitable losses that are part of every personal life and career, he couldn't handle them. He took them as direct blows to his self-esteem, and so accelerated his downhill course of alcohol and drug abuse. But now, after twenty years of going down the wrong track, he was giving it all up to start over again as an autonomous person. That takes courage. But Howard assured me that Bob was at peace with himself. He was excited by the idea of starting all over again—going back to school as if he were just out of high school.

The latest news is that Bob is now the kind of person you can sit and have a nice conversation with, without feeling anxious because he's hyper, or trying to sell you something, or manipulate you, or dominate the conversation. Today Bob is an agronomist. Well, actually, he does landscaping and gardening, but he likes to describe himself as an agronomist because he is, after all, an Adaptive Aggressive. But the point is that he is no longer living on the low side of his energy. He's in the middle of the range of his life energy, and could even reach the high end if he added a spiritual element to his life. Bob has smoothed out the rough edges, become less aggressive and more constructive. He's come to terms with who he is, letting go of problems created by his conditioning. He does landscape work for the rich and famous, getting gratification from his connections with celebrities, and generally living a satisfying life. There's no more conflict within him.

So no, this is not a tale about someone conditioned to be an Adaptive Supportive waking up one morning and realizing that he's really a Dynamic Aggressive and going on to become president of the United States. Real-life personal growth is not usually that dramatic. But the picture is still a positive one because here we have someone who was able to fine-tune where he was in the natural life energy picture, jettisoning the low side of his Adaptive Aggressive nature, and improving his life in the process. And ultimately, improving one's life is the goal of self-understanding.

Dynamic Aggressives: The Ultimate Go-Getters

There's a bit of folk wisdom to the effect that any child can grow up to become president of the United States. That may or may not be true, but it sure helps to be a Dynamic Aggressive!

Dynamic Aggressives are society's leaders and policymakers. They are competitive, action-oriented individuals with the ability to motivate and lead others. They actively seek to control people and even influence the course of history. Social change would not be possible without the leadership of these powerful and effective people, who take every opportunity to actualize their visions. They rise to the top of their professions, and can be found in the upper echelons of government, industry, and the church. They're the ones who lead us as presidents, prime ministers, CEOs, heads of religions, and self-employed businesspeople and entrepreneurs. On the seamier side, they're the ones who take advantage of us as con artists, religious charlatans, and dictators. In short, Dynamic Aggressives are the people who, when put in an environment, will organize that environment, and sometimes exploit it.

These leadership "naturals" tend to be outgoing, intelligent, single-minded, self-reliant, and politically aware. They can also be self-centered and egotistical, and they sometimes hate to lose so much that they focus on winning at all costs. Thus they can be insensitive, manipulative, stubborn, and arrogant. They are driven people who may be too heavily focused on amassing power and money.

The day-to-day lifestyle of Dynamic Aggressives is not like that of most of us. Of course, they tend to be richer than most of us, and to live in more opulent surroundings, but a more essential difference is that relaxation is never a goal for them. You're not going to find these people watching television—unless they are on it. They're generally not into novels or drama, because their drama is their own lives. They do not seek out peace and quiet; they don't like it. What they like is action—specifically, action that they're generating. And you'll often find them surrounded by an entourage of people who help them do so.

Gathering such an entourage is not difficult for Dynamic Aggressives, who are so charismatic that they attract other people without even trying. Their ability to command the loyalty of others seems almost effortless. People believe in Dynamic Aggressives, they trust them, and they are willing to work with them. This loyalty can be attributed, in no small part, to the visionary drive of this group. They see the big picture in life and generally have designs on changing it. So on their up side, these people can make the world a better place.

Dynamic Aggressives have gestalt minds—everything is instantly seen. If you show them a lake, they visualize what could be done to develop it. If you show them a hill, they see beyond the obvious cluster of trees and develop an immediate picture of its possibilities. Once they see the whole picture, they work backwards to figure out how to implement their vision. Then they rally others to help realize that vision, since they are poor at detail work themselves.

In fact, many Dynamic Aggressives are not highly educated people for this same reason. The educational system, especially at the doctorate level, requires too much detail work and follow-through for the Dynamic Aggressive. These are impatient people who want things to happen now, and they don't want to get bogged down in the process. It's not that they're afraid to dig in and work, but rather that skipping the details and delegating them to others is how they can keep their own momentum going full throttle. And Dynamic Aggressives are excellent at motivating others and forming teams to get a job done.

However, they tend to be more competitive than cooperative, and their first loyalty is to themselves. They have strong egos; they want to win, and they want to be right. They don't go around any obstacles they encounter; they go over them. Still, on their up side Dynamic Aggressives can be compassionate people with little pretense. When their natural charm and dynamic energies are put to use, they can be very beneficial to the world. After all, they're the ones who take risks that no one else would dream of taking, and do things that no one else would dream of doing. They're opportunity-grabbers. And that's the kind of activism that real progress is made of.

A Dynamic Aggressive on the down side is another matter entirely. At this end of the spectrum, Dynamic Aggressives are extremely demanding and can push others to the edge with their criticism. Emotionally, they may be cold and unengaging because they are shut down themselves. Surprisingly, this lack of emotion can create a sense of mystery that attracts others. There's a certain appeal about a person who is not an open book—although some of these people seem to have reached the extreme of having their pages permanently glued together! They continue to attract, though. Many people who are not otherwise passive will simply accept a Dynamic Aggressive's hostility and negative energy because they are drawn to their powerful qualities.

Power is everything to a Dynamic Aggressive, and vulnerability is something to be swept under the rug. So this group generally doesn't talk about pain; they suffer quietly. As for drug abuse, this is not an issue for Dynamic Aggressives, because drugs would make them lose their all-important control, or at the very least, side-track them. Also, it's rare that one of these go-getters is slowed down by illness. Nor are they slowed down by poverty. They thrive in it—briefly—until they work themselves out of it and get as far away from it as possible, ultimately establishing themselves as the complete antithesis of poverty in some grand setting or other.

The Dynamic Aggressive's dominant role among people is mirrored in other areas of the animal kingdom. Even in a group of animals that dominates others, you will find one that rules the other dominant types. One lion will lead other lions, for example. Dynamic Aggressive people operate in much the same way. You will never see two Dynamic Aggressives with equal control; one is always the dominant member of the group. Other people seem to sense who is the strongest member of a group and acknowledge that power.

What would happen if we had no Dynamic Aggressives? We'd have no societal growth. Their energy leads the quest for change in every part of our social fabric. Someone who's not infused with this particular energy will not go out and start a reform movement or a corporation—at least not successfully. It takes a certain measure of stamina, courage, and self-confidence—egotism, actually—to face adversity and get to the top.

Once at the top, the Dynamic Aggressive faces enormous challenges—in the case of political leaders, for instance, the challenge of creating a greater vision of society and then actualizing it. To do these things, the leader has to inspire confidence and trust, and, given some charisma and good handlers, this part of his task is highly doable. In fact, we as a nation seem quite ready to blindly follow our leaders, banking our trust in them the way we leave money in the bank—unchecked for long periods.

The trouble comes when there is competing leadership that

prompts us to face the fact that our trust has been betrayed. Examples abound: We were told by the presidential candidate that taxes would be cut, but now that he's president, they've been increased. We were told that he disliked PAC groups, but now we find that he's accepted vast sums of money from them. These examples of misplaced trust, part of Bill Clinton's political problems now, are typical of how the Dynamic Aggressive politician can get himself into hot water.

No Dynamic Aggressive simply wakes up one day and finds him- or herself in a position of leadership. Our societal heads go through enormous battles to get there. The average person would find these battles too overwhelming and the game too tough to play, but the true Dynamic Aggressive does not. They become combatants to reach their positions: being a warrior is a rite of passage required of all leaders in our society.

Therefore, society must be careful of Dynamic Aggressives when they are on their down side, because these are practiced warriors who seek to control everything in their environment, including other people. A predatory Dynamic Aggressive will seek out relationships and environments that can be controlled to his or her advantage, no matter what that control means for others. And the Dynamic Aggressive is like the great white shark—without natural predators. So they can be extremely dangerous.

Consider the nature of corporate takeover artists. These people didn't learn to be takeover giants in school. If that were the case, then the millions of people who got more degrees than they did would have done the same. They did not, for the simple reason that they don't have the type of charismatic energy possessed by Dynamic Aggressives—charisma that allows them to attract other people and work through their energy. Dynamic Aggressives are masters at using the power given to them by others. Machiavelli wrote the book, and other Dynamic Aggressives follow it.

On their down side, Dynamic Aggressives have no loyalty at all. They assume that loyalty is due to them, not the other way around. In fact, they can be quite sensitive about the issue of loyalty. They'll pay for it if they must, by giving power and prestige to their loyal supporters. Unfortunately, they fail to recognize that loyalty can never really be bought, that it's not a commodity to be given and taken away.

Why, then, are we continually drawn to Dynamic Aggressives? The reason is that we get something important from them: a deeper understanding of the meaning of life. Throughout history, Dynamic Aggressives have interpreted the larger meaning of life for other people. So rightly or wrongly, we choose to follow them and live by their teachings. The best example of this phenomenon are the many priests and spiritual leaders who are Dynamic Aggressives.

This energy group has some very skilled orators, although their charismatic communications skills are generally one-way; that is, they're not great listeners. But because they speak so well, Dynamic Aggressives can develop a large following. The question is: What do they do with their magnetic and visionary qualities? At one extreme, they may treat others with benevolence and focus on making the world a better place. At the other end of the spectrum, they may be utterly ruthless and deceptive people, such as Adolf Hitler, Julius Caesar, and Genghis Khan. Either way, the rest of us will change our way of thinking—even our whole way of looking at the world—at their say-so. They're the paradigm-makers and -breakers.

In this regard, a fascinating example of a Dynamic Aggressive was Jesus Christ. Christ was not merely an Assertive who sought power and control over his own life; rather, he sought to influence the lives of others. So he was a true Dynamic Aggressive, albeit not today's money-and status-hungry type. But he, too, had an up side and a down side. In the latter, he experienced pain, denial, guilt, and fear. He did learn from those periods and returned to the high side of his energy. Likewise, Martin Luther King, Jr., was a Dynamic Aggressive who actively sought to change our society. He had strength and vision, and he developed the allegiance of others and put it to his use. His down side was characterized by the marital affairs that others used against him.

There are fewer examples of female Dynamic Aggressives, probably because society suppresses the mechanisms of this energy type in women. Those who do surface, much like their male counterparts, may be destructive in manifesting their energy. They can be self-interested and controlling—witness Margaret Thatcher—but their charisma is not forced. They come by it naturally and express it at a very high level. The average woman could never evolve into a Margaret Thatcher. If you took the most educated woman and made her prime minister of England, she would not have the same effect. The missing element? Margaret Thatcher's natural Dynamic Aggressive energy.

Female Dynamic Aggressives must overcome considerable odds to express their energy. Throughout history, these women have not been given the same opportunities as men to demonstrate their unique characteristics, with the rare exception of a few heroine warriors. For the most part, women have had to express their Dynamic Aggressive qualities through socially acceptable channels, such as writing. And even as writers, women were not at all acceptable until the mid-1800s.

By withholding the opportunity to excel from many women, society may be especially repressive of female Dynamic Aggressives. The ones we do see may seem at times particularly pushy and obnoxious. But they probably have to be in order to get anywhere. Remember, in the top levels of society these women are competing in a male milieu, so they may have to take on typically male characteristics and ways of doing things to get anyone's attention. And there's a double standard about what's considered pushy and obnoxious in a man versus in a woman.

By the way, if you're having trouble conjuring up a mental image of any Dynamic Aggressive, male or female, whom you know personally, you may not know one. In fact, there's a good chance that you've never even met one, because this is the smallest energy group: only about 0.5 percent of the population is Dynamic Aggressive. Actually, the majority of the population does not belong to any Dynamic energy group at all, but is, rather, Adaptive. Yet it's part of the go-getter mentality—or perhaps mythology—of this country that we're all "supposed to" be like the Dynamics. But this is just not human nature for the majority of us.

At any rate, the rarity of this particular energy subcategory is a good thing; if we had too many Dynamic Aggressives milling around in society, the conflict level would be incredible. These highly territorial people—and those they got to follow them—would be destroying each other right and left, and the environment would be more of a shambles than it already is. Plus nobody would be willing to deliver the mail, to drive a cab, or to farm the land—what was left of it! So it's a good thing this group is not more prevalent.

Of course, if you *have* met a Dynamic Aggressive, you no doubt remember the occasion. When one of these people enters a room, everyone else in it sits up and takes notice; there's just no way you can miss one. It's not that Dynamic Aggressives necessarily have hyperactive mannerisms or a loud, attention-seeking demeanor. On the contrary, they are often quiet, calm, methodical people. But they radiate an unmistakable energy that can only be described as intimidating.

How do Dynamic Aggressives get to be the way they are? Neither conditioning nor heredity are particularly relevant; it's a matter of a special energy that lies within. So it doesn't matter how they were taught, or what school they went to, or what their parents were like, or what foods they ate. Instead of the old saw "Blood will tell," we should think of the phrase "Life energy will tell," because this is certainly true in the case of society's leaders.

Up Side/Down Side: A Whole World of Difference

Because the Dynamic Aggressive is the most powerful of energy types, the difference between his up side and his down side can be tremendous. Indeed, the chasm between the two sides of this energy can have serious implications for the rest of society. On their up side, Dynamic Aggressives can be great spiritual leaders who galvanize an organization or an entire nation. On their down side, they have the potential to become a Hitler or a Stalin. And here's a scary thought: You and I might not want to be in a war, but if the two people who head our governments are Dynamic Aggressives on their down side, we may end up shooting and killing each other for reasons that are totally absurd. It's happened—too many times.

Think about politics, and the Dynamic Aggressives who run government. I find it interesting that these people generally tell others that they subscribe to traditional values. In many cases, though, this statement is merely a tool that allows them to attract the loyalty of Adaptive Supportives and maintain control. In reality, the Dynamic Aggressive's values are all his or her own. If left unchecked, the Dynamic Aggressive will exercise a compulsive, almost addictive need to influence others. As leaders in politics, industry, and religion, they will use whatever dogma exists in society to control others. Witness the ability of the church to thrive on conformity, dogma, and ritual.

Dynamic Aggressives on the down side are prone to gross depression, acute anxiety, and a hostile attitude toward anyone who stands in their way. If they fail at an endeavor due to these obstacles, they will start again, but remain extremely vengeful. Dynamic Aggressives never forget the people who played a part in their failure.

One of the most harmful forces known to man is a Dynamic Aggressive motivated by hate, someone such as Saddam Hussein, whose charisma and negative energy, combined with his ability to make policy, has led to the death of many people.

On a higher side of their energy, Dynamic Aggressives will convert their negativity into pragmatism. They have a realistic view of life that allows them to move beyond the cynicism that mires other energy types in negative inactivity. Many people can never see the good in life because they are consumed by what is bleak, disturbing, and wrong in the world. The Dynamic Aggressive can overcome this cynicism, take an optimistic view of the world's chances for improvement, and work to that end. Look at Jimmy Carter and his work to house the homeless and mediate conflicts. Dynamic Aggressives make excellent mediators, by the way, if only because they're so practiced at the art of the deal.

On the high end, Dynamic Aggressives who are connected with their spiritual sides are conscientious and balanced individuals, and their aggressiveness becomes a positive, constructive quality. A Dynamic Aggressive operating at this level can improve the environment, uplift people spiritually, make a company operate in a more responsible way, and change the world for the better.

A Dynamic Aggressive may evolve from the low side of his or her energy to the higher-end qualities. Early in life, many of this country's robber barons were ruthless in their treatment of the environment and other human beings. Through a metamorphosis of some sort, they later came to understand that they were abusing their power. These people, such as Carnegie and Rockefeller, then tried to make amends through philanthropic works and foundations.

Unfortunately, though, history shows us that, in general, Dynamic Aggressives do not operate from their higher energies. Since civilization's beginnings we have had only 230 years of world peace, in part because those with Dynamic Aggressive energy seek unconditional power and control. They lose their connection with the world around them and begin to believe that all others are there to serve their needs. Thus politicians are bought, judges are bribed, and anyone in their path becomes a manipulable object, to the point of becoming cannon fodder.

The Work of Dynamic Aggressives:
Moving and Shaking

One way of describing the Dynamic Aggressive is simply to say that this is the type of person who "goes after it"—and gets it. You (unless you are a Dynamic Aggressive) and I would never go after it to begin with; it's not part of our energy. Even if we were forced to go after it, we wouldn't feel good about it, and we wouldn't be going for it with the same passion that Dynamic Aggressives do. But they're the ones with the predatory passion, and in a broad sense, getting what they want is their life's work. In doing so, they move and shake the world.

In terms of occupation, Dynamic Aggressives are only satisfied with policy making positions that allow them to manifest their energies, whether in politics, business, banking, or religion. In any of these fields, they tend to rise to the top and become leaders. If a particular position does not have the promise of power and control, the person with this energy moves on to something else. Staying in one place for a long time is not something they're good at; in fact, it's not unusual for Dynamic Aggressives to make a dozen career changes along the way. When they finally solidify their position of power—say, in the real-estate field—others can see that their background is all over the place, in areas that have nothing to do with real estate.

In many cases, Dynamic Aggressives start off as careerists in their chosen field and then give that field up totally to pursue other interests. For example, a Dynamic Aggressive who becomes a doctor may tire of the politics involved in the profession and decide to do something else instead. They're not afraid of loss, and they rarely worry about their ability to make money, a task that is not usually a problem for them.

Generally, the Dynamic Aggressive's ultimate professional goal is to work for himself or herself. At the start of their careers, they will do a lot of job-hopping—for example, from industry to government and back to industry again—to gain the skills they need to strike out on their own. Eventually most Dynamic Aggressives will end up working for themselves. They are entrepreneurial by nature, and they dislike working for others. They rarely last in corporations unless they rise quickly to the top, because they don't want to join the club and follow the policies of others for long. They want to be the policy-makers themselves.

Still, on their up side, they *can* work in harmony with others. They have constructive ideas about what needs to be done, and they work hard to achieve those goals. If the hard-driving leadership qualities of the Dynamic Aggressive are balanced with the high-end qualities of other energy types, a lot of positive work can be accomplished. The thing to remember, though, is that the work of the Dynamic Aggressive is always to some extent self-directed, in the sense that these people are individualistic careerists who work on themselves as much as they work on the projects at hand.

Once they're in charge, Dynamic Aggressives tend to have Adaptive Aggressives working at the level right beneath them—witness Reagan and Oliver North, or Hitler and Goebbels, for some non-high-end examples. The Adaptive Aggressive group doesn't have the charisma of the Dynamics—which is good because there's no challenge there—but they do have the drive and know-how to implement the Dynamic Aggressives' policies. And the Dynamic Aggressive does need good implementers, because detail work is not his forte. Indeed, not taking care of details can be a real problem for these broad-stroke visionaries.

I can illustrate this from personal experience. I have a Dynamic Aggressive friend who has a beautiful house. But since he never takes care of anything, none of the doors work. It's a nine-million-dollar house, and yet you go out to get a newspaper in the morning and none of the doors works to let you back in! This happened to me when I was a houseguest, and since the bell was non-functional and my friend was asleep, I decided to jog down the road to a service station to phone him so I could get back into the house. But the electric fence didn't work, so I couldn't get off the property! What I finally did was to climb in a window, which I could do because it was broken.

I got my friend up and we decided to have brunch out on the terrace. Of course, the table was cracked. We decided to take a sauna, but the sauna board broke; we landed on the floor. The Jacuzzi had some kind of scuzz in it; I wouldn't even get in it because no one had thought about throwing in anything to kill the bacteria. The swimming pool hadn't been skimmed, and I could just visualize the phantom of the black lagoon coming up, or some rare and exotic snake that happened to have been in the neighborhood crawling through the electric fence deciding to go for an uninterrupted swim. I myself decided not to.

And this was just his house. Another time, we went to a castle that he owned in France—a magnificent eleven-hundred-year-old castle that he'd bought for a song and that even came with its own village. This is typical of how a Dynamic Aggressive operates; they always make great deals. The only thing was, the castle needed extensive repair. There were four walls to the place, and that was about it.

"I've got all the paint here," my friend said.

"I think we need more than a few gallons of paint," I pointed out. "I think we need a construction engineer, carpenters, and contractors. I think you need to completely rebuild the entire place, because all you really have is the walls."

It turned out that he had to spend some three and a half million dollars to get the castle ready for occupancy, but then, of course, he forgot a few little details, such as provisions for turning on the heat. No, detail work was not his strong suit!

As bosses, while Dynamic Aggressives are often aloof and even hostile, when they pepper that general tone with a little positive feedback now and then, people respond very gratefully. Dynamic Aggressives seem to sense just how much partial reinforcement to sprinkle into their interactions with underlings to achieve optimum benefit.

You will rarely find a Dynamic Aggressive having a long

conversation on the telephone. Whatever it is, they want to get it said and get on with it—even in the case of a personal call. If you want to meet with them, fine, but it's like this: where, when, why, good-bye. It's nothing personal, but chatting is just not on the Dynamic Aggressive's agenda. You could say that "Time is money," but you could also say that "Time is life," and the Dynamic Aggressive's life is just too full of action for aimless talk to be part of it.

One of the most important people a Dynamic Aggressive needs is a spokesperson or "interpreter." Dynamic Aggressives tend to react with anger, and they rarely edit themselves. In a crisis situation, they will come in, take charge, and get the job done. But they don't want the public to see or hear the process, so they hire a buffer—a spokesperson—to handle communications. This approach is not necessarily negative; it's simply part of what it takes to get the job done.

An interesting characteristic of Dynamic Aggressives' modus operandi is that they know how to use other people's money and influence to get what they need, while most of the rest of the world has to chance using their own. So when Dynamic Aggressives lose, they don't generally lose as much.

And when they win, they win plenty, sometimes at a huge cost not just to other people, but to the environment itself. They use the environment to their advantage, whether that means strip mining, overfishing, or digging deep wells in the ocean that cause pollution. Think about who controls environment-damaging companies. It's not the average guy, the Adaptive Supportive. It's not millions of Adaptive Supportives who have banded together. It's always a relatively small number of Dynamic Aggressives who control millions of other people, and ultimately the fate of the land.

Success and the Dynamic Aggressive

In the end, most Dynamic Aggressives define success by the amount of power, control, and money they amass. A Dynamic

Aggressive at the helm of a corporation does not want the business to remain small and stable; he or she may keep extending the company until it eventually ends up in financial trouble. Perhaps the core business makes money but the subsidiaries do not, and thus the process of stripping it back down begins. The point is, these achievers par excellence are not satisfied with one company and a few products. They always want more and will overextend themselves to achieve their goals. Success for them is an ever-expanding thing.

An interesting aspect of this energy type, which is generally seen as the most successful group, is that Dynamic Aggressives actually fail more than most others would ever fail. The difference is that when most others fail, that may be it—they won't try again—but Dynamic Aggressives consider dropping down and failing to be just one part of the larger process of getting where they're going. And Dynamic Aggressives *always* get there, even if we sometimes have to pay by learning the kind of lesson you later read about in history books.

Dynamic Aggressives like to do things on a grand scale, so once they have it made, they often acquire magnificent homes. The house becomes an extension of their power, boosting their self-esteem and satisfying their need to be recognized. You never see the chairman of the board of a big company living frugally. But despite all they own—the yachts, mansions, and expensive goods—Dynamic Aggressives don't know how to relax and enjoy their possessions. Instead, they fill the house with people—their entourage—every minute of the day.

In fact, Dynamic Aggressives rarely spend time alone; they need people around them at all times. Their lives are achievement-oriented, and they get depressed if people don't know about their successes. They'll hire publicists to plaster their names on billboards and in newspapers to make sure the world knows about them. Call it insecurity-motivated, which it no doubt is to a large extent, but publicity is a vital component of success for this group.

Relationships

If you are in a relationship with a Dynamic Aggressive, you'd better be careful, although if you are an Adaptive Supportive, you probably don't have to worry—you're not going to be having much of a relationship with a Dynamic Aggressive, unless you want to go into slavery! Generally, the Dynamic Aggressive seeks out people like the Adaptive Aggressive, both at work and in relationships. These are people who share the drive of the Dynamic Aggressive, but who, lacking their charisma, do not pose a threat.

Actually, it's difficult for Dynamic Aggressives to get into any kind of deep relationship. To them, life is the relationship. That's their first obligation, their first loyalty. Their loyalty to individuals is secondary.

Generally, Dynamic Aggressives will develop a relationship with one highly trusted person in whom they confide. They want a relationship that makes them feel safe and protected because they thrive on loyalty—the kind that is given *to* them. So you could say that these are the type of people who, rather than falling in love, fall in need. If a Dynamic Aggressive is threatened by a relationship, he or she will abandon it in a second. But the same quality that allows them to do this can also make them exciting partners. Dynamic Aggressives are not burdened by feelings of jealousy and possessiveness because they are used to having things and then moving on. Whereas most other people don't get off the starting block, the Dynamic Aggressive has already been there and back.

In lieu of true friendships, which they rarely develop, Dynamic Aggressives associate with people who have positions of power similar to their own. They acknowledge only those people they believe to be their equals, and intentionally avoid anyone who does not serve their needs. They may be cordial to others, and they will surround themselves with Adaptive Aggressives for purely practical reasons—these people help them to function. But when it comes to developing real friendships,

Dynamic Aggressives generally fall short because they will not reveal their true selves. They fear vulnerability and want to minimize the risk that others will take advantage of them.

Dynamic Aggressives always have an agenda, and this is true in the relationship arena as well as that of work. As long as the other person meets those expectations, the Dynamic Aggressive has no reason to end the relationship. But they bore easily and are rarely monogamous. They often have multiple—if shallow—relationships, and they believe that all other people are there to meet their needs. It's as if they view their partners as "service" people of some sort.

Thus the men may have mistresses. And some use call girls—interestingly, not so much for sex, but as confidantes. These leaders of society, who seem to have everything, often have absolutely no one to talk to, in the sense of revealing their innermost thoughts and feelings. They can't appear vulnerable to those who are part of their circle, and this includes their wives, who are often Adaptive Aggressives who might take advantage of any revelations. Often the Dynamic Aggressive can't even talk to a psychiatrist or psychologist because the fact that they needed one might leak out and jeopardize a run for public office.

Do you have a Dynamic Aggressive neighbor? That's good, not because it brings up property values, but because if he has any problem with you, he'll confront you directly in a straightforward way, at the outset. He won't play any silly vengeful neighbor games, whereas some members of other, less busy energy groups sometimes seem to thrive on these.

In general, the only people Dynamic Aggressives really need to stay away from are other Dynamic Aggressives. Together, two members of this energy group would attempt to control each other, leading to high-level competition and constant conflict.

On the other hand, Dynamic Aggressives can form strong relationships with Adaptive Aggressives, who will provide them with protection, carry out much of their work, and remain loyal. An Adaptive Aggressive can also handle the volatility of a Dynamic Aggressive. Whereas other energy types might take a Dynamic Aggressive's outburst personally, the Adaptive Aggressive does not.

Female Dynamic Aggressives may have some problems in their relationships with men. If the man is too passive, the Dynamic Aggressive woman may quickly become bored with him. But these extraordinary women can have a hard time finding men who are not intimidated by them or obsessed with possessing them. And they may experience a lot of clashing and competition with another charismatic energy, such as a Dynamic Assertive or Dynamic Aggressive man.

A Dynamic Aggressive man and woman, in fact, are likely to have an intense and tumultuous relationship. The union would be lacking in a couple of vital elements: a sense of calm and an ability to relax. Imagine these two on a tropical island for a week of vacation. Within days, they would select a site for a new home, open up a tennis court, and figure out how to buy the island and finance the purchase with cheap bonds!

Life with a Dynamic Assertive man can be difficult for the Dynamic Aggressive woman, too. This would be a tough relationship because both have a difficult time compromising, apologizing, and acknowledging mistakes. A better bet for the Dynamic Aggressive woman would be the Dynamic Supportive man, who would be intelligent, worldly, and trustworthy, but not highly competitive.

The Parent Trap—Dynamic-Aggressive Style

In the area of parenting, an unfortunate energy combination would be a Dynamic Aggressive father and an Adaptive Supportive mother. The children would see again and again that their mother does not stand up to their dominating father—a pattern that will in no way benefit them.

But whatever the parental combination, it's not easy being the child of a Dynamic Aggressive; these children are apt to get caught in the trap of excessive parental expectations. Dynamic

Gary Null

Aggressives are tough on their offspring; they tend to demand that the children be every bit as ruthless and successful as they are. There's an aggressive nature to the family dynamics. And the children may be raised in an austere fashion because the Dynamic Aggressive wants them to work for what they get—just as he or she had to do. The ultimate goal is to ensure that the children have the same material success as the parent.

Thus Dynamic Aggressives will support their children, but that support is usually conditional. The kids are acknowledged when they do what the parent expects of them, or, better yet, when they do something that makes the parent feel good about who he or she is. But the lack of unconditional love in these children's lives can lead to tragic results. They may become alcoholics, drug addicts, or even suicidal. They feel constant pressure to succeed and to fulfill their parent's expectations. If they don't, the Dynamic Aggressive will let them know that something must be wrong with them. How could they "fail" when the parent gave them so much? This cynical view of life can lead the child to the mistaken belief that all people are equally emotionally ungiving.

Growth and Transformation

Dynamic Aggressives have a rich, full personal life in the sense that they have a lot of peak experiences. That's because they're the ones willing to take the risks, and with risk-taking comes the opportunity for self-actualization. So if you want to point to a particular beauty of the Dynamic Aggressive life, you could say that these people are exquisitely attuned to their capabilities and use them to live life to the fullest.

While individuals in this group are astute enough to be attuned to their natural energy, they may be lacking a connection to their spiritual self. But nothing improves in life unless we pay attention to our spiritual energy. When that attention is composed of decency, ethics, and morality, our natural energy will manifest at the highest level. We might create products that benefit society or, at the very least, do not hurt others.

As Dynamic Aggressives begin to earn money and get ahead in life, they may forget the spiritual part of the equation. Indeed, the equation can become strictly intellectual. If they are smarter and faster than those around them, they can get ahead early in life by making better deals. But they may fail to consider what is good for others as they pursue their goals.

On the other hand, many Dynamic Aggressives use their power to support important causes but keep a low profile about this aspect of themselves. Some examples are Armand Hammer, the former head of Occidental Petroleum; Walter Annenberg, the founder of *TV Guide*; and several members of the Mellon family. Without such people, many of the greatest art collections in the world would not be available for the rest of us to see.

In some cases, Dynamic Aggressives learn the lessons of giving early on and support such causes throughout their lives. In other instances, a Dynamic Aggressive may realize toward the end of his life that he has overlooked certain values. He then decides—perhaps out of remorse, or a fear of death—to give something back to society by supporting a cause. But the fact remains that there are many great monuments we can enjoy today due to the direct action of Dynamic Aggressives.

So Dynamic Aggressives are capable of transforming their energy dramatically. They can become less interested in wielding power and more concerned with achieving greater harmony in life. They may not go out and better the world, but they will try to understand their place within it. This can be a humbling experience that changes a Dynamic Aggressive's perspective on everything. They may finally accept that all of their money, power, and prestige does not make them immortal.

If You Are a Dynamic Aggressive

Although fewer than one in two hundred people is a Dynamic Aggressive, there is a chance that you are manifesting this energy. If so, there's something important that you should do: examine the role of your childhood conditioning in your behavior today. I say this because, as a Dynamic Aggressive, you can have an enormous impact on the lives of others. Therefore, you must strive to be as self-aware as possible.

Start by considering the type of early conditioning your own parents received. If their parents or grandparents treated them as commodities—to be influenced and used to serve their purposes—then your parents may have passed that same conditioning on to you. If so, you may be lacking in compassion and emotional rapport as an adult, which would lead you to view other people as mere objects. Dynamic Aggressives who receive unconditional love as children still have an aggressive energy, but it is tempered by their parents' acceptance of them.

If your parents were especially strict, recognize that you may be a difficult person to get along with. No doubt you expect a herculean effort, if not perfection, from everyone around you. Because you are determined to work through a problem, you want everyone else to exhibit the same sense of commitment and discipline.

Dynamic Aggressives who did not receive unconditional love as children tend to distrust other people. If this is true of your upbringing, the unfortunate reality is that you may ultimately distrust yourself as well. Dynamic Aggressives are often fearful that they will one day be exposed as shams; this is the case for so many leaders and power brokers in our world. While they need the attention and adulation of the public, they are terrified of any real intimacy with people because of this underlying feeling of inadequacy.

In an ideal world, Dynamic Aggressives would use their charismatic energy as a catalyst—a lightning rod of sorts—to make other people more conscious of their own potential. Rather than spend all their time on their own projects, these charismatic leaders would apply their energy toward motivating others and moving them toward constructive change.

If you want to work in this constructive way, you must be aware that your energy can swing from high to low at any time. Actually, all of us must recognize that there is a duality to our energy that continually challenges us. If we ignore this challenge, we're never happy and we're never healthy. Putting our energy to good use is an active process that we must constantly reaffirm if we are to avoid the cycles that can lead to negative and destructive results.

Finally, recognize that some events in life—such as a serious illness—will not be assuaged by a long list of accomplishments. You need to develop your resiliency, and thus your ability to handle such life events, by becoming more flexible and more open to others. Learn to acknowledge your own mistakes as well as the accomplishments of others. Show some gratitude and loyalty to those who assist you in life. These changes will not only strengthen your relationships but will also set the stage for your own transformation.

The Mind-Powered World of Dynamic Assertives

They're the ones who show us the way. Like Dynamic Aggressives, Dynamic Assertives seek to guide us, but they do so by using only their highly developed powers of the mind and of self-expression, never by force or coercion.

Dynamic Assertives are rare people in our society. They have a forceful personal magnetism and an energy of mind that distinguishes them from all other energy types. They may represent a small percentage of the population (I'd say about one in a hundred people is a Dynamic Assertive), but they transform existing systems for everyone by challenging the status quo. Without them, society would not progress.

Above all, this powerhouse of an energy group is engaged with life. They try to live it to its fullest, all the while pondering its meaning in a lifelong quest for understanding. Dynamic Assertives see the big picture in the world around them and identify areas in need of constructive change. When manifesting their energy at its highest level, Dynamic Assertives will challenge the injustices that oppress us all. They will achieve break-throughs and set trends in their chosen field, be it business, science, education, literature, or philosophy. They are spiritual, ethical, and intellectual illuminators, human beacons lighting the way to social change.

Here's a thumbnail description of a Dynamic Assertive: *the kind of person you could have a conversation with and then write an article about it.* These are free-flow, stream-of-consciousness people. They take an idea and go with it, not recognizing boundaries or limitations. Talking with them can be a sort of awakening—if you can deal with it. Dynamic Assertives can be intimidating because they don't recognize barriers—social, sexual, economic, or any other kind. So you might begin talking with one and then say to yourself, "What am I getting into? Can I handle this?" If you can, you're in for an exciting ride.

Since limitation is not part of their gestalt, Dynamic Assertives thrive on change. They believe in the very idea of change and in the limitless possibilities it implies. Ultimately they serve as the "correctors" in society, the people who can identify wrongs and have the courage to correct them. Think of Mahatma Gandhi, Robert Kennedy, Nelson Mandela, Margaret Mead, Thoreau, Spinoza, Plato, and Socrates. These are people who held a mirror up to society and said, "Take a close look. Do you like what you see? Is what you see, what should be?" In asking these kinds of questions, Dynamic Assertives break the ground for new roads upon which everyone else will eventually travel.

Dynamic Assertives are found in every stratum of society; they don't necessarily rise to the top of businesses and organizations the way the more goal-oriented Dynamic Aggressives do. So these people are not necessarily names in the news—in fact, most aren't. Some are—Ralph Nader, Dr. Benjamin Spock, and Eleanor Roosevelt are Dynamic Assertives we've all heard of—but there are also people in our midst who hold regular jobs, and are not in the least famous, but who definitely manifest this life energy. Have you known any? If so, you'll probably be able to count them on one hand. You'll surely have vivid memories of them because they tend to be, in the *Reader's Digest* phrase, our "most unforgettable characters."

Many Dynamic Assertives distrust authority, which they believe operates from a self-interested agenda. They will sacrifice all to challenge such authority and facilitate change. As a result, Dynamic Assertives are a threat to established power and often end up being booted from institutions, discredited in their fields, locked away in prison, or even killed. They're martyr material. Consider Nelson Mandela, who spent nearly three decades in prison in South Africa for opposing the policies of a ruling class that oppressed millions. He was a danger to these rulers, so they attempted to silence him by sweeping him out of the way.

In fact, Dynamic Assertives generally are the first to be destroyed in a revolution of any sort. The authorities want to stop these nonconformists before they can cause a critical shift in perspective among other energy types, particularly Adaptive Supportives, who have the strength of numbers but rarely challenge authority on their own initiative. When enough Dynamic energies get together, they can focus the consciousness of many into a mass call for change; consider the Declaration of Independence and the genesis of the American Revolution. More recently in our history, consider how a small core of Dynamic Assertives sparked the movement to end the Vietnam War. And on the socio-ecological front, you may remember the time when concern for the environment was not part of any political or educational agenda. It took Dynamic Assertives such as Rachel Carson and others to forge the paradigm change that made environmentalism an acceptable mainstream stance in this country (retrograde radio talkshow hosts notwithstanding).

Dynamic Assertives differ from Dynamic Aggressives in that the former serve as catalysts for change without seeking to control other people. They are opinion-makers who can look beyond themselves to the common good, but their mission is to inspire and motivate other people, not to gain power over them. So Dynamic Assertives lead mainly by sharing ideas that others can use. Gandhi is an excellent example. He did not want to control other people, nor did he ask the rest of the world to live as he did. Through his own evolution as a human being, he simply showed others that change was possible. He chose to provide a model for society, not to run it. By the way, Gandhi is also an example of the fact that you don't have to be outgoing to be a Dynamic Assertive. You can be a quiet person. Mind power does not require high-volume projection to make itself felt.

More than any other energy type, Dynamic Assertives live in the moment. They are spontaneous and fluid people who respond to their circumstances. If they like something, it shows. If they dislike something, that also shows, and they don't pretend to be engaged in something when they're not. They may be lighthearted one moment and serious the next. In addition, they have a childlike curiosity that leads them to explore all aspects of life, so they would be the first to go to the moon or the bottom of the ocean.

The Dynamic Assertive's disregard for limitations is one of his or her most distinctive qualities. Whereas others might view fear, failure, or adversity as insurmountable roadblocks in life, the Dynamic Assertive views these as challenges. It's not that this group doesn't have fears, but rather that they face those fears and go through them. When Dynamic Assertives make mistakes—and they do so plenty of times—they pick themselves up and go on with their lives. Failure and disappointment become a part of their lifelong learning process rather than reasons to abandon their dreams.

The joy of creating often outweighs the adversity a Dynamic Assertive may face. Consider George Washington Carver, who overcame slavery and racism in the South to develop into a self-educated man and become one of this country's most important horticultural scientists and inventors. He created new uses for peanuts, sweet potatoes, and soy plants, which he helped develop in the South, where the soil had been increasingly depleted from overcultivation of cotton and tobacco. His work ended up providing a big boost for the economy of the region, and Carver went on to become the head of the agriculture department at Tuskegee Institute in Alabama, where he instituted a "school on wheels" that traveled around the state to teach farmers the principles of soil enrichment. He was a true Dynamic Assertive manifesting the high side of his energy; he had the talent, intelligence, and charisma to transcend immense society-imposed handicaps.

A problem Dynamic Assertives may have is that of being misunderstood by others. One reason is that, as intellectually honest people, they reveal their true reactions to things. So when they like something, they tend to show it, and when they dislike something, they show it too. There's no equivocation; you don't have to second-guess them. But this makes a lot of people nervous because it goes against the social convention of being falsely agreeable. This is especially so in the case of women, who are generally expected to be polite dissemblers in the cause of pleasing others. So Dynamic Assertives can be called rude or uncaring when in fact they're just trying to be upfront with people.

They can also be called just plain weird! And they *are* different in that this is a very inner-directed group. We have to respect the fact that any time we're in the presence of someone who is very charismatic and intellectually strong, he is not going to be functioning in the same way that most people around him are. For instance, a Dynamic Assertive may be very quiet and calm when everyone else is excited. Or he may be very excited when other people are calm. He doesn't act based on how everyone else is acting. He acts based on how he feels at the moment—and is therefore labeled strange. (By the way, substitute *she* for *he* in this paragraph to get a feeling for how women Dynamic Assertives may have an even harder time being accepted than men!)

An interesting aspect of Dynamic Assertives is that they tend to be less limited by the aging process than other people are. First of all, as independent thinkers, they don't buy into how a person is "supposed to" act at any particular age. Second, they're just not interested in slowing down for one second. I know some Dynamic Assertives who are in their eighties. When you're with them, you forget immediately that you're dealing with octogenarians. Whereas another person may have only their youth, looks, and body to excite someone, these people have far and away more than that. They have a dynamic, high-velocity energy to share, and that's not an age-dependent gift.

In short, members of this energy group are the most exciting to be around. They've got the vision and drive of the Dynamic Aggressives, but without that group's need for control, they're more generous, and—to use a plain word but one that says it—they're generally nicer. And their intellect-generated charisma can be such a magnetic force that you remember time spent with a Dynamic Assertive your whole life.

From Idealism to Hedonism: The Up and Down Sides of Dynamic Assertives

From the high end to the low end of a Dynamic Assertive's energy there's a big swing, and some people in this group do go to each extreme during their lives, sometimes repeatedly. Dynamic Assertives have the potential for high-end qualities such as selflessness and compassion, and they also have the potential for self-absorption and an egotistical perspective. When they get distracted from the ideals that give meaning to their lives, they may lose their focus on constructive change and become self-destructive.

On the up side, Dynamic Assertives have the patience to listen to others and see issues from their viewpoint. But they lose that essential balance on their down side. Then they may become self-righteous and attempt to persuade others that their beliefs are the only correct ones. And they can be highly successful at this endeavor! People who interact with a Dynamic Assertive must take care to evaluate the validity of their belief systems, because sometimes charisma can lead them down the wrong path.

Ascending their energy curve, Dynamic Assertives can be exceptionally giving and compassionate; they express their heart energy better than any other type of person. But on their down side, when their vision narrows and they become self-centered, compassion disappears. Dynamic Assertives can become selfish and full of pride; they may exaggerate their own importance to generate attention.

When Dynamic Assertives pursue their beliefs, they can become overzealous and compulsive. In some cases they no longer share their ideas constructively with society because their manner puts people off. They may cease to communicate in a balanced and reasonable way that allows other people to understand their message. Or, they become like racehorses going at breakneck speed; other people can't keep up and eventually become exhausted by the effort. And the Dynamic Assertive himself can burn out.

In fact, Dynamic Assertives must be especially attuned to the need for balance in life. They can become such workaholics that they deny other vital aspects of living, such as developing their relationships, health, and spirituality. They may surround themselves with a lot of parasitic people and meaningless activities, such as partying and entertaining, to compensate for a mounting sense of insecurity and loneliness. And, sadly, they may abandon their pursuit of ideals for the pursuit of material wealth.

But such greed isn't the rule. In general, I've found that the most generous people in the world are Dynamic Assertives, and if this generosity is not taken too far, it is definitely an up-side trait. There are a couple of reasons that Dynamic Assertives are so generous. One is that they usually don't have problems making money. However, even when they are living quite modestly, Dynamic Assertives will often be extremely magnanimous with what they do have. You see, money and possessions are not the be-all and end-all for Dynamic Assertives; this group is much less status-conscious than Dynamic Aggressives. The be-all and end-all for Dynamic Assertives is *ideas*, which they like to share—and so their things, and even their homes, just kind of become part and parcel of the sharing process. This is the second reason Dynamic Assertives are often so magnanimous: To them, mind and spirit supersede the material. You might even say that, to a Dynamic Assertive, the material is immaterial!

An amazing level of hospitality may be part of the Dynamic Assertive's magnanimity. They make it extremely easy for you to be in their environment. In fact, in the case of some Dynamic Assertives I know, their house is basically an open house—a place where you, and many other friends, too, are free to just *be*. There's no constricting "guest" feeling in their homes because you're not really a guest—you're a participant in the experience of life that you and your Dynamic Assertive friend are sharing. The phrase "My house is your house" rings very true when you're in the home of many a Dynamic Assertive.

This up-side picture of Dynamic Assertive generosity is a beautiful one, but of course there can be problems with it—big problems. For one thing, sometimes a Dynamic Assertive won't be financially well off, and yet he'll continue to—almost literally—give friends the shirt off his back, and severely impoverish himself in the process. For another, friends who are not of the same energy group just don't have it in them to reciprocate at the Dynamic Assertive's level of generosity, and if the Dynamic Assertive expects this, he or she may at some point become quite disappointed and hurt.

Third, even if a Dynamic Assertive isn't financially wiped out by being overly generous, he or she is prone to being egregiously used. A Dynamic Assertive friend of mine falls into this category. He's got a large house that's forever filled with guests. But what are some of these "friends" doing? They're making long-distance phone calls from his house for hours on end and not paying for them. They're eating meal after free meal at his table and never offering to cook, much less pay. They're even stealing things out of his rooms. I've tried to tell him that his generosity has gone from an up-side trait to a problem, but sometimes one Dynamic Assertive talking to another has trouble getting through!

Dynamic Assertives on their up side are quite capable of relaxing, unlike their energy cousins the Dynamic Aggressives, who don't know how to rest. This facility in the art of relaxation is a big plus in terms of health. On the down side in the health area, Dynamic Assertives, when they are manifesting their energy at its lowest level, can lose control—and fast. The respect they have for their minds and bodies on the high end may simply disappear. If they are not careful, they can become highly self-destructive and hedonistic, often developing addictions to junk food, alcohol, and drugs, as well as gambling. Their bodies may become polluted, increasing their susceptibility to disease. This begins a downward spiral, and a Dynamic Assertive can become mentally and physically ill very quickly on the down side.

A difference between a down-side Dynamic Assertive and a down-side Dynamic Aggressive is that the former tends not to destroy other people, but rather him- or herself. The damage is directed inward, although, of course, those who are very close to a downward-spiraling Dynamic Assertive would be negatively affected as well.

Understand, Conceptualize, Lead: The Work of Dynamic Assertives

Dynamic Assertives are highly functioning people when they operate from the high side of their energy. Place them in any new environment, and their first impulse is to organize it and make it work. Note: they don't have to own it or preside over it. But they do have a keen sense of order and can envision the best way to make a place or a situation function well.

One of the distinguishing characteristics of the Dynamic energies is that they are conceptually creative.

Dynamic Assertives, in particular, love to bring their new ideas to fruition. They're certainly not the type to sit around and let good ideas slip by. They take advantage of every opportunity to turn their ideas into reality, enthusiastically explaining to others what they're up to and how they can help.

Dynamic Assertives generally do not focus on personal achievement goals. For them, the point of any endeavor—and of life, for that matter—is not to win or to gain control, as in the case of Dynamic Aggressives, but to arrive at new levels of understanding. As a result, they believe the process is key. Dynamic Assertives are motivated to explore the processes of their lives. This orientation also applies to their work and to their interactions with others. The Dynamic Assertive is a systems person who designs solutions to problems and determines how a job should be done. At that point, he or she often turns the project over to other energy types, such as Creative Assertives, to devise the actual mechanics, and Adaptive Aggressives, to see that the work is implemented.

Sometimes Dynamic Assertives will have Adaptive Supportives working for them—which is fine—but will expect them to perform in a visionary or creative way, and then become disappointed when they don't. I've seen this happen with several of my friends who are Dynamic Assertives; they end up yelling at people in their offices because these workers are not thinking along the same lines they are. It's unfair, and Dynamic Assertives have to guard against such unrealistic expectations.

Dynamic Assertives often like to work for themselves. In this way they can pursue the issues that have meaning to them and maintain responsibility for their own lives. Given their sense of independence, Dynamic Assertives generally do not fit into established institutions, which can make them feel constrained and controlled.

Dynamic Assertives have tremendous raw energy, and sometimes it seems as if they do in a week what other people might do in a year, or even a lifetime. But while all this get-up-and-go is commendable, sometimes sit-down-and-stop is a good thing, too, and Dynamic Assertives often forget this. They'll work twenty hours a day without setting aside time to rest their minds and bodies. Another pitfall: Dynamic Assertives can be highly critical of themselves and others. Perfectionism, in that it demands the highest level of performance from oneself and one's assistants, can be a good thing. But the down side of perfectionism is that one can become opinionated, judgmental, and intolerant of other people's weaknesses.

Dynamic Assertives can swing between cooperation at one end of the spectrum and competitiveness at the other. When they are ascending their energy curve, they will work in harmony with others to actualize a vision. But they may become competitive with other Dynamic Assertives and, on the low end, this competition may result in unnecessary rivalry. In extreme cases, Dynamic Assertives will become territorial, protecting their turf by negating the accomplishments of others.

Beyond that, Dynamic Assertives must be constantly aware of the potential for spiritual burnout. All of us can identify people who had wonderful ideas to share and who could have made a great difference in the lives of others. But if their ideas are not accepted—always a danger for Dynamic Assertives because others misunderstand them—they can become disillusioned and bitter. Why do they have a gift, they ask, if others will not accept it? This question cannot be answered intellectually, and Dynamic Assertives must turn to the spiritual realm to put such disappointments in perspective.

Success is important to Dynamic Assertives because it validates their beliefs and ideals. They want other people to accept their ideas and respond to their creations; thus they measure their success according to that acceptance. But they may come to resent the things that accompany success—the many people in their lives, the demands of the public—or they may become arrogant. As for the monetary aspect of success, on the high end, money does not define the lives of this group or play a significant role in motivating them. Many Dynamic Assertives make a lot of money and spend it just as easily. They generally are not the type to play the stock market or otherwise invest their money. They would rather spend it on living. The down side is that Dynamic Assertives may use their money totally selfishly, rather than support charities or other causes that go beyond themselves.

Despite all the problems that Dynamic Assertives can have vis à vis the world of work, when they do make their mark, theirs are the most meaningful and inspiring contributions. I'll give you a good example: someone I've had the privilege to know, Bob Guccione. Yes, he's the editor of *Penthouse*, but he's an unsung Dynamic Assertive hero, as far as I'm concerned. I'll tell you why.

Several years ago I had written an article on the politics of cancer, the first major article of its type in America. Back then, nobody in any major medium would take on the cancer establishment. A tiny newspaper called *Our Town* did publish that first article, though. Then, an editor at *Forum* magazine, Al Freedman—a longtime friend of Guccione—read the article and called me. "Why don't you meet Bob Guccione?" he said.

I didn't know either of them, and I'd never read *Penthouse*, but we set up an appointment and I went over to meet Bob.

He turned out to be a very soft-spoken, quiet man. But this is what he said: "I like what you're doing, and I like what it means. I'm going to help you. I'm going to take your articles and put them into my publication so sixteen million people can read them." And that was the end of the meeting.

Then, a week later, there was another meeting, but this time, all of the lawyers, editors, salespeople, and everyone else from *Penthouse* was there. And every one of them was coming down against the articles. "We're going to have lawsuits; we can't defend ourselves against the lawsuits. Sponsors are going to withdraw their ads because these multinational corporations, including drug cartels, own all kinds of advertisers that we use in our publication." Everyone was dead set against the articles.

But Guccione said to me and to the whole group, "If I have to go without a single advertiser and take every nickel to put this out, I'm going to do it. If I lose 20 million dollars an issue, I'll lose it." He said, "We're going to save some lives and we're going to take on the cancer establishment. That's my promise." The man was going against the advice of his entire staff.

Here was an example of an inner-directed man who believed in a cause and then acted on it. He believed in taking on authority, and was fiercely independent and autonomous. Yes, he also promoted sexuality and freedom of sexual expression; he promoted erotic fantasy fulfillment. This was within his rights, and part of the needs of other people.

But when it came to social commitment, he was more determined than any other person I've ever met in the United States, and he took people on while incurring a tremendous potential for loss. He really could have lost it all. As it turned out, he did lose a lot. You see, he did print the articles, and he offered free article reprints to anyone who objected to his magazine, so that they wouldn't have to buy it to get the information. But then 1.3 million free reprints were given out. He also lost about seven pages' worth of advertisements, which meant that he probably lost, over a period of a year, 11 million dollars. Now, what kind of person would willingly give up 11 million dollars to have an article or series of articles published?

A Dynamic Assertive would. Many people over the years have requested reprints of, or have been affected by, those articles. They've no doubt saved a lot of lives and changed a lot of lives, but none of this would have happened without the dynamism of Bob Guccione.

Relationships—For the Here and Now

The Dynamic Assertive's first relationship is with life. This group wants to experience all that life has to offer, and so living—not relating to one other person on a daily basis—is the priority. Consequently, their relationships tend to be measured; Dynamic Assertives may share only certain aspects of their lives or a certain amount of time with a partner. They generally do not form the all-encompassing, long-lasting type of relationship that society has stamped with approval. Once again, they are not comfortable with the mold our culture has cast for them.

For most people, the idea of having measured relationships is an alien concept. You're either in a relationship every day, or you're not in it at all. But Dynamic Assertives have a more fluid sense of life. They generally do not value permanency as much as the ability to live in the moment. Thus they can share time with someone one day, but not see the person at all the next. Given their highly independent nature, they're happy to be loners at times and they simply do not have the same need for permanent relationships that other people do. This can be a real problem because, since Dynamic Assertives are exceptionally magnetic, people tend to *want* to have a permanent relationship with them. But wanting won't necessarily make something happen when it goes against a person's natural life energy. So if you happen to be in a relationship with a Dynamic Assertive, remember: It's not going to be always, and you're not always going to come first. It's nothing personal, though!

Compared to other energy types, Dynamic Assertives are more discriminating in the relationships they form. They look for people who are enjoyable to be with but who are similarly independent and open-ended in their approach to relationships. They can be supportive of others but also impatient. They don't want to be a caretaker for someone who is merely trying to cope with life, as opposed to experiencing it to the fullest.

Dynamic Assertives are spontaneous; they do whatever comes to mind. If there's anything that will unsettle them, it's a person who attempts to regulate their lives by setting boundaries in a relationship. So again, if you're in a relationship with a Dynamic Assertive, it's nothing personal, but they're not going to take well to your trying to rein them in with restrictions. Think of having a relationship with a Dynamic Assertive as being along for the ride. It can be a real joyride, but you're not going to be too popular if you keep putting on the brakes.

More than any other energy type, Dynamic Assertives have a difficult time being monogamous. They can be fiercely loyal, dedicated, and sensitive to the people in their lives, but they generally recognize that one person cannot meet all of their needs. What's more, they want to dedicate their energy to the life process, not to maintaining a relationship within the narrow framework that most people set. The confines of a monogamous relationship can make them feel bored, frustrated, and angry. And ultimately their spouses are likely to end up angry, too. I'd say that if you're looking for a picture-book, long-term romance, complete with country cottage and white picket fence, a Dynamic Assertive is not the way to go. There are other energies better suited to live happily ever after behind that fence.

Dynamic Assertives tend to have a lot of people coming into, and out of, their lives. Their natural charisma and constructive energy attract people who want to share in the excitement, and Dynamic Assertives can have hundreds of acquaintances and friends with whom they interact regularly; they feel comfortable with many different types of relationships and levels of sharing. A problem sometimes arises, though, with juggling these multiple relationships, and finding time to spend with the people who are most important to them. Some of these people, wanting more, will get tired of waiting for the Dynamic Assertive to get around to them, and will drop from the scene. This contributes to the high turnover rate in the Dynamic Assertive's social circle.

Most Dynamic Assertives have no interest in controlling other people. But if they are not careful, they may influence others unduly without realizing they have done so. The danger is that another person will become dependent on the Dynamic Assertive, and he or she may feel suffocated and bogged down by the relationship. To protect themselves from this scenario, Dynamic Assertives often seem to keep others at a slight distance.

Dynamic Assertives are especially wary of insecure people. Since they don't feel possessive of their partners and friends, they expect the same in return. When a Dynamic Assertive becomes involved with someone who is jealous, there is likely to be a great deal of conflict. Undoubtedly, the other person will feel threatened by all the activity and people in the Dynamic Assertive's life. Many Dynamic Assertives respond to this jealousy by ending their other relationships with friends. But this stopgap measure, intended to keep the peace, is hardly a healthy or satisfying way to handle the problem. If a Dynamic Assertive must deny his or her natural energy to appease the jealousy of another, then the value of the relationship is questionable.

I've seen this jealousy scenario happen. I had a male friend who was one of the finest Dynamic Assertives I've ever met. He was the type who was up for anything. He would, for instance, call you up out of the blue and say, "Let's go to the museum!" and you would get there and somehow find yourself eight floors below ground level looking at the priceless manuscripts the museum had in storage. I'm still not sure how that one happened, but that was the kind of zany outing that was his style.

Anyway, my friend married an Adaptive Aggressive who was very threatened by his other relationships. She asked him to give all that up so that they would only have "safe" relationships with other couples.

He complied; the non-couples and spontaneous activities were gone from his life. But the pizzazz was also gone and his life became a deflated, tamed, comfort-seeking thing. There were no more spur-of-the-moment adventures, just living-room, married-couples socializing.

I think we all know—regardless of our energy group—that these socially acceptable couples relationships can be excruciatingly boring. I mean, face it: Four people being mutually interesting to each other is a condition that's almost impossible to fulfill. And for the fast-paced, mind-driven Dynamic Assertive, an entire evening of Mr. and Mrs. Smith plus Mr. and Mrs. Jones—well, let's just say that this is not likely to be his or her favorite activity! My friend didn't complain, but in my book he lost a lot—too much, in fact, considering his extreme Dynamic Assertive nature.

More than any other energy type, Dynamic Assertives need time alone for introspection, away from their relationships with friends and partners. For most of their waking hours, they give an enormous amount of their energy to other people. In a sense, society runs off the energy that Dynamic Assertives provide. But periodically they have to withdraw from society and give themselves time to re-energize if they're to keep giving at the same level. When they do withdraw, others should understand that they're doing so out of personal necessity, not out of unfriendliness.

As fluid, spontaneous types, Dynamic Assertives are not the most predictable of folk. This can be upsetting to others attempting to have a relationship with members of this energy group. Unpredictability is a paradox. People are attracted by it, but they're also put off by it. Unpredictable people are like firecrackers—you don't know if you really want to play with them all the time.

It's worth noting that Dynamic Assertive women face particular problems in forming relationships. These women have all the same qualities as their male counterparts—they're intelligent, challenging, and highly engaged with life—which makes them threatening to the average man. A Dynamic Assertive woman has to be an equal in any relationship, and she must find a partner who is not threatened by her charisma and self-assuredness. That's no easy task, and many Dynamic Assertive women end up with partners who try to prove that they are superior by competing with them, often in childish ways.

As a result, many Dynamic Assertive women find that their relationships are draining, or even impossible to sustain. Some men simply won't accept these women for who they are, and attempt to "tame" them by bringing their energy under control. For example, a Dynamic Assertive's partner may want her to downplay her career. But, of course, trying to suppress a Dynamic Assertive's energies is not going to make for a good relationship in the long run.

Despite their problems with romantic relationships, Dynamic Assertives can be terrific friends. They are extremely loyal; they never forget a friend, and will go to great lengths to help the people they care about. One Dynamic Assertive I know was in England when he heard that a man who had worked for him fifteen years earlier was dying of cancer in the United States. This Dynamic Assertive did not have any money, but he used his credit cards to fly to Miami, that same night, to visit the former employee. That type of loyalty and sensitivity is typical of Dynamic Assertives on the high side of their energy.

As parents, Dynamic Assertives may not be so successful. Parenting a young child requires constancy—not often the Dynamic Assertive's strong point. But when they are in touch with the higher self, they can do an excellent job in some aspects of child rearing. For example, they will encourage independent thought in a child and share all their insight about human nature as well—both highly valuable gifts to the young. And they tend to speak to their children with respect. This is an idea that does not seem to have occurred to some people in our society, but Dynamic Assertives usually respect the mental and spiritual potential of others, regardless of age, and even of species; members of this energy group can be true friends of animals. On the down side, however, Dynamic Assertive parents can be so self-absorbed and impatient that they distance a child. Even worse, they may fail to devote time alone with the child—a cardinal sin of parenthood—because they are so preoccupied with their work and the other people in their lives. If the child must compete with throngs of people for the parent's attention, he or she will resent it mightily.

Energy Combinations

To form healthy relationships, Dynamic Assertives must be given the freedom to be who they are. The energy types most likely to create this space are Creative Assertives, other Dynamic Assertives, and Dynamic Supportives, provided they are operating from the high side of their energy. These people understand the Dynamic Assertive's devotion to the life process, while other types may not be able to tolerate it.

A Dynamic Assertive and a Creative Assertive can make a beautiful combination, especially when both are ascending their energy curve. They can forge a wonderful, trusting relationship that allows for an exciting exchange of ideas. The Dynamic Assertive sees the big picture; the Creative Assertive knows how to execute the details to complete that picture. Because they are caring and sensitive people, Creative Assertives will be cooperative and supportive of a Dynamic Assertive. They will make sacrifices to help bring the Dynamic Assertive's vision to life, and benefit other people.

Two Dynamic Assertives also can have a spectacular relationship. If both are on their up side, they will share their strengths and their love of life, creating an exciting and spontaneous relationship. It's like two meteors traveling side by side: They brighten the sky wherever they go. The beauty of this relationship is that both will be living and sharing in the moment; the relationship doesn't anticipate tomorrow, or seek to set boundaries, or attempt to establish a permanent commitment. It simply allows the passion of the moment to exist without looking to define and encode it.

Two Dynamic Assertives can have a good business relationship as well, as long as they avoid the natural tendency to compete. They can accomplish a lot together and even help to pace each other so that neither one burns out. For the relationship to work, though, each Dynamic Assertive has to respect the other and recognize that the relationship has its limitations—the fact that they are business partners does not mean that they can meddle in the other's personal sphere.

One of the finest friendships possible for a Dynamic Assertive is with a Dynamic Supportive. They have a lot in common—their high level of energy, love of life, and creativity, for example—but they won't feel the constant need to compete and prove themselves to one another. It would be an easy and highly enjoyable relationship for both.

A relationship with an Adaptive Aggressive is trickier. It could be fine if the Adaptive Aggressive does not have ulterior motives. The Adaptive Aggressive may be quite effective in implementing the Dynamic Assertive's vision, and the two may genuinely enjoy being together as well, appreciating each other's very different types of energy and ways of interacting with the world. But there can be problems. Given their opportunistic nature, Adaptive Aggressives may join with a Dynamic energy to better their own condition or to learn what they can from the Dynamic Assertive before moving on. What's more, the Adaptive Aggressive might attempt to tie up the relationship by establishing boundaries for the Dynamic Assertive, something the Dynamic Assertive will come to resent.

Another danger is that an Adaptive Aggressive will assume all the qualities of a Dynamic Assertive—his or her openness, assertiveness, and experimental approach to life—to appear to be just the right person for the Dynamic Assertive. This mimicry is a specialty of the Adaptive Aggressive, and it can be appealing to Dynamic Assertives who are looking for someone to agree with them, compliment them, and do what they want to do. Think of Elvis Presley, a Dynamic Assertive who surrounded himself with Adaptive Aggressives. These people spent more time feeding off his stardom than providing him with true friendship.

With this type of relationship, the Dynamic Assertive is not dealing with the Adaptive Aggressive's real self. The Dynamic Assertive may do certain things for the pure joy of it, while the Adaptive Aggressive is merely configuring him- or herself, chameleon-like, to the present environment because he or she expects to gain something from it in the end. In this case, the relationship between a Dynamic Assertive and an Adaptive Aggressive can turn explosive.

Danger: The Betrayal Trap

A disturbing phenomenon I've seen too much of lately is the tell-all book, in which an Adaptive type who's been trusted by and living or working with a Dynamic Assertive turns around and writes an unflattering book about him or her. This is the in-print manifestation of the problem of betrayal that Dynamic Assertives often face.

Dynamic Assertives are particularly prone to this backstabbing phenomenon because of the kind of lives they lead and the kind of people they are. Both Dynamic Aggressives and Dynamic Assertives lead unusual lives and accomplish extraordinary things that others like to hear or read about. And both groups depend on many people around them to implement the details of their work. But Dynamic Assertives, who tend to be the more forward-thinking and unconventional of these two energy groups, as well as the less cagey, can supply a potential bad-mouther with more material. What's more, Dynamic Assertives' tendency to share—everything from ideas to feelings to their means of sustenance and shelter—means that others can really get involved in their lives. Then, if these others are less than scrupulous, they can use what they've learned to make a profit, or simply to create gossip or bad feeling. So Dynamic Assertives should always be on guard against the danger of betrayal, although for those living a fully engaged life, being betrayed at some point is probably inevitable.

Openness to Personal Change

Dynamic Assertives have a tremendous potential for growth. Unlike some of the other energy types, they thrive on change and take a fearless approach to achieving it in their lives.

Personal growth is always based on self-knowledge, and one thing that can be strongly said about Dynamic Assertives is that they know who they are. Introspective souls, they've spent hours pondering themselves, their ethics, and their places and missions in the world. They're not generally religious but they are spiritual, certainly in the sense that their own spirit is known to them, having been examined so closely and so often. Other energy types, without a similar feeling for their own personal core, can fall prey to following false or dangerous gurus. A radio demagogue or shock jock, for instance, or a TV evangelist, can provide an attractive, ready-made belief package to those who, lacking their own sense of identity, need one to latch on to. But Dynamic Assertives don't fall into this category; in fact, they're often the ones who point out to others the foolishness of being a sheeplike follower.

Dynamic Assertives have an innate sense of what it takes to grow; they recognize that growth is possible only when one is vulnerable. Vulnerability leads to openness, spontaneity, and fluidity, all of which provide fertile ground for positive change. Because Dynamic Assertives are willing to live in the moment, they can turn on a dime and take advantage of opportunities to change, and to have peak experiences in the process.

The best example of this ability of Dynamic Assertives to "go with the flow" and opportunistically learn from the experience is their perspective on failure. Dynamic Assertives can fail time and again without allowing failure to break their resolve. When they fall down they simply pick themselves up again. They don't revel in the pain of the fall, and they certainly don't listen to naysayers who advise people to back off and play it safe once they fail. The Dynamic Assertive uses failure as a tool for learning, at times turning negatives to positives in an amazing way.

One obstacle to growth for Dynamic Assertives is their childhood conditioning. Many Dynamic Assertives feel conflicted throughout life because they were conditioned to be another energy type, such as an Adaptive Supportive. They may get a lot of negative input during childhood from parents who do not understand their Assertive energy and who squelch their dreams. As they become adults, they sense that their life is not as fulfilling as it should be, but are terrified of allowing their true self to shine through.

When a Dynamic Assertive's early conditioning exerts a negative influence on his or her life, it's something like gravity pulling at an ascending star. And in fact, at any point in life, they are in danger of being pulled back into the conformist world by someone who expects them to fit into society's mold—to take a nine-to-five job, perhaps, or to form a permanent relationship that requires them to deny vital aspects of their natural energy.

The Dynamic Assertive woman, in particular, may have strong conditioning to be an Adaptive Supportive; indeed, women are rarely conditioned to be a Dynamic energy of any type. As a result, they may have to go against the grain their entire lives, fighting to overcome people's perceptions of who they should be and how they should live their lives. And even those who overcome this obstacle to express their true energy may face another problem. Given their strength, individuality, and high level of functioning in relation to others, there may be very little impetus for them to grow. Some of them get caught in a circular pattern of growth, focusing all their energy on one area of interest until they conquer it and become bored. In the process, they fail to identify and explore other avenues of growth and transformation.

Dynamic Assertives and the Need for Renewal

More than anything, members of this energy group need to establish a balance in their lives. They can't run at full speed for long periods of time, pursuing the process of life and their visions relentlessly, without taking time out for introspection. Remember, if you are a Dynamic Assertive, your charisma will draw many people to you, but if you're the type who just "cain't say 'no,' " you're going to be surrounded by such a mob all the time that the people whom you really care about will not be able to get through to you, and they'll eventually be repelled. Also, you can unwittingly repel people with your potential for self-absorption and self-destructive behavior.

To balance your energy and use it constructively, you need to clear some space in your life for meditation and reflection. Give yourself a chance to renew, and you will have the fuel to manifest your energy at its highest level. Many Dynamic Assertives lose this ability because they allow themselves to become perpetually busy. They get so carried away by their own creativity and energy that they create a terrible imbalance in their lives. If you work so hard—even at something you truly enjoy—that you deny other aspects of living, you will alter your perception of life and your ability to relate to others.

The danger, then, is that you will forget to plant the seeds of growth in your life, allowing yourself instead to be consumed by work, overexpansion, and by the many conflicts that pepper our day-to-day existence. Learn to delegate authority so you have time to renew, and to be patient with others who have their own pace and approach to completing a project.

Remember, too, that there are negative consequences to a self-sacrificing commitment to any cause, no matter how worthy. If you are not careful, you can develop a "martyr complex" that ultimately makes you self-obsessive, overly intense, and boring. This can kill your spontaneity, joy, and creativity—the driving forces in your life.

Be aware, too, of the tendency to pursue new projects for the wrong reasons. Perhaps you are just chasing money or trying to prove yourself to other people. Be sure to pull back from time to time to check your motives and avoid these traps. These are the times when you can say, "I don't need more money right now. I don't need to compete with others by starting another project. What I need is to reflect on my deeds and allow myself to grow." If you "de-clutter" your workload in this way from time to time, the work you do take on will be more rewarding.

A final challenge: Be more selective in the people you bring into your life. Like many Dynamic Assertives, you probably have a tendency to form dozens of relationships that have no real meaning. They may simply be byproducts of the constant activity in your life, not a recognition by both parties that you have something to share. Such relationships can be draining, and they take time away from those that really are important in your life. Again, de-clutter, and give your best qualities a chance to shine.

The Bridge Between Energies: Dynamic Supportives

It takes a while to appreciate some people, but if you meet someone who's immediately likable, there's a good chance that he or she is a Dynamic Supportive. People with this energy have a genuine affability that comes through right away, making them instantly easy to relate to. What's more, they can relate to all different types of people. While a high-powered Dynamic Aggressive might have nothing to say to a down-to-earth Adaptive Supportive, or a Creative Assertive, on a bad day, might have nothing to say to anyone, the Dynamic Supportive usually can communicate on a positive level with everyone. You could say that, like the sun, he or she casts warmth on all people, without regard to group or status.

Indeed, Dynamic Supportives are particularly warmhearted. This compassionate, charismatic group includes many healers, conciliators, teachers, and clergy. Dynamic Supportives have stability, an energetic balance, and an inner sense of what is genuine. Other people are drawn to them, but Dynamic Supportives are not oriented toward making changes in others or in their environment. They do have a definite set of values, but they do not force these on anyone. Instead, they quietly set standards, by their actions, warmth, and presence. In other words, they motivate others by example.

Dynamic Supportives are sensitive to the emotional energies of their environment. They are energetically and intuitively attuned to other people, and they naturally engage on an emotional level. They have an empathetic nature, which means that they identify more easily than others do with what they see or contemplate, becoming, at the extreme, like sponges for whatever vibrations surround them. They have inner vision, and they sense the broad schemes of nature. Dynamic Supportives are independent people who have a strong will and character and an especially strong sense of self. Other people and situations do not intimidate them.

On their up side, Dynamic Supportives establish a healthy psychic coming and going as they connect emphatically with the external world and return home to the self. On their down side, they may absorb outside conflicts and feel troubled, unbalanced, and physically ill. Their distress and concern for other people can cause them to lose sight of their own plans, and they forget to take care of themselves.

Many Dynamic Supportives might be considered "unfocused dynamics" because they have a lot of charisma but do not necessarily know where or how to use it. They may meander in life and fail to actualize their abundant potential. In many cases, in fact, they can be unmotivated, lethargic, and even lazy in realizing their full potential.

This tendency can be enormously frustrating for other people who recognize the untapped potential in a Dynamic Supportive. Imagine Fred Astaire deciding not to pursue a film career because he thinks no one really wants to see him dance anyway, or Einstein deciding not to solve the puzzles of the universe because it's too much hassle. That's the kind of situation the people around a Dynamic Supportive sometimes perceive, and it can drive them crazy. But all the cajoling, prodding, and encouragement in the world won't change the basic nature of the Dynamic Supportive.

When others try to force a Dynamic Supportive to realize his or her potential, it's like blowing up a balloon halfway and then expecting it to continue on its own. It simply won't happen. The balloon deflates again, because it is not self-starting. That's why other people must accept that a Dynamic Supportive's potential will be actualized in the context of his or her own life, not according to their own expectations. They have to respect that the Dynamic Supportive is often doing a great deal of good in his or her own way.

Likewise, it would be a mistake to look to the Dynamic Supportive for leadership, as we do with other charismatic people. Dynamic Supportives generally have no interest in directing others. However, they do have a singular ability to bring people together in understanding. Their ability to view life from a broad perspective and to empathize with others allows them to draw disparate energies into a working whole. They know intuitively what works and what does not. They can facilitate a dialogue in a nonthreatening and noncompetitive way. They understand both the Dynamic energies, typically the initiators in society, and the Adaptive energies, who help put initiatives into effect. Thus the Dynamic Supportive can serve as a bridge between the two, facilitating communication and cooperation.

Dynamic Supportives sometimes do not take the initiative to make social or personal change for several reasons. For one thing, they are simply content to be who they are. They have nothing to prove to anyone and are not easily externally motivated. Second, they take on the problems of others at their own expense when they do not set limits on their empathy. They can be so drawn into other people's inner conflicts that they live outside themselves psychologically. As they identify with these emotions, their minds may become restless and unfocused. And finally, even though they do plan for the future, Dynamic Supportives can become absorbed in the present. In doing so they adapt to their circumstances, sometimes a little too well. It's not that they don't see the big, long-term picture; they do. But the down side of their seeing the broad picture can be a negative relativism: "Nothing in itself really matters, so why bother?" This gives them an excuse to forget about the details of life and to let things go.

For Dynamic Supportives who want to make personal changes, the tendency to lose focus can be disheartening. As potentially capable planners, they recognize that they have not followed through. They have a tendency to melancholy and may become depressed on their down side. This, in turn, can make it even more difficult for them to keep track of details and to follow through. The result can be that they find themselves in a negative cycle.

On their up side, Dynamic Supportives have a natural optimism. They are easygoing, joyful, and accepting people. They may have trouble sticking with their long-term plans, but they keep the blues away by doing things for others and making more plans. You can't keep them down. As is the case with the other Dynamic energies, a Dynamic Supportive can experience a major failure in life that would devastate someone else, and yet be back in the game the next day. They approach each endeavor— in both their personal and professional lives—with sincerity and a strong sense of commitment. They are stable, reliable, and extremely responsible in fulfilling their obligations.

Dynamic Supportives are also direct, self-aware, and self-sufficient. If something gets in the way of doing what they believe is right, they address the problem head-on. A Dynamic Supportive will not let personal fears drive his or her life. They don't dance around problems and avoid them; they deal with them directly and face their fears.

While Dynamic Supportives don't back off from their convictions, they do have a softer approach than do other energy types. Their observations and comments are usually relevant and funny because they have a terrific sense of humor. On their up side, they're thoughtful, spontaneous, and unafraid. Part of their charm is that they have a lot of self-confidence, but they don't necessarily do anything earthshaking with it. You won't see them getting into a workaholic rut by slaving away twenty hours a day. In fact, the term "laid back" sometimes seems custom-made for the Dynamic Supportive.

Interestingly, some "Dynamic Supportives" aren't—that is, some people who seem to display Dynamic Supportive energies are not really doing so from a natural inclination, but because of a role inherited from childhood. Many children grow up with caregivers who have not learned to appreciate themselves or who have personal problems with which they cannot cope. When a child is asked to parent the parent—to interpret, facilitate, and keep the peace at home—he or she may later appear to have a natural supportive energy. In some cases this may really be so; in others, the child's conditioned energy may overlay his or her natural energy.

As adults, ostensibly Dynamic Supportive people have to ask themselves if they find joy in the benevolent actions they perform for others. A natural Dynamic Supportive will truly enjoy being helpful and supportive. But the question is tricky, since even the natural Dynamic Supportive may experience stress and depression until he or she has learned to protect the inner self.

A key to identifying false Dynamic Supportives is this: They seek out the helping role more than they are asked to take it on. Natural Dynamic Supportives are sought out, and they tend to be more effective than the next person in motivating and helping others precisely because people are drawn to their charisma and ask for their help. Also, unlike conditioned Dynamic Supportives, people who are naturally of this life energy do not feel lost or without purpose when they are not functioning in a helping role.

Strong, Gentle, Accommodating
. . . *Too* Accommodating

Dynamic Supportives have a natural balance, but they are so emphatically attuned to their environment that they can easily be drawn outside themselves and into other people's energy. And when these other people are troubled, chaotic, or negative, the Dynamic Supportive's own balance may be upset.

Indeed, this energy group's concern for other people can lead to trouble if it's not tempered by good judgment. Dynamic Supportives are the group with a lot of members who are often just plain "too nice." They may try to help people who will not help themselves, and spend an enormous amount of time doing things for others. As a result, people may take advantage of these "Mr. or Ms. Nice Guys" if they have not learned to set limits on their empathy and re-center themselves.

The other Dynamic energies—the Aggressive and the Assertive—sometimes rub people the wrong way because they can be opinionated, driven, and rude. The Dynamic Supportive, by contrast, is more likable because he is more mellow—more likely to smile, to agree, to be helpful. But herein lies a problematic aspect of the Dynamic Supportive's life. If a person is agreeable and helpful all the time and then one day, for whatever reason, he doesn't agree, or help, those around him have a tendency to resent it.

"Why aren't you helping me?" they ask.

"I ran out of money."

Or, "Why aren't you agreeing with me?"

"I've come to a different conclusion than you have."

"What kind of an excuse is that?"

Indeed, those are no excuses to people who have been spoiled by a Dynamic Supportive's support. They come to expect things from a Dynamic Supportive that they would never expect from anyone else. So people in this energy group have to take protective psychic steps to make sure others don't take them for granted and then act offended when the Dynamic Supportive steps "out of character."

If Dynamic Supportives do not take these protective steps, they are often prone to disease. On the down side, in fact, Dynamic Supportives may use illness as an excuse not to achieve. Their rationale tends to be something like, "I'll be right there just as soon as I'm well." The problem is not that they fake illness. It is that they do not take responsibility for their own lives. They have a hard time saying no to others and giving themselves equal time.

A Dynamic Supportive on the down side can get set up quite easily. Other people see that they are strong but gentle, an appealing combination that makes others latch on to them. They sense the potential and think, "Gee, this person is really going someplace." Chances are, the Dynamic Supportive does not live up to this observation when he or she is on the down side. They can get lazy and not project their energy into anything worthwhile. There is too much being and not enough doing. You can come back ten years later and they haven't even done the dishes. In many cases they simply do not direct themselves.

The Dynamic Supportive's attention to detail also swings from one extreme to the other, depending on whether they are on the up side or the down side. On the high end, they pride themselves on their ability to handle the details of life. Their home life is organized, with everything in its proper place. If you were to visit their attic, you would find everything neatly sorted, packed, and labeled by date. On their down side, by contrast, their life has no details. All the small things that make up their daily existence seem to slip away. At this point, they don't even know if they have an attic, let alone what's in it.

On the up side, Dynamic Supportives have positive and flexible energy. But their tendency will be to simply accommodate to a situation when they are on the down side; they neither learn from it nor transform it. Still, most Dynamic Supportives are very strong about standing up for the truth. They are responsible people with excellent character, and they would not let another person take the blame for them. In many respects they are models for character development.

Helpers Par Excellence

Dynamic Supportives are well suited for careers that focus on helping others. They have a giving nature, and they love to deal with other people's energies. These traits can make for good therapists, medical doctors, chiropractors, and social workers. All of these occupations require intelligence, intuition, and communication skills, which Dynamic Supportives generally possess.

It's a cliché that when young people just getting out of college are asked what kind of job they want, they usually say, "I'd like to work with people." But to really work well with people you have to have a certain flexibility, and it's members of this group, the Dynamic Supportives, who have it. They know how to bend. Dynamic Supportives have the wisdom to analyze a situation fully while realizing that there may be several approaches to it. They have the intelligence to decide on a best approach, but they will not force their conclusions on others. They are good listeners, they have a value system, and they think as much with their hearts as with their minds. These qualities, along with their charisma and willingness to help others, make people pay attention to them.

It's interesting to see the flexibility and mellowness of the Dynamic Supportive reflected in his or her habitat. Their houses tend to have that lived-in look that tells you that the housekeeper is more interested in enjoying life than in keeping the art books arrayed just so on the coffee table. In fact, you might not even be able to *see* the coffee table under what's accumulated on top of it—newspapers, coffee cups, take-out menus, toys, and the like. This is not to say that the Dynamic Supportive is always a slob. On the high end, he or she sometimes gets quite organized. But organization and cleanliness are not the driving forces that they are in the lives of, say, Adaptive Assertives.

Because of the Dynamic Supportive's relaxed attitudes, in housekeeping as well as other areas of life, his is a comfortable house to visit. If the Dynamic Supportive has teenage children, for example, it will probably be his or her house that the neighborhood kids like to hang out in. They'll know they can grab something good from the refrigerator and even put their feet up on the furniture without the parent having a fit. What's more, the visiting kids will probably be able to actually *talk* to the parent in a meaningful way, without any unpleasantness resulting from having dyed their hair pink, failing algebra, or even coming from the wrong side of the tracks.

I have a theory that you can tell where a Dynamic Supportive lives by looking at his yard. Take a walk through a middle-class suburban neighborhood. Everybody's got their picket fences crisply painted a blinding white and their lawns neatly mowed and edged. Then you come to a yard that's a little different. Not only is the fence paint yellowing and peeling, but a picket or two is gone. And the lawn—well, it couldn't be edged because it has no edge. It just sort of fades into mud because the Dynamic Supportive hasn't gotten rid of the shade trees and replaced them with tiny specimen trees the way everyone else on the block has. The Dynamic Supportive likes big, shaggy trees the way he or she likes big, shaggy dogs. The trees rain leaves all over the place in the fall, but this doesn't bother the Dynamic Supportive. His neighbors are tempted to hate him, only they know him, and he's too nice to hate.

The thing is, the neighborhood kids love him. Actually, they love his yard. I have a friend I've discussed my yard theory with, and she believes that it's not so much the front yard that identifies the home of a Dynamic Supportive as the backyard. She offers her own backyard as an example, explaining that her husband is a Dynamic Supportive.

When people are over, she reports, and they look out the back windows, they usually ask, "What is that large hole over there? The one with the mud surrounding it and all those old planks crisscrossing it at odd angles?" They can't help asking because it looks as if some sort of explosive device has landed in the back of her yard, blowing apart a wooden picnic table and Adirondack lawn chair in the process, and it seems as if this event has somehow escaped the whole family's notice.

"Oh, that's my son's fort," she has to explain. She has to reassure the guests that there was no explosive device involved; it's simply that her young son likes to dig, and to build, and so her husband (the Dynamic Supportive) has given him a corner of the yard in which to do both to his heart's content, even to the point of sacrificing a couple of pieces of lawn furniture. On closer inspection the guests see that the fort incorporates stray bits of fencing, a beat-up blanket, and some rope, and that it looks like an eight-year-old's paradise. Indeed, other kids are always coming to play in her yard, preferring it to their own well-manicured little versions of Versailles. The point is that, as a Dynamic Supportive, her husband is involved in helping his son develop his interests, and he is independent enough not to care about prevailing suburban standards.

At work as well as at home, Dynamic Supportives tend to be independent. While they may not be assertive with their independence, they do like to work on their own, rather than be supervised. As a result, they can be especially effective salespeople—not the stereotypical obnoxiously aggressive kind, but the kind who knows how to communicate in a more low-key way and really inform and help the customer. They love to get out there and talk and work with people. Other qualities—including their patience and concern for others—make them excellent teachers. Dynamic Supportives are articulate communicators, and they pride themselves on their capacity to teach others. They can develop a bond of trust between the student and themselves.

Members of the clergy tend to be Dynamic Supportives as well. They will sacrifice for others and tackle important issues, as illustrated by clergy in Central and South America who have battled against human rights violations, and even been sentenced to jail for helping people find homes in the underground. The same was true during the Vietnam War, when many members of the clergy spoke out against the ethical atrocities of the war.

In an ideal world, all Dynamic Supportives would be considered a resource to be tapped as catalysts to inspire acts of human decency and as arbitrators to help resolve conflict. Not only are they objective, but they can cooperate with anyone, under any circumstance, to manage a conflict. They are effective in this way because they know how to put their own egos aside and help others save face and even build self-esteem. Their own performance is important only to the extent that they want to do well at something they care about.

And Dynamic Supportives can deliver a superb performance. When they are motivated to do a job, they do it extremely well. What's more, because they are good people, they will often go out of their way to do a good job, putting in extra time for little compensation.

Given their sensitivity, Dynamic Supportives do not like to be criticized, but they will allow it. On their down side, they may lose their motivation to continue working. That's why many Dynamic Supportives cannot actualize their desire to work for themselves, even though they are unhappy without independence.

The Ideal—and Universal—Friend

Dynamic Supportives develop relationships based on trust, respect, and unconditional love. Their fine qualities—including loyalty, selflessness, and dependability—can make for an excellent relationship. Dynamic Supportives are also insightful. They have an understanding of the person they are with and will look after his or her needs.

Their willingness to sacrifice adds to their appeal as a partner or friend. Dynamic Supportives won't hesitate to give a loved one anything they have. On the up side, they are forthright partners who will show their feelings openly. They do not hold back. They are loving and affectionate—and they're not afraid to demonstrate their emotions, no matter what the consequences.

Their friendships, too, last a lifetime. If you're looking for a friend who will stick with you in good times and bad, the Dynamic Supportive is it. Even on their down side, Dynamic Supportives will remain good, supportive friends. However, they tend not to be spontaneous or in the moment. They are planners who want to know when and how something is going to happen.

A Dynamic Supportive woman can be a wonderful partner and friend. She will be flexible, understanding, patient, and nurturing. Men find Dynamic Supportive women extremely attractive. They are a fountain of wisdom, and they have great strength. Many men value the energy of a Dynamic Supportive woman more than any other energy type because she is stable and nonthreatening. The woman will not bring so many needs into the relationship that the man feels overwhelmed, as if he must be Superman to maintain his standing in the relationship.

Dynamic Supportive women will not be subordinated in a relationship; they require that a partner treat them very much as an equal. Of all the energy types, none is more willing to go out of her way to help others. But they must be appreciated, and they will take it quite personally if their trust and confidence are betrayed. They hurt deeply, more so than others who may be more callous or indifferent. But they are more willing than other types of women to let go of problems.

The Dynamic Supportive woman generally looks for a strong, monogamous relationship. At the same time, she may have many male friends. Due to her giving and understanding nature, she will not want anyone she likes to disappear from her life. In fact, one danger for Dynamic Supportives—females and males alike—is that they may end up in a bad relationship because they do not like to push anyone out of their lives. They do not detach easily, and it may be hard for them to remove someone from their lives once the relationship is formed.

Dynamic Supportive people are intuitive. They might not change the world, but they understand it. They might not change themselves, but they understand who they are. These qualities make them enormously accepting of other people, warts and all. Dynamic Supportives accept their own weaknesses and the failings of others without criticism. They can be the best of friends and partners because they do not demand perfection from everyone around them. More than any other energy type, they are willing to overlook the flaws and negative aspects of their friends and partners.

Dynamic Supportives can be great parents as well. Their tolerance means that they generally give children a lot of unconditional love. They don't place excessive importance on winning or losing, and they have the constancy and wisdom to provide children with guidance. They're also patient, easygoing, and giving; they're the type of parent who actually looks forward to sitting down with the kids to do homework, or to taking them camping. They foster independence in their children, who often manifest an amazing self-sufficiency at an early age. And their children are usually respectful, despite any outwardly outrageous dress.

Within their family, community, and work environments—their three basic orientations—Dynamic Supportives will try to live according to high ideals. They do not tolerate destruction or injustice. They would be the first in a community to rally others to clean up their block or to challenge an unfair practice in the school system. Dynamic Supportives will always confront such issues, but generally with a more tempered passion than some other energy types. Dynamic Supportives are not vengeful people who want to inflict harm on others.

They are also humble and kindhearted. When you're around a Dynamic Supportive, you recognize them by these qualities. Chances are they will not achieve national recognition for their work because they lack the motivation to do so. But they can be counted on to play a vital role in any group or organization to which they belong, providing the vital equilibrium which balances the extremes within the group.

As for energy combinations, a beauty of the Dynamic Supportive is that he or she can blend in with just about anybody. No matter what type of energy they join with, their natural charisma will shine through. Dynamic Supportives are happy people, and other energy types will be drawn to that quality. And whereas other energies may be too intense and self-absorbed, Dynamic Supportives will reach out to relate to all types of people. They are patient and understanding, and their lifestyle is comforting and familiar to others.

To zero in on a particularly promising energy combination, a Dynamic Supportive can have a terrific friendship with a Dynamic Assertive. In fact, this is one of the easiest and most enjoyable of all relationships because both parties understand what it means to have strength. Neither has to compete with or prove anything to the other. It's a hassle-free relationship.

A Dynamic Supportive can also form a permanent and loving relationship with an Adaptive Supportive or a Creative Assertive. The Dynamic Supportive and Adaptive Supportive share a vivacious personality, while the Dynamic Supportive and Creative Assertive have their creativity and intellectual qualities in common.

There is, however, a combination that the Dynamic Supportive should be wary of, and that's a relationship with an Adaptive Aggressive. Given their generosity and kindness, a Dynamic Supportive may be taken advantage of by an Adaptive Aggressive. They could end up doing everything for this person, to their own detriment, if they are not aware of their tendency to put others before themselves.

Seeking the Spiritual

For the Dynamic Supportive, emotional and spiritual growth generally supersedes the material. Therefore, transformation is possible for them if they can learn to stay focused and channel their dynamic energy. A positive environment is especially helpful to this energy type. It can make all the difference in a critical period of transition.

When Dynamic Supportives receive unconditional love, they blossom into strong and unique people. In fact, because they are strong in spirit and character, they tend to blossom no matter what. Unfortunately, many Dynamic Supportives will encounter a spiritual awakening but fail to reach out and grab it. They understand it, but they don't embrace it.

For the Dynamic Supportive, everything is a concept—an idea that does not necessarily have to be actualized. In that context, then, spirituality is just another idea. Dynamic Supportives are moralistic, but they generally are not assertive enough to accept that they can and should live according to a spiritual definition of life.

When the proper conditions exist for their psycho-spiritual transformation, Dynamic Supportives can become regenerated people, truly joyous and energetic. Their transformation will often have some sort of mystical aspect attached to it. When this group becomes enlightened, their natural intuition and deep vision become enhanced, new energies are released, and they apply their gifts to benevolent service and selfless action.

Set Limits, Keep Focused

If you're a Dynamic Supportive, you face some particular vulnerabilities due to your energy type. Other people may find your capacity for empathy and attunement so pleasing that they encourage you to play a supporting and mirroring role regardless of whether you want to. And you may have an even more difficult time if your parents did not help you set limits as a child and encourage your other identities to take shape. Throughout life you will find again and again that others expect you to provide support, and you may not be able to extricate yourself from this role.

As a Dynamic Supportive, you must learn to set limits on these natural inclinations. Otherwise you are susceptible to becoming de-centered, disturbed, and overwhelmed by negative emotional energy in your environment. Your energy may lead you to bond with others on whatever psychological ground is available, even if these other people are involved with inner phantoms, attachments, and complexes. So you can become attached to many types of energy, but your level of stress may increase as you move away from your own and other positive energies. The danger is that you will live too much outside of yourself and then lose track of the way back to tranquillity and balance. Eventually this imbalance may make you vulnerable to disease.

Like many Dynamic Supportives, you may become so absorbed in other people's energy that you lose sight of your own plans for the future. In a worst-case scenario, this loss of focus can cause distress by combining with the negativity you internalize. At that point you may be susceptible to depression, which means you are even less likely to act on your intentions. A vicious cycle begins.

Learn to set limits on your empathy and to withdraw as needed. The world won't stop turning because you are not there to push it, although people may try to make you think it will. Remember that other people are drawn to the energy of a Dynamic Supportive because they sense his or her strength. They will ask you for help and advice, but you must distinguish between those who are motivated to use your help and those who are not. This process may very well eliminate 90 percent of the people who ask you for help. Be honest, with yourself and others, about your need for time to yourself. You must learn to participate and then retreat.

There's no doubt that Dynamic Supportives have the inner resources for transformation. Your strong sense of self will allow you to be introspective in a productive way because you are not afraid to contact the inner self.

Of course, Dynamic Supportives do need quiet time to be in touch with this voice. Meditative approaches can be of benefit to you, but you must have the discipline to make time for such reflection. Then—and this is most important—you must push yourself to put your plans into action. It's a difficult task, but you have to overcome the Dynamic Supportive's tendency to fill notebooks with dreams, interpretations, and wonderful insights—and then let them lie to gather dust. Begin to put these insights to use in your life.

Finally, to avoid the tendency to drift, keep in mind that the time you have is a finite commodity, and the effort you can put forth is limited as well. So take a hard look at how you spend your time and effort, and ask yourself where you can pare down. What sorts of interventions are you best at carrying out? What requests can you refuse? Which people will actually use your help?

With the answers to these questions, you can decide which actions to stick with and which to drop. Don't try to help everyone. Schedule time for your personal renewal—and protect that time.

Creative Assertives, Life's Interpreters

Some people create when they're encouraged to, and some when they're paid to. But when a person creates simply because he or she *has* to, because it's *in* that person to paint, write, act, dance, or make music, and he needs to do so practically as much as he needs to breathe, then that individual is a Creative Assertive.

Creative Assertives are the artists who interpret life for the rest of us, and tell us, through their art, how they see things. (Because asserting one's view of the world, in some medium or another, is what art is all about, Creatives manifest only as Assertives.) The Creative Assertive group is the one that gives color and definition to our experience on this planet and beyond, helping us to perceive implications, nuances, beauty, laughter, and pathos where we might otherwise see only facts— or nothing. So this group enriches our lives greatly. These are the people who think as much with their hearts as with their minds, and one can't help but admire the quality of their high-end energies. They are thoughtful, giving, gentle, loyal, and idealistic. And they're not afraid to stand up for their ideals, even when that means challenging authority.

Through their art, Creative Assertives continually remind us of what's right and wrong in life. They reflect our social mores, showing us what is beautiful—and not so beautiful—in society. As philosophers, artists, writers, and the like, they look at society and make a statement about the human condition through their artistic expressions. While some of these receive widespread exposure—examples would be the work of popular filmmakers and authors—some never see the light of day: the poems of a "desk-drawer" poet, for example, or the soliloquies that an unemployed actor can perform only in front of his bathroom mirror. But whatever their level of societal acceptance, people with the creative urge tend to be sensitive and caring. Without these people, the world would be bleak indeed.

Creative Assertives live in a state of high involvement with their environment. They are sensitive to ambient energy and can react emotionally even without knowing exactly what has hit them. As a result, their sense of self can be precarious. Perceptually, they are especially acute and will perceive more than the next person. Where one person sees a tree and a dog, they see a tree and a dog and a hundred other objects and scenes.

Their heightened sensitivity and perceptual ability give them a lot of information to deal with at once, and they sometimes feel they don't know what to make of it all. They absorb a lot from the outside and then reflect back. Sometimes, because they are in a sense conduits for sensation and energy, their feeling for their own identity is weak.

Early on, Creatives must negotiate some potential pitfalls. Given their particular energetic qualities—and society's less-than-understanding reaction to them—they may have childhood experiences that leave them vulnerable as adults. Their energetic and perceptual openness can lead them through a maze of unexpected emotional twists, turns, and flare-ups, and it can make them feel more sensitive than the rest of the world, and inconsistent in the ways in which they cope with life.

The Creative Assertive child may have it even harder if his or her parents and teachers are inconsistent and negative in their mirroring. Parents may feel at a loss to stay attuned to a child whose imaginative life and emotions are so unpredictable and different from their own, and may find it impossible to experience and mirror joy in the child's efforts.

Thus Creative Assertives tend to be low on joy, and to lack confidence in their inner resources. Since their work must stem from creativity, they may continually fear that they will no longer be able to produce or that others will reject them or their work. They often look outside themselves for solutions, self-definition, and guidance. They may throw themselves into someone else's belief systems, for example. These are the people who join New Age cults and other transformational groups by the millions.

Creative Assertives can be so busy searching, analyzing, and seeking themselves in the reactions of others that they miss the opportunity to live in the moment. They spend a lot of time planning for the future or holding on to things that went wrong in the past. In fact, they cling to negative experiences more than any other energy type—and they can exhaust others with an ability to talk about these experiences endlessly. Until they learn, as we all must, to let go and trust the inner self, they can exhaust themselves with constant activity and questions about their essential nature.

The problem is, a person who's always thinking is not necessarily always thinking productively. A Creative Assertive may dwell on issues and questions that do not allow him or her to resolve anything. The same question asked a thousand different ways does not help Creative Assertives become any smarter about themselves. In some cases these superanalytical people must learn to surrender their all-encompassing need to understand life. They have to trust in the process of letting go. They question life more than any other energy type does—and perhaps more than they should.

After all, the real lessons of life are not the ones we are taught; they're the ones we learn through the process of being in the world. Consider the student who asks a Zen master for the answers to a thousand questions so he can be a thousand times smarter. The Zen master says, "I can't answer even one of your questions, and you wouldn't be any smarter if I answered questions for the rest of your life." In essence he is telling the student that we do not understand life through questions and answers. To master life, we must learn to live it. That's the concept Creative Assertives must come to understand.

More than any other energy type, Creative Assertives tend to identify with their persona—that is to say, the identity they consciously fashion for themselves to present to the world. Creatives are the type who wake up in the morning and ask themselves not just "What will I do today?" but also "Who will I be today?" "How will I act?" "How will I seem?" "How do I want others to see me?" They have to plan everything out in terms of the face they will present to the world. It can be a charming face, but at times it's almost as if it's been laboriously pasted on.

Creative Assertives will go out of their way to be helpful and generous to others, wonderful qualities that can work against them if they are overly motivated by a need for acceptance. Creatives swing between intense involvement with others and aloofness—and the latter attitude often predominates at a deep emotional level. They may pretend to themselves that they are powerful, but they are always vulnerable to discovering that they are not strong and perfect. They tend to avoid people and situations that would awaken them from this fantasy.

Male or female, the Creative Assertive has a gentle and sensitive nature. Unlike the Dynamic energies, who would just about bounce back even if you threw them off a cliff, Creative Assertives can break easily. They hurt when they feel unappreciated, and any episode of disrespect or betrayal is like a stab to their heart. Because Creative Assertives are self-sufficient and giving, others may take them for granted or fail to acknowledge their needs. They can be the best of friends and partners, but they must be understood and respected for who they are. They are the roses of life, these creative thinkers and artists, but you would not hold a rose the same way you would a hardier plant.

The Creative Assertive woman can be like Isadora Duncan— not afraid to show the color of her spirit, and frequently perceiving herself to transcend physical, emotional, and mental boundaries. She is extremely attractive to men but also quite volatile. As a result, she is the least likely energy type with whom a man will want to have a relationship. Most men like people they can control, and the Creative Assertive woman is uncontrollable because her emotions vacillate so much.

She may become completely immersed in her work for periods of time, and then decide to focus more on relationships because she believes she is missing out on that aspect of life. But she brings the same volatile energy to her relationships that she does to her work. Other people may not be able to handle the intensity of the energy she shares. She can be creative, constructive, vibrant, and joyful, and she has an enormous stretch of mind. But those very qualities will scare off men who want a predictable relationship. A man may be drawn to the energies of a Creative Assertive woman, but her ephemeral quality makes it difficult to find a point of connection. The man goes here, and she's over there. It's an intimidating experience.

Other women are also intimidated by the Creative Assertive woman. She represents the freedom they have not experienced in their own lives. Thus other women will be drawn to the Creative Assertive, but they may not want to form a close friendship with her. Indeed, they may criticize her for being flighty, immature, unstable, or hyperactive. So acquaintances may attend the Creative Assertive woman's performances or invite her to their parties, but they don't necessarily want to live next door to her or invite her to their church or synagogue. After all, she might dress strangely and want to talk about the rabbi in the middle of the service.

The Creative Assertive male also has an unbridled desire to express himself through poetry, writing art, dance, filmmaking, and the like. He perceives things intensely, with all the definition, nuance, and color that give life its dimensions. Where we see a simple field, for example, he sees an entire landscape and a vast tableau of design. Creative Assertive men, like their female counterparts, are born with a visionary energy that one cannot develop. You either have it or you don't. Those who do can then enhance that energy with education and craftsmanship.

Woody Allen is a Creative Assertive. He's not dynamic or charismatic, but he certainly expresses his view of the world through creative forms. However, he is also an example of how the Creative Assertive's ever-erupting insecurity makes him want to please everyone—that is, as a comic, he became less funny when he started playing to the critics rather than to "plain folks." Interestingly, even Allen himself recognized this dilemma in *Stardust Memories*; in that film one of his characters becomes more involved in pursuing acclaim than in making people laugh.

Unfortunately, the Creative Assertive male is often considered unmasculine. Other men seem to fear that he will threaten their own masculinity. After all, the Creative Assertive male is not likely to subscribe to the stereotypical measures of manliness, such as muscle-flexing or handiness with a football. They express the concept of manhood differently. In fact, they generally are more interested in their role as a human being than in being a "man."

Because the Creative Assertive is not—to put it mildly—society's most highly rewarded type, and because it's often difficult for males, in particular, to manifest their creative sides, many Creative Assertive males in our society are subtly or not so subtly conditioned to be other energy types. Even if a child is not told, "Don't you dare be a poet," he can pick up on the cues. He notices that it's the "artsy" cousin whom family members talk about in somewhat hushed tones, as if he's different, and not quite acceptable. Of course, if the cousin becomes extremely successful with his art, the tones may become less hushed, but there's still that taint of going against the normal, "all-American" grain.

I think of a childhood friend I had who went on to become a small-town football coach with a family and a very normal, responsible kind of life. About ten years ago I went back home to see him, and he said, "Let me show you something."

Now, I'd lived across the street from him, and we'd been the best of buddies practically from the cradle, but what he showed me came as a complete surprise. He pulled out from beneath his bed a big bundle of poems, articles, and book manuscripts he had written. I read them all that day and that night, and I said, "Tom, this is beautiful work! Why are these sitting under your bed?"

He said, "Well, you know, I didn't want anybody to think I was queer and a writer." His conditioning was so strong that he was denying his own creative self. He was living as a conditioned self, as an Adaptive Supportive, and he was not realizing his potential.

I've also seen seeming Dynamic Assertives who are really Creatives at heart. These are people who do everything to be assertive, and yet feel insecure. They're people who should be spending time introspectively creating, but instead they're out there trying to be major honchos because they were told this image was the one for them.

All in all, society seems to be sending mixed messages to Creatives. Most aren't paid well, if at all, for their creative efforts. They're considered a little strange. But we laud a few highly and tolerate the rest, making allowances for their unorthodox behavior because they're artists. They're the ones who reveal the full breadth of our emotional lives, interpreting it and displaying it before us. So we need them.

Reach *In* and Touch Someone: The Up and Down Sides of Creatives

There's an old saying about how easy it is to be a writer—all you have to do is slice open a vein and let everything flow out!

This is actually a graphic illustration of how the work of any Creative comes from deep within the person, and while using a razor blade is not the method of choice, accessing one's inner core is always necessary if one is to be a real artist. And herein lies the up-side/down-side dichotomy for Creative Assertives. On the up side, when a Creative is in exquisite touch with his or her innermost reserves of memories and feelings, he can produce great work and be fulfilled doing so. But if a Creative goes one step further and gets *too much* in touch with his inner memory and feeling bank, he can end up living in the past, rehashing old problems, and forgetting to buy the groceries. This "super-in-touchness" is the down side of the Creative type.

Because they live so much in their minds, Creative Assertives may have trouble making their way in the world. They seek out ideal environments that do not always exist. Also, they often swing between extremes in their emotions and levels of activity, and tend to become narrowly focused on certain aspects of their lives, to the exclusion of equally important other areas.

To be healthy, all things must be in balance. One cannot focus strictly on work, relationships, exercise, relaxation, or any other area of life for a long period. Yet all of these things must be tended to, in turn, on a regular basis. On their down side, Creative Assertives may work obsessively and ignore the need to do these other things. When people work excessively, even if they love what they are doing, they deny the other facets of life to their own detriment. They lose sight of the fact that they're part of a larger world, and forget how to relax, mellow out, enjoy the company of others, and enjoy life.

When Creative Assertives are on their up side, they will deal with stressors appropriately. But on their down side, they may have an inordinate number of physical ailments because they do not always give themselves time to heal and nurture wellness. They may use illness as a rationale for not achieving their goals or even as a way to gain the attention of others and draw more energy toward themselves. Indeed, some Creatives seem to find in hypochondria a way of gaining needed succor, and being chronically ailing can become a way of life for some.

A sure sign that a Creative Assertive has not developed a strong connection to the inner self is a preoccupation with his or her reputation. Some Creatives need constant reaffirmation that what they've done is good; there can never be enough applause and accolades. Consider the actor who gets depressed if the public is not adoring, or the author who can't take even one bad review. Sometimes, if the Creative Assertive was not mirrored joyfully as a child, he or she becomes afraid to make contact with the inner self for fear there is nothing good—or nothing at all—to discover within. Thus the outside world's reaction to his work becomes the only thing that provides him or hev with a feeling of self-worth.

Part of Creative Assertives' down-side picture is that they can get into power drive, trying to control every aspect of the environment in an effort to banish uncertainty. Their energy is channeled into action and appearances, and they may become flashy and shallow. And if they can't keep up the façade, they often become morose and self-absorbed. Nothing matters but their own pain and problems. They can't see the future.

This moroseness and self-alienation interfere with their ability to create, and with the quality of their work. When nothing exists except their own world, their art and their connection to others suffer. Soon they spend all their time talking about their problems and pain. They hang on to that pain and ruminate about their limitations and fears. At some point they may try to find themselves at a spiritual or transformational center, but they are generally disappointed with the process because it does not meet their high expectations.

Creative Assertives are always looking for something in life. But they tend to look in the wrong places because they focus on themselves. Rather than look at how they can use life, they look at how they can improve their skills and talents to enhance their creativity. They will take class after class to improve themselves, for example. But in the process they receive false nourishment and avoid the really intractable problems in their lives. It's as if they say, "When I perfect myself, then I'll get into my work, get my work into the world, get into a relationship."

Creative Assertives have a hard time simply being in the world. To enjoy the moment, they would have to let their brains relax. That's tough for them. For instance, if you hand them a rose, they won't simply accept it for what it is. Instead they will analyze the rose, compare it to other roses they have had in the past, and connect it with other events in their lives. The mind never shuts off, and they're always someplace else, not in the moment. They are, in fact, the world's biggest worriers. They worry about *everything*. It's probably a result of their highly developed imaginative abilities, but they can imagine all sorts of awful things happening, and sometimes seem to think that keeping these images in their mind will somehow prevent them from actually coming to pass!

Creative Assertives may rationalize their weaknesses into strengths. "I could be in the present, in the body, but I'm too spiritual for that," they may say, or, "I'm not running from the world; I'm just independent." If you ask a Creative Assertive why he or she can't lighten up and enjoy life, a typical response might be that it's impossible to do so in a world filled with suffering. But their seriousness may be taken to extremes and can turn into self-pity.

The Up-and-Down World of Creatives At Work

It isn't easy being a Creative Assertive and working in the real world at the same time. One problem stems from the area of motivation. People are motivated to work by many things—money, prestige, the need to subsist, a feeling of satisfaction. Creative Assertives can be motivated by all of these, but they have another fuel behind their work—the absolute *need* to do whatever they're doing. In other words, a true Creative Assertive *has* to paint, make films, dance, do stand-up comedy, write, sculpt, or whatever. The need is nonnegotiable, really, and sometimes it gets in the way of "normal" functioning.

The complicating factor here is that this need to engage in one's art tends to wax and wane, which means that the Creative Assertive tends to be on a more erratic schedule than the rest of us. Let's say that he's a painter. The nature of the creative urge is such that he may find himself inspired for a period of several days, and feel impelled to paint straight through. At another point he may be all "painted out," and not want to look at a canvas for weeks. The irregularity of the creative urge can be a problem in terms of taking care of other life responsibilities, which tend to be constant. Creative Assertives, and those they live with, have to keep in mind that you can't regulate artistic output the way you can other types of work. You can try, and obviously there are deadlines that have to be met in any real-world endeavor, but it's going to be difficult at times.

Another problematic aspect of being a creative person, especially if one is making a living from one's art, is that, if it's all coming from within, there always seems to be the chance of everything just drying up, in which case the artist will be completely out of luck. So for Creative Assertives, there's always that worry in the back of their minds that the artistic gift may suddenly and mysteriously desert them, just as mysteriously as it appeared in their lives. Thus the movie star fears that he'll never be invited to do another film; the author, that she'll never publish another book; the painter, that this will be her last painting that's worth anything. The question, "What if the well runs dry?" is a scary one to live with.

Nevertheless, Creatives have to live with this question, and the world has to live with Creatives, because we need them. A lot of what sparkles and shines in our world, and a lot of what inspires people and makes them think, and laugh, and even takes their breath away, is the work of Creative Assertives. The plain fact is that there's no one better for creative work than a Creative Assertive! But in terms of the nitty-gritty of their working conditions, you have to be careful. You have to give them a lot of space to work independently. Otherwise they will burn out and become angry, and they won't want to work with you anymore. I often hire Creative Assertives for short-term projects, for example. To keep the relationship healthy, I give them all the autonomy they want and acknowledge their work. I would never take one of these people and tie them down in an office.

Also, I wouldn't make a Creative Assertive a manager. While members of this energy group are natural doers and creators, you're not likely to find them in positions of authority, because this isn't their forte. Not that they seek out management positions. They generally are not interested in management functions or supervising other people, in part because they are sensitive and do not like to judge others or be judged themselves. They are motivated by the need to create and have their work accepted, not by a desire for money or for control of people or systems.

Creative Assertives aren't necessarily the best choice for ongoing, long-term jobs either, because they tend to be inconsistent. I learned this lesson when I hired a Creative Assertive as a caretaker. He would feel good one week and bad the next; he would milk the cow one week and not the next. This volatility is often part of their nature; after all, if they were consistent, they would also be predictable, which is contrary to the creative energy, in which spurts of enthusiasm and energy contribute to the process.

For ordinary projects that don't require major inspiration, the Creative Assertive works well under pressure. In fact, this group often needs pressure to perform because they tend to procrastinate. Without a deadline, they tend to put off work as long as possible and avoid bringing anything to completion. This problem can be compounded by their perfectionistic tendencies. They will continually rework a product because they are never satisfied with the results. At some point others simply have to tell them, "Time's up!"

Creative Assertives tend to measure their self-worth with everything they do, a propensity that can be both positive and destructive. If they don't like something they've created, or if they do not succeed with a project, they take it personally. Any barriers they encounter will be taken personally as well. It's as if the barrier were made exclusively for them, and they can become very frustrated and overly focused on the barrier itself.

In short, the world of work can be a roller coaster for Creative Assertives. They're intermittently motivated. In a good mood, they're productive dynamos; in a bad mood, they become despondent. They accelerate as they get involved in their work, then gradually decline into apathy. The continuity found in other energy types, and in most of life, may be lacking in the Creative Assertive. They have trouble determining if their creative ebb and flow result from psychological blocking or a natural process. So they fret and analyze some more.

Relationships—Cyclic, Complex

When it comes to getting close to others, Creative Assertives can be skittish if they have not yet learned to appreciate themselves. They will be alternately intense and distant; they approach and avoid. They can drain another person of energy with their need for mirroring and appreciation, then retreat into an aestheticized aloofness.

Creative Assertives also tend to idealize a few special people and populate their lives with nonequals. They may seek out people with strong personalities who they imagine can guide them through life, or people who can enhance their self-esteem. Thus they may end up with few true friends who will challenge and support them in a constructive and realistic way. Until the Creative Assertive learns to actualize his or her creative gifts in the world, he or she will squander energy in fantasy accomplishments and relationships.

Creative Assertives generally know a lot a of people, but they may not have a lot of friends or lasting relationships. Even so, Creatives leave a legacy with those who have known them.

Others may have a hard time bonding with a Creative Assertive because they can't move fast enough to meet his or her many expectations, but they will undoubtedly remember something about the person. They'll remember his or her creativity, vitality, or unusual view of the world; however, they may not remember the Creative Assertive as someone they wanted in their life, because the relationship was so draining.

Indeed, Creative Assertives often have intense and volatile relationships. They will bend over backwards to be supportive and encouraging, but once they are comfortable in a relationship, their energy may change if they dwell on problems from the past. They may spend a lot of time focusing on their problems—and relating them to a partner or friend over and over again—because they don't know how to resolve conflicts. They don't know how to let go and move forward. Creative Assertives ask questions that do not need a resolution. They lay a hand where there is no need to be touched. It's as if they finish a recipe and then start all over again. They have a difficult time letting things be.

Creative Assertives also tend to find faults in everyone, including themselves, their friends, and their partners. When that happens, it doesn't mean they don't love you, and it's not a sign of rejection. They simply cannot accept things as they are, and must analyze everything and everyone around them. But they will never be as tough on others as they are on themselves. Creative Assertives are tougher on themselves than are any other energy types. They continually challenge and punish themselves. But they are the only energy type that will use self-criticism as an avenue for change.

Their sensitivity can make them quite defensive. Therefore, others who interact with Creative Assertives must be constantly aware of the little emotional mine fields they have planted all around them. If a partner or friend triggers one of these mine-fields—for example, by asking about their work, their motives for doing certain types of work, their inability to let go of pain—the Creative Assertive may very well respond with an emotional explosion. And if asked to sweep away these defensive minefields, the Creative Assertive may not be able to do so.

On their down side, Creative Assertives have a fear of failure. Their self-esteem can be badly damaged if they fail at an endeavor or do not succeed to the degree they anticipated. Their inability to bounce back from a failure can affect other aspects of their life. Real, perceived, or anticipated failure can leave them stuck in a rut. Then, their fear of being hurt by others only complicates the picture, and with these two fears at work, the openness a Creative Assertive brings to his or her art may be lacking on a personal, human level. Underneath the charming exterior, the Creative Assertive has taken cover in emotional distance. What you get is the persona.

Consequently, the relationship can be boring because on the Creative Assertive's end it does not come from the self. His or her emotions do not come from the moment. The relationship may become unnecessarily heavy and intense, and eventually one or the other can't take it anymore. Once they separate, Creative Assertives generally will distrust relationships for a while. They throw themselves back into their work. Eventually they may reenter a relationship and start the cycle again.

Relating with Creative Assertives requires patience, because their needs are not simple, and they change. Members of this group appear to be quite independent, but it's more complicated than that. They need time alone to focus on their creative spirit. And while they need others periodically, they also may fear they will be overwhelmed by the strong personalities to whom they often gravitate. They want to be admired, but their fear of failure may send them off into their corners, where they can hide their imperfections.

While Creative Assertives are indeed giving, supportive, and cooperative people, they may have a tendency to do things for others simply to be recognized and to enhance their self-esteem. They will help another person in any way possible, thereby showing that they are giving; in return, they expect that person to acknowledge their efforts. If he or she does not, the Creative Assertive will be hurt by the experience and withdraw.

Many people hesitate to get close to a Creative Assertive because they have a tough time handling their periodic need for space and their volatility. If you were to come across a log, for example, you probably wouldn't do anything to change it. You would simply sit on the log and let it be. The Creative Assertive, on the other hand, might decide to dance on the log or to paint a picture of it; he or she might write a poem about it or even whittle a carving out of it. The point is that you never know what they will do, which can be disconcerting.

Creative Assertive men may have a difficult time with women. Not only are relationships of secondary importance to them, but they also have an intense need, at times, to be alone to create. During this phase they may work twenty hours a day, seven days a week, for months on end. Think of Hemingway, Faulkner, Joyce, Picasso, or Renoir. They put this type of intensity into their work, while neglecting other aspects of their lives, because they were fueled by passion.

At some point, though, the Creative Assertive man will shift to the other extreme and experience an intense loneliness and need to bond. He'll want to mellow out and balance his life, but he may burn out the woman in his life because he puts the same energy into the relationship that he puts into his work. He wants the relationship too much, and his emotions are volatile. His tendency to swing between the two extremes of intense work and intense relationship, never staying at either end for very long, does not make him that desirable a partner, at least to those with more conventional expectations.

Female Creative Assertives are similar. They generally have one-on-one friendships. They may appear shy and hesitant at first, but will eventually come to trust someone once they are comfortable with the relationship. But they, too, may swing between being distant and involved in their own energy and being too closely involved with the other person's energy.

Creative Assertives are reluctant joiners, which affects their ability to develop relationships. They're often secretive and reclusive. And they may not be able to connect with others because their ideas are unique and difficult to share with people who are not of similar mind. Consequently they may feel most comfortable with others who share the same energy and can appreciate their lifestyle and way of thinking. While another creative person may be involved in a totally different field, at least he or she understands what it is to create and to be alone in the process.

Family life is problematic for Creative Assertives. Their intense need for emotional support surfaces in the safety of the family, which they tend to use and to blame. They may not make ideal parents or relatives for that reason. They can be particularly difficult parents if they have not learned to contain their emotional highs and lows, confusion, and neediness. They can be easily distracted by their search for meaning in life, and they may not give quality time and attention to the people around them, including their children. While it's not their nature to intentionally hurt another person, unintentional neglect can create uncertainty in the family setting.

Energy Combinations

On their up side, Creative Assertives are capable of quiet, harmonious relationships. If they pair with someone who has the same energy or a complementary one, they can be content and productive. But they can have tortured relationships as well if they end up with the wrong partner. And even if they are miserable, they may stick with it and feel martyred.

An energy pair with promise is that of the Creative Assertive and the Dynamic Assertive, who can make a beautiful combination, especially when they are both on their up side. They can have a wonderful, trusting relationship and a dynamic exchange of ideas. For example, they may both work for common causes that broaden the perspective of other people's lives and enhance the quality of their own.

One has the vision; the other has the creative skills. Bring these two qualities together and you have the big picture and the ability to carry it out. The Dynamic Assertive can identify an important issue and bring it to the public's attention, while the Creative Assertive can produce the campaign—the posters, documentaries, or movie scripts—that brings the issue to life and promotes change. It's one of the best combinations you can have. All Dynamic Assertives, in fact, should work with a Creative Assertive to see a project to completion. They are not only patient, but also supportive, cooperative, and loyal. They're sensitive, and they truly care about others.

However, a Creative Assertive may be drawn to a Dynamic Assertive for the wrong reasons. For example, if a Creative Assertive woman has not yet found fulfillment through her art, she may identify with the creative quality of the Dynamic Assertive and form a relationship with that person because she wants to discover his "formula." She assumes the Dynamic Assertive is fulfilled, and she wants to find out how he's doing it. But the Dynamic Assertive may be moving forward at such a rapid speed that the Creative Assertive, who is usually more past-oriented, feels overwhelmed and frustrated.

Two Creative Assertives could have a wonderful relationship if both are on the high end and are manifesting their creativity. The results won't be the same as with the Dynamic Assertive/ Creative Assertive combination, because a Creative Assertive does not involve other people the way a Dynamic Assertive does. But the relationship can be beautiful because each respects the other's expression of life through art. Both will tend to be trusting, giving, and sympathetic, and the relationship will be fulfilling as long as they can deal with their problems. The newness that automatically springs from the mind of a Creative Assertive will be injected into the relationship. One caveat about a Creative/Creative pair: If they're both in the exact same field, the inevitable competition could be a big problem. The relationship has a much better chance of survival if the two are in related or divergent artistic fields.

A Creative Assertive can have a good relationship with a Dynamic Supportive, and with an Adaptive Supportive as well. Both can provide the unconditional love and support the Creative Assertive needs. A possible problem is that the Creative

Assertive's tendency to fret and complain will eventually wear on the Adaptive Supportive, who is likely to be a more relaxed and calm person.

The Challenge: Let Go of the Past

Creative Assertives are drawn to peak experiences. They go out and search for these experiences through their creativity, performances, and dialogue with other people. However, because they look for these experiences "out there," rather than within themselves, they don't always find them.

A down-side tendency evident in many artists is that they look inward for artistic material but not for ways to grow spiritually. So they live with old pain. Yes, they make feeble attempts to escape the pain, but since these are not vigorous enough, it's like trying to get out of quicksand by moving up and down rather than moving forward. They're stuck in the quicksand, and their relationships may be stuck as well.

Creatives tend to thrive on their bad experiences, which can keep them locked and prevent them from making changes in their lives. They will try to achieve change by taking one step forward. They'll grab on to every guru, ashram, book, and New Age process they can find. The problem is, one foot is still planted. Despite all the motion, they haven't really changed. They *could* change. Creative Assertives certainly have the intellect to do so. But, strangely, it's often as if they have learned the lessons of the desert so well that they avoid the oasis just ahead.

Transformation comes only when the body, mind, and belief system change, when one truly gives up the past. By relinquishing the past, Creative Assertives can free themselves to be in the moment. Then their responses, attitudes, beliefs, and values can be created in the present. If I was a racist yesterday, it doesn't mean I have to be a racist today. If I didn't exercise yesterday, it doesn't mean I can't exercise today.

The power of any person—not just Creatives—resides only in the present; that is, a person can only do things *now*; no one on earth can do things yesterday. But when people surrender the power they possess to remembrances from the past, then their pain, guilt, fears, and insecurity will dictate the moment. They won't be comfortable with the here and now; they'll be in the past and, no doubt, resenting the fact that they are.

What's missing for many Creative Assertives is a forward momentum. It's frustrating to take a step ahead but never really get anywhere. They've got all this motion going, but they're really not moving forward. Creative Assertives spend a lot of time trying to figure out why this is so—why they are not moving forward, why they are not more dynamic, why they cannot enjoy life more. They can become like the Woody Allen character in movies—the type who's had his problems analyzed for so many years that he's the world's most highly educated neurotic. But he's still got the problems because he hasn't let go of them. Woody Allen manages to make this situation seem hilarious on screen, but for Creative Assertives stuck in this rut, it's not really funny.

What Creative Assertives don't realize is that the answers generally lie with their failure to disconnect from the past and to believe in their own efficacy. They are limited by their attachment to guilt, previous experiences, and supposed rights. The irony is that Creative Assertives aspire not to have limits, but in many cases they are held back by self-imposed limits.

Creative Assertives have trouble trusting in themselves, unless they are at the high end. They will question their previous values—and analyze them ad nauseam—but they will not change those values. It's the same barrier they face again and again in life—a fear of truly looking inward.

The process of growth for Creative Assertives is complicated by their inability to deal with confusion. If something confuses them, it stops them cold. They have to spend time analyzing it. And it's usually an issue in their own life that confuses them, such as the nature of their relationships, the nature of their work, the reasons for their work, the reality of their life, the reasons people either accept or reject them. These questions stem, in part, from the sense of personal unreality that can permeate their lives. They conjure up position statements to replace the answers that would come from listening for guidance from within. They're afraid that nothing will come if they let their intuition take over, and they can't bear the anxiety of anticipation.

What's more, the disappointments of life often cause depression in Creative Assertives, more so than in any other energy type. They generally lack the emotional wherewithal to overcome disappointments, so they stop themselves from progressing. They put their life and their energy on hold, even as they go through the motions of living.

Go with the Flow—and the Ebb

If you're a Creative Assertive, you've probably known it for a long time. But you may not have known that the idea of the "tortured artist" is not something that has to apply to you. The key is understanding yourself, and understanding and managing the creative process you engage in.

First, you have to learn to tolerate your creative ebbs and flows, so you don't interpret them as signs of personal strength or failure.

The ebb and flow of creativity are natural parts of your being. It's like a natural circadian rhythm, with low energy, high energy, and low energy again, although the cycle may last much longer than a day; it could extend over a week, a month, or more, and contain mini-cycles within it. The point to remember is that if you try to sustain the high energy at all times, you may fall prey to artificial stimulants such as drugs. You'll burn out as you try to force a creative mood beyond its natural limits. Likewise, you need to move beyond the low energy and pull yourself out of depression—not necessarily by resuming the creative process, but by doing other things for a while.

You'll probably only feed the depression if you think you have to be heavily involved in creativity at all times, because you'll be disappointed to discover that this is impossible.

It might help to think of your creative force as a pendulum. Rather than going up and down, it swings from left to right—from a period of creativity to one of rest and renewal. Think of the latency period as a seasonal change; the tree is not always in bloom. You can't be creative every day. You need time to reflect and engage in life, just as a dedicated athlete must have time to rest and rebalance between competitive events. Indeed, many of our great artists have gone out into the world, experienced life, and then returned to interpret it through their art. So go out and experience life, then come back and interpret it. After all, you may have nothing to express if you do not engage in life yourself.

An important task for Creative Assertives is to develop a real sense of self. This is a difficult task if their self-esteem has taken a beating over the years. Their particular energy makes them feel self-inconsistent. As a result, they look outward to find out what others want them to do and be. They don't know who they are, and they spend too much time immersed in fantasies about being special. They don't deserve the same hardships as other people, they think. There must be some mistake. I'll just go find that nice creative high, and that way I won't have to think about these problems anymore. In this way they tend to run from the person or situation that will drag them back to earth.

As a Creative Assertive you must learn to appreciate yourself. Find the courage to be truthful about who you are, develop a set of values, and then put them to work. Otherwise you will never be able to bring your work into the world and you will feel too much pressure in relationships. You will spend your time coming and going, embracing and fleeing.

The goal for the Creative Assertive is self-discovery, under the guidance of the inner self. Inner-directedness must be developed, and the imagination must be gotten under control. If not, all your energy will be dissipated by feel-better fantasies, and the imagination will remain superficial. Stop running around and start listening to yourself. Don't waste your energy envying others and looking for praise. Stop doing things to make yourself liked by others. The accolades you seek must come from your own ego admiring your own self.

Once you create a relationship with your inner self and find your creative drive, you can take it out into the world. Many Creative Assertives get stuck in the first stage and remain forever in a state of dreamy self-absorption. Your work has to pass from thought to form.

Learn to recognize what's going on in your creative life. If you feel restless and unproductive, but still enthusiastic about what you're doing or plan to do, don't worry. Small blocks such as these are part of the creative process. Conversely, if you feel as if you don't care, that nothing's happening, you need to work on yourself. But don't run off to take a course or buy another book. Don't start questioning yourself, asking if you're really talented, and don't make excuses for not working. Instead, learn to experience the moment. It will invigorate you. Try to manifest your thoughts in your work; if you fail, try again.

If you're like the typical Creative, you also have to let go of yesterday. Loosen your mutual stranglehold with the past. It's not that you have to reject the past completely, but you have to take a step away from it. Use your memories for your work, but then step away from them so you can really relate to the person you are with at the moment. In that way you'll be giving the person you are with—and that includes your present self, too!—a fair shake.

A final challenge for the Creative Assertive: You have to learn to manage your special energetic openness and perceptual acuity. You have to shut down your perceptual Venetian blinds, as it were, withdraw, and take time for yourself. Thus you can renew your spirit as you prepare to enjoy your creativity once again.

Most of the People You'll Ever Meet: Adaptive Supportives

The various Dynamics and the Creatives, interesting though they are, actually comprise only a small segment of the population. Let's look now at the natural life energy group that includes most of the people you'll ever meet—about 90 percent, in fact. This NLE group's numbers, and the volume and type of work it gets done, make it arguably the most important one of all. What is this single largest energy category in our society? It's the Adaptive Supportives. And in a lot of ways, when we talk about "our society" or "our culture," it's the Adaptive Supportives we're referring to. Because there are so many of them, their values and way of life pervade our culture, and this is true not just of the United States, but universally.

Adaptive Supportives have many positive qualities—as a rule they are loyal, giving, and easygoing in their approach to life. What's more, they can be very hard workers and highly conscientious about their work, both in terms of doing a good job and providing for their families. And since these are the people who tend to work at society's more menial and physically demanding jobs, sticking with a job year after year sometimes constitutes an unrecognized act of heroism on the part of members of this group. After all, working fifty hours a week managing a corporate department or writing novels might, in certain respects, be considered hard, but working fifty hours a week cleaning people's houses or putting together cars on an assembly line is *hard work*.

Despite hardships, this is a group that knows how to grasp opportunities for happiness. They do so in the best, most realistic way—by enjoying the small, common pleasures of life. So a family picnic, going to the drive-in movies, going to the shopping mall on a Saturday, sending a Christmas card, participating in a charity bake sale—all these things can bring a lot of joy to an Adaptive Supportive.

And note this well: Being able to extract joy from everyday things is a gift not everyone has. Not to denigrate the energy groups we've looked at so far, but consider how some of them would approach a family picnic. A Creative Assertive might not want to go because she'd be mentally rehashing a fight she had with another family member half a decade ago, so the picnic would be too traumatic. A Dynamic Aggressive wouldn't be able to go because her appointment book would be completely filled for the next year. Besides, there wouldn't be enough important people at the picnic; you can't network with toddlers and elderly aunts. A Dynamic Assertive might actually show up, but end up haranguing everyone for bringing along a portable TV, or for using too many Styrofoam cups and despoiling the environment. An Adaptive Supportive, on the other hand, would actually enjoy the whole event—the anticipatory fun of the preparation, the picnic meal itself—complete with demanding toddlers and the football game on in the background, the camaraderie of the cleanup.

Again, the joys of this group are not grandiose; they don't involve elaborate schemes. They're little, subtle things. And this is all part of the picture of Adaptive Supportives at their best; when they're on their up side, there's a genteelness to these people, an order to their lives and a functional balance to them that make everything seem as if it's exactly the way it should be.

The Malleable Mainstream

In another area, though, this group has a problematic aspect that can't be ignored. In fact, the history of the world rides on this aspect, and it always has—sometimes in the wrong direction. The problem is that this group can be manipulated by authority figures. Adaptive Supportives are the followers in life—the vast majority of the people, who adapt their lives to prevailing belief systems, and live a narrowly defined existence. Rarely do they challenge those in power, no matter how wrong their belief systems may appear to be.

The irony is that Adaptive Supportives could be a tremendous force in society, simply by virtue of their numbers. But most Adaptive Supportives fail to recognize the power of the individual in effecting constructive change, and instead seek the security of anonymity. By conforming to the expectations of the majority, they relieve themselves of responsibility for their own lives. Of course, this approach to living is a trade-off, requiring them to give away their power to others. If Adaptive Supportives were to recognize their power and band together as a collective force, they would, like a tidal wave, wash over the people who control them.

Unfortunately, that scenario is rarely a threat to the people in power. Adaptive Supportives are motivated, in large part, by a need to be accepted by others. Their whole lifestyle is supportive of the status quo, and they thrive on the sense of belonging that comes from "fitting in." But to do so, they must deny their individuality and independent thought. Once they take this route in life, which they're conditioned to do from childhood on, they become dependent on the approval of others. Adaptive Supportives need to know that they are part of a larger group, and they derive their identity from their relationship to the majority.

They generally have a fixed notion of what is right or wrong, and so, throughout life, Adaptive Supportives resist any challenge to their belief systems from the nonconformists in society. They don't like to change, and they certainly don't want to accept anything that is new or different. Adaptive Supportives conform to group standards in all situations—their homes, workplaces, places of religion, and so forth. By doing so, they get the reinforcement they need from others and buttress their sense of belonging. They make a statement that they are like the others with whom they are aligned.

But the desire to be like others exposes us to some pitfalls. For one, we lose our sense of the uniqueness of individuals. By creating a collective concept of themselves and submerging their identity in that of the group, Adaptive Supportives deny the qualities that make individuals different. They suppress their own individuality, and they expect others to suppress theirs for the sake of the group. That philosophy can lead to some perverse cultures. Consider Japan, where the concept of "I" has little meaning. The needs of the company take precedence over the needs of the individual. As a result, independent thought is discouraged, and the masses become obedient and intolerant.

The real danger with Adaptive Supportives is that they will cling to faulty belief systems. They have a strong need to trust in one authority, and they feel vulnerable and threatened if an idea or person challenges that authority. When Adaptive Supportives are presented with alternatives to an established paradigm—in politics, religion, or even something as practical as approaches to health care—they have a difficult time rejecting their original belief and shifting to another. In essence, they don't want to hear both sides of an argument, they don't want to consider an opposing viewpoint, and they don't want to change how they think and feel.

The crux of the matter is this: The process of change threatens Adaptive Supportives' sense of security, which is of utmost importance to them. They place great value in feeling secure—in their homes, jobs, and relationships. This is the group that often stays for decades with jobs that offer a steady paycheck, regardless of whether the work is satisfying or even threatens their health. They tend to stay in bad marriages as long as these make them feel secure. They remain obedient to authority figures who acknowledge and meet their need for security. Adaptive Supportives pride themselves on permanency; they derive comfort from knowing in advance exactly how their lives will be played out.

But when security becomes paramount, the chances are good that other vital issues will not be addressed. In fact, Adaptive Supportives may ignore such issues when they pose a threat to their sense of security. If you work in a corrupt government agency, will you challenge that corruption and jeopardize your job security? If you work in a company that pollutes the environment, will you question its policies and put a regular paycheck at risk? For most Adaptive Supportives, the answer to such troubling questions is no. They choose to support that which keeps them secure.

It's not surprising, then, that Adaptive Supportives often live with a feeling of powerlessness. They relinquish control over their own lives, giving more power to authority figures than they do to themselves. This gives them a myopic view of life and closes off many avenues of growth and transformation. For example, Adaptive Supportives rarely challenge doctors on the treatments they prescribe, no matter how questionable those treatments may be. If you were to provide Adaptive Supportives with evidence that a particular type of surgery does not correct the problem it supposedly helps—and that, in fact, it harms many of the people who undergo it—most would still have the operation themselves if the doctor told them to.

The tendency of Adaptive Supportives not to question authority goes hand-in-hand with their having structured their lives within narrow confines. They let society define the parameters of their existence, and as long as they stay within the socially prescribed notions of what is right and wrong, they feel happy and safe. The problem is that their belief systems can become a kind of false mini-reality, an intellectual island of sorts that contains everything they consider necessary for survival. Paradise could be a hundred feet away, but Adaptive Supportives will stick with what they have been conditioned to accept. And if that particular reality causes them pain—in a relationship or job, for example—they do what they must to adapt and survive. They resist change even when the current situation creates discomfort or pain.

It's not that Adaptive Supportives don't recognize an injustice or feel angry about it. They are intelligent and giving people who most certainly empathize with the pain of others. But they tend to hitch their social consciousness to that of a Dynamic Assertive spokesperson, and if none is available, they won't act. Theoretically, no one should need a leader to stand up to an injustice and demand change. But Adaptive Supportives do. So they will adapt to negative forces they encounter, be it pollution in their water or toxic dumps in their backyards, until a Dynamic leader or leaders show them that protest and change are possible. Sometimes they have to be shown again and again before they will act. In addition, it helps if many other Adaptive Supportives are getting on the bandwagon at the same time. Members of this group are joiners by nature, and the safety that seems to come with numbers appeals to them.

Sometimes Adaptive Supportives may seem blind to the possibilities of protest and change, but it's not usually as simple as that. It's an anxiety issue. These people may know intellectually that something in society needs to be corrected, but they don't want to stick their necks out to get the job done. They're caught between what they know should be done and what they are fearful of doing. They're comfortable enough where they are; and even if they're not, they fear that change will cause even more discomfort. "Why risk it?" they think. "I'll just make do with what I have."

The reality, of course, is that life is changing all around them anyway. The world doesn't stand still because we deny the need for change. But Adaptive Supportives may let others do the hard work of change for them. In East Germany, all it took was about seventy-five thousand people to bring the government down. Where were the tens of millions of other people who stood to benefit from democracy? Why weren't they protesting in the streets, helping to bring about the process of change? They weren't because they were not of a change-oriented life energy.

When Adaptive Supportives do change, it's usually because an authority figure has given them "permission" to do so. When the authority in their lives changes, they'll shift course and go along with whatever the leader expects of them. If the Pope were to allow women to become priests, the masses would adapt to the change and support it. If the president of the United States were to become a vegetarian, tens of millions of Americans would follow suit and become vegetarians as well. Unfortunately, this approach to change is not the best, since authority, and not independent thought, is still the driving force.

Adaptive Supportives consider themselves to be an extension of authority—and they operate from the assumption that since the authority figure is always right, they, too, are right. This attitude not only causes them to avoid change but also makes them highly obedient. They entrust so much power to authority figures that they may fail to challenge the most obvious wrongs committed by those figures. Throughout the Vietnam War, there was never a demonstration of more than three hundred thousand. The Adaptive Supportives did not show up, even though they, ironically, were the very people that the authorities sent off to do the fighting.

The inescapable fact is that Adaptive Supportives can be easily manipulated, given their obedient nature. They'll obey to the extent of killing people—even to the extent of killing total innocents and children—and even killing themselves—if an authority figure tells them to do so. After all, it wasn't mainly the higher-ups who killed more than six million Jews and many additional millions of others during World War II. And think about this: Thousands of Iranian children died on one summer day when their mothers sent them walking across a minefield. The reason? The Iranian army didn't want its tanks to be destroyed, so someone had to go across first. The mothers gave their children little prayer books and sent them off to die. They did what was "right" according to their religious beliefs and their doctrine of obedience to the law. They were "just following orders."

Granted, episodes such as these are extreme. But they do point out the dangers of the collective mentality. In everyday life, this mindset can slowly wear away at Adaptive Supportives. By following the dictates of others—by doing what is asked of them—Adaptive Supportives eventually come to mistrust themselves. Their conditioned beliefs become all-important, and they deny the real self. They become disengaged from life and detached from their true feelings and thoughts. The ultimate outcome is that they may deny responsibility for themselves—for their physical, intellectual, emotional, and spiritual health.

From Heroism to Hedonism: The Up and Down Sides of Adaptive Supportives

When Adaptive Supportives operate from the high side of their energy, they have many positive qualities. Foremost among these is their giving nature. These are the people who give to charities, answer phones at telethons, and volunteer their time to all sorts of worthy organizations. On their up side they recognize human suffering and do what they can to help others. Adaptive Supportives can be extraordinarily generous in all the small ways that have meaning—cooking food for a fund-raiser, for example, or sharing what they have with a neighbor in need. They can be a great force for good when they are properly guided.

They also have, as we've mentioned, a wonderful ability to

appreciate the subtle joys in life. Adaptive Supportives don't need cruises to exotic ports or visits to pricey restaurants in order to experience pleasure. They can find joy in the seemingly small experiences, such as that family picnic we discussed, or a class play, or an evening of bowling. Their capacity to recognize the simple joys in life suggests a sensitivity that everyone should strive to achieve, and the other energy types could take a lesson from Adaptive Supportives in this area.

Adaptive Supportives possess what you might call a soft energy—that is, there is a delicate quality to their interactions with others. They often have a quiet attitude and a natural shyness. In fact, one of their finest qualities is humility—a characteristic that is sorely lacking in some energy types. Adaptive Supportives can be humble, sincere, and trusting. They also have an easygoing approach to life, a lightness of attitude that makes them pleasant to be around. They have a nice sense of humor, and can be playful. Nevertheless, when push comes to shove, this is one tough group of people, who know how to activate their survival skills. For instance, in recent years, as job opportunities have disappeared in the eastern industrial states, many Adaptive Supportives have migrated with their families to the Sunbelt to seek new employment. It takes gumption to pick up and move to a new region, especially when there's no guarantee that things will work out there.

Adaptive Supportives' sense of loyalty is another fine quality, provided they are able to withdraw their allegiance from someone or some entity that no longer deserves it. (The phrase "My country, right or wrong" comes to mind here. Supporting one's country when it's right is one thing; however, considering the history of the twentieth century, loyalty to one's country when it's perpetrating wrongful deeds is a morally bankrupt concept whose time has gone.) But on the positive side, Adaptive Supportives are unsurpassed in their capacity to be extremely loyal to a friend or mate. The part of the traditional marriage vow that refers to the partners remaining faithful to each other whether they're richer or poorer, in sickness or in health, is not just a bunch of empty, flowery words for many an Adaptive

Supportive. They mean what they say with this vow, and many provide shining examples of dedication both to the ideal of marriage and to their own spouses.

Adaptive Supportives can have tremendous courage as well, especially when they are acting according to the higher ideals of their belief systems. They will sacrifice their lives for the values in which they believe. Adaptive Supportives are the first to charge into battle to fight an enemy or support their homeland in a just cause. They're the first to rush into a burning building to save the life of another human being. When they use their courage properly, Adaptive Supportives are to be admired greatly.

On the low end of the energy spectrum, the Adaptive Supportive is another person entirely. They close down inside, shutting themselves off from the world around them. They lose their vital connection to the issues that have meaning for themselves and others. In this phase, many Adaptive Supportives are completely oblivious to their environment. They will sit by idly as their water, air, and soil are polluted with toxins—and do absolutely nothing about it. They don't speak out against the polluters themselves, and they don't even lend their support to others who attempt to bring about positive change.

Another down-side tendency of Adaptive Supportives is that they do not consider issues in depth. Their goal is to avoid potential conflict, so they hunker down in the security of their homes, their jobs, their day-to-day routines. All of their respect and loyalty are channeled to one authority, and any new idea that challenges that authority only confuses them. So Adaptive Supportives will position themselves on one side of an issue, then stay there no matter what kind of evidence or logical exposition proves them wrong. And if fear is thrown into the mix, then logic has no chance whatsoever with most Adaptive Supportives. That's why the really shrewd demagogue always peppers his rhetoric with a good amount of fear-mongering. There may be nothing to be afraid of, but he'll make something up just to keep the Adaptive Supportives in line.

At their worst, Adaptive Supportives will do whatever an

authority figure tells them to do. They operate from an un-thinking, unfeeling sense of obedience that allows them to take part in highly destructive acts. Adaptive Supportives will carry out the orders of others without ever considering the morality of what they are doing. As long as the person in control acknowledges their need for security, they will remain obedient. What's more, they can degenerate into a mob mentality; Adaptive Supportives are the ones who will boo a performer off the stage or throw beer cans at a baseball player.

Adaptive Supportives tend to have more health problems than any other energy type. On their high end, they will take some steps to improve their health, such as eating organic produce, taking vitamins, or exercising. More often, however, their diet is terrible—full of junk food, chemical-laden refined foods, and fat. When their health suffers as a result, they often use illness as an excuse not to participate in life. Their sickness becomes a crutch, and they refuse to make constructive changes in their diet and lifestyle.

Many serious disorders and diseases—such as arthritis, heart disease, and cancer—seem to be especially prevalent among Adaptive Supportives. This phenomenon stems, in part, from their tendency to repress their thoughts and feelings, to avoid resolving the conflicts in their lives, and to toe the line by remaining obedient to authority. The connection here is that obedience is often accompanied by a silent rage, and repressed anger has been shown to have deleterious physical consequences.

In fact, Adaptive Supportives are masters of sublimation on their down side. They go for every kind of escapism society has to offer—television, spectator sports, junk food, alcohol, drugs, and supermarket tabloids. Adaptive Supportives are the armchair quarterbacks who overidentify with a sports team, reliving all the intricacies of a game for days afterward and living vicariously through the athletes' victories, defeats, and—perhaps most important—their exciting risk-taking, which is part of each game, but not usually part of an Adaptive Supportive's day. They are the people who see Clint Eastwood movies so they can identify with the forces of good against evil. These diversions give them a momentary reprieve from the predictability and boredom of their lives.

More damaging, however, is the Adaptive Supportive's use of addictive products to quell the pain he or she feels—the pain of a bad relationship, of doing unsatisfying work, of not being appreciated by others. Rather than identify the source of the problem, resolve the issue, and move forward with their lives, many Adaptive Supportives suppress the pain by escaping into addictions. They distract themselves from any potential conflict in their lives with caffeine, alcohol, cigarettes, cocaine, tranquilizers, and other medications.

These addictions often stem from their sense of powerlessness. On the down side Adaptive Supportives feel a loss of control over their own lives. But rather than take steps to regain control, they become anxious, cynical, and despondent. That's when they turn to products such as alcohol to take their minds off the problem at hand. The Japanese offer a classic example of this. Because their society does not recognize the importance of the individual, many Japanese "company men" spend their evenings in a state of intoxication. Getting drunk allows them to escape the stringent expectations of society and release some of their natural energy. Drunk, they can act as they wish, rather than as society tells them they must.

Relationships—Strong Bonds, Even Lifelong Romance

The single most important element in an Adaptive Supportive's life is often family relationships; everything else in life revolves around these. This group tends to establish secure, long-lasting, and monogamous relationships. They take their emotional bonds seriously and value the stability of their home lives.

It's not unusual for Adaptive Supportives to marry at a young age, even in their teens, and to stay married for the rest of their lives. In many cases, they marry young because they want to wake up in the morning and know they have the love and support of their mate. That assurance in life has more meaning to them than any momentary thrill they might get from a more exotic lifestyle. Adaptive Supportives want stability, and they are willing to forgo some of life's adventures to attain it. But many marry young for another reason as well. They lack the aspirations that drive dynamic energies, and thus they escape into marriage and the family unit at an early age. Rarely do they strike out on their own in an exploration of life.

Nonetheless, Adaptive Supportives have some fine qualities to contribute to a relationship. They are easygoing and sensitive people who will open themselves up to others. It's as if they are waiting to be experienced by another person and willing to be explored. They are capable of living in the moment and enjoying it, so they can be very sensual. What's more, there's no harshness or aggressiveness to their natural energy when it comes to forming relationships. Adaptive Supportives are willing to give a partner love and respect, and they want to receive the same in return.

In addition, Adaptive Supportives are utterly loyal to their partners—a positive quality that generally serves them well in life. Of course, this same characteristic can lead a person to stay in a bad relationship and end up with a lifetime of heartache. So Adaptive Supportives have to be careful, or they can become trapped in a relationship with an abusive mate. Their sense of obligation—and overwhelming need for security—can keep them in some awful situations.

Another potential problem for Adaptive Supportives is that their partners may attempt to change their natural energy. Some people have a hard time accepting Adaptive Supportives as they are. For example, an Adaptive Supportive's partner may consider his or her shyness to be a personality flaw, and then try to "correct" it by drawing him or her out. These people don't recognize that an Adaptive Supportive's energy can serve as a moderating force in the relationship. In addition, a person's true energy should be respected, not fought.

Adaptive Supportives who find the right partner often form highly symbiotic relationships. Their relationships become truly equal in that each person's needs are fulfilled and each is contributing all he or she can to the good of the marriage. If one partner is working outside the home and one is working within it, this doesn't matter; the important thing is that both are contributing in the best ways they can to the relationship.

Sometimes you'll see a couple who are both Adaptive Supportives who have a relationship that lasts a lifetime, and yet they don't seem to communicate. Other people may not understand how this can be—how, they ask themselves, can a couple be married and never say anything of any importance to one another? But outsiders don't grasp the essence of this relationship. This man and woman *have* communicated. Now, they know each other. They're comfortable with each other. That's what's important to them.

Now if I as a stranger come in and say, "Well, hold on a minute. What do you mean, you're comfortable with each other? That's not enough! You should be experiencing the interchange of new ideas! Why don't you have some meaningful conversations?" the couple might answer, "We have nothing to say to each other. But we're comfortable."

"Yes, but that's not right," I might say.

Well, it *is* right—for them. The point is, who am I to come in and say that these people should be changing their relationship, or that they should be experiencing this, or doing that? At least they go to bed at night and sleep a good sleep. They know that when they wake up in the morning, they have the support and love of the person beside them, whether they talk about something new or not. That person is *there*. And while they don't have the highs that some relationships do, they don't have the lows either. There's something to be said for this kind of steady, secure, long-term bond. After all, think about what it would be like to have all your relationship-related pain gone, as well as all the insecurity, anger, and depression. Even if, in the process, you had to give up all your relationship-related superhighs, the idea might still be tempting.

This kind of trade-off is what makes some Adaptive Supportive relationships so long-lasting. They don't really have the lows or the highs. They're just kind of driving along at fifty-five miles per hour. They don't go fifty-six, and, even if you took away the speed limit, they never would. Nor do they ever have to pull over to the side and stop because they've broken down, or because they feel an urge to ask themselves why they're on this journey in the first place. No, they just keep tooling along with the kind of steadiness that constitutes part of the strong undergirding of the Adaptive Supportive world.

When it comes to friendships, Adaptive Supportives form strong and long-lasting ones. They are honest enough to tell a friend what they are thinking and feeling. And they demand very little of their friends, except for the trust and loyalty that they so readily give themselves. Those who can return these qualities will have a friend for life in an Adaptive Supportive. On the high side of their energy they are caring, supportive, giving, and concerned. While these qualities may be somewhat hidden if an Adaptive Supportive is not actualizing the high side of his or her energy, the friendship can still be very solid if the Adaptive Supportive has a good sense of self. The friendship will be comforting and noncompetitive, allowing both parties to relax and be themselves.

Relationships with family members can be more complex. The family unit is important to Adaptive Supportives, and they devote a lot of their time and energy to family members. They can be loyal, giving, and highly protective parents. The problem is, their sometimes rigid view of life can make them especially judgmental of the people closest to them. Adaptive Supportives want to pass on to their children the same conditioning they themselves received, and they expect their children to share all their beliefs without question. As a result, the children may feel there is little room for them to explore different avenues in life. Eventually, they may rebel against the family to break free of its rigid doctrines and escape their parents' preconceived notions of how they should live their lives.

In fact, children who grow up in an Adaptive Supportive

home may end up taking a radically different approach to life than their parents did. As teenagers they start to sense that their family life is not dynamic in any way—their parents are not challenging authority, for example, or attempting to make positive changes in their lives. The children start to feel that they are in a cultural, political, or religious prison. When they break free, the new route they choose in life may depend entirely on the influence of their peers.

Energy Combinations

As for life energy combinations, Adaptive Supportives tend to be happiest when they're not overwhelmed by the other party in the relationship. So a Dynamic Aggressive, in particular, would not be a good bet for a relationship with a member of this soft, easily manipulated energy group. In fact, in the long term, a kind of slavery might result from this pairing. Nor would an Adaptive Aggressive be a terribly promising partner. These are the people who figure out all the angles and then go on to use them, and there's just too much of a chance that the more naive Adaptive Supportive would be opportunistically used—and as a result hurt—especially when you're looking at a many-years-long relationship, which is the kind that Adaptive Supportives generally want.

A relationship with a Dynamic Assertive has some possibilities. The Adaptive Supportive can live vicariously through the activities of the Dynamic Assertive, and the latter can gain needed love and support from his or her quieter partner. The dangers here: The Adaptive Supportive may find the whole thing too intense, and the Dynamic Assertive may get bored. So it's good if the two don't spend too much time together!

Of course, since Adaptive Supportives tend to place a premium on togetherness, at least in terms of physical proximity, this might be a problem. Thus members of other, less intimidating energy groups are generally the best candidates for partnership with an Adaptive Supportive. Prime among these are

Adaptive Supportives themselves. Two Adaptive Supportives together, and on their up side, can form a beautiful, uncomplicated, decades-long relationship that comes as close to the "happily ever after" image of fairy tales as anything else on this planet. Such a relationship satisfies the needs of both partners for security and permanence, and what's more, it can produce some well-adjusted, happy children—no small feat in today's world. Other realistic possibilities for the Adaptive Supportive are the Dynamic Supportive (that most "laid back" of the Dynamics) and the Adaptive Assertive. An Adaptive Supportive and a Creative Assertive sometimes do well too, although the Creative's mood and activity swings may not be easily tolerated. With this particular combination you have two people progressing through life at completely different rhythms. The Adaptive Supportive tends to plod along, while the Creative leaps, bounds, races, and then stalls. So these two, together, would not be exactly synchronized!

The World's Most Important Workers

Adaptive Supportives generally do functional work. They may be clerical-level employees or blue-collar workers in government agencies or factories. They may work at the checkout counters in retail establishments or at construction sites. Rarely do Adaptive Supportives seek out positions of responsibility. Instead, they may look for ways to exercise some control over their immediate work environment.

Sometimes other energy types make the mistake of judging Adaptive Supportives by the social status of the work they do. They make value judgments about people based on their position in life, the number of degrees they have earned, or the amount of money they have accumulated. But to do so is to ignore the fact that any given job, when done correctly and with pride, is equal to all others because it contributes to society. All the parts work as a whole, creating an essential balance that makes life better for everyone.

For instance, postal workers are generally not found on the cover of *People* magazine; they're not "important" enough. But a post office worker is suddenly very important when you need your mail. Likewise, a construction worker is important when you need a building to live in, and a sanitation worker, who toils to keep your environment clean, could be the most important person to you in terms of your health. In fact, he's probably a lot more vital to your life than many of the faces on magazine covers.

Indeed, Adaptive Supportives play an absolutely essential role in our culture, as in any. Without them, the inner workings of society would simply cease to function. Those who denigrate functional workers have a limited understanding of value, and they grossly downplay our mutual need and interdependence. The Dynamic energies need the cooperation of Adaptive Supportives, just as Adaptive Supportives can benefit from the leadership of Dynamics and the artistic efforts of Creative Assertives.

On their up side, Adaptive Supportives are conscientious and responsible workers who take their jobs seriously. Many, in fact, are highly skilled and talented craftspeople. They take great pride in the quality of their work, and they continually seek to improve and perfect their skills. What's more, they respect the notion of excellence in general, and appreciate it in others' work as well as in their own.

A strength of this group is that if you show an Adaptive Supportive the right way to do a particular job, once he or she masters it, that person will continue to do the job at the same high level consistently. I've seen this phenomenon with such workers as gardeners and school crossing guards, who will continue to put themselves out week after week and year after year to make every element in the garden fit exactly into specifications, or to make sure that no child crosses the street until all traffic is at an absolute standstill. With Adaptive Supportive workers on the high end of their energy, slacking off is a concept that just doesn't apply.

Of course, the Adaptive Supportive gardener will not be the one to try unusual color combinations or let the hedge grow to some unorthodox height in order to experiment with a new sun/shade pattern. You'd need a Creative Assertive gardener for that. Likewise, the Adaptive Supportive crossing guard won't be the one to launch a campaign for a town bike path, whereas a Dynamic Assertive might. The thing is, if you put members of these other groups in the respective jobs, they probably won't stay with the work as long as an Adaptive Supportive will. Nor will you have the same measure of self-administered quality control.

But on the down side, Adaptive Supportives often erect artificial barriers to the personal growth that would give them more opportunities in the workplace. They may dislike their jobs, but they won't seek the education, training, or experience needed to do something more interesting. In many cases they simply do what they must to get by and earn a paycheck. In essence they trade off opportunity for job security—an aspect of work life that has tremendous value to Adaptive Supportives.

A pitfall for this group is that their desire to explore life will peak early on, generally in high school or soon thereafter. Many then lose their motivation to grow professionally and personally. They begin to dwell on past achievements as a way to sublimate their frustration with the boredom of their present life. Adaptive Supportives often gather to talk about the "glory days" when they excelled at a sport in high school, for instance. They can become consumed by these remembrances, repeating the same stories tirelessly to a group of close friends. But rarely do they want to look at their present situation to identify opportunities for change and growth.

As a result, Adaptive Supportives can become spectators in life. They begin to live vicariously through others, by watching soap operas and movies, or reading tabloids. It's as if they believe adventure is something to be created and experienced by others, not something available in their own lives. Adaptive Supportives even begin to identify with other spectators who share their interests, such as the fans of a particular sports team or famous personality. In essence, they look for positive reinforcement and a sense of self in such spectator groups.

Personal Change Is Not Comfortable

Adaptive Supportives have a difficult time with change, and this is true just as much on an individual level as on a social or political one. Many are so attached to their beliefs and lifestyle that they cannot conceive of questioning those precepts, let alone moving beyond them for a new direction in life. They may change the circumstances of their day-to-day existence—their jobs, houses, or even family and friends—but they don't change themselves.

There's no denying that personal growth requires awareness, effort, and commitment. It requires a willingness to consider all sides of an issue; to take chances in life; and, in the end, to make constructive changes. While Adaptive Supportives may perceive that there is more to life than they were led to believe, they're generally afraid to jeopardize what they already have to go out and pursue it. That would mean stepping outside their models of belief—an action that is sure to cause some discomfort.

Indeed, Adaptive Supportives tend to deny their capacity for intellectual growth, particularly as they age, and particularly when they are on the down side of their energy curve. They don't trust their ability to grow because they might have to deny what they currently are in the process of doing. It's all a little too difficult and frightening, so self-awareness is not something they move toward. The end result is that they may deny responsibility for themselves in every way—for their emotional health, their spiritual health, and their physical health as well. This is the group that says about death, "When your number's up, your number's up," convinced that there's nothing they can do to forestall that. After a certain number of years of this kind of fatalism and denial, any capacity for personal change or growth dwindles to nothingness.

To revive this capacity, Adaptive Supportives must recognize that there is nothing intrinsic about them that prevents personal growth. Despite all their beliefs and fears, which can indeed be stifling, they—just like everyone else—are capable of change. But they have to take charge of their own development. They can't wait for some big boss figure to give them permission to change, to say it's okay. This waiting for permission is a major stumbling block for many Adaptive Supportives. They wait for a signal from some higher-up before they begin to make any major transition.

The few Adaptive Supportives who do break through this "big-boss barrier" become very excited about their own untapped potential. Once they start the process of personal growth, they open themselves up to new experiences and new ways of viewing their lives. The catch is that they may need someone to work with them—generally a more dynamic personality—to keep them motivated and to supply structure and direction. Provided they have that guidance, they will continue to develop their potential.

Who Are You? Only *You* Know

In the end, Adaptive Supportives are capable of substantial transitions when they break out of society's mold and reach the high side of their energy. With the right catalyst to encourage them, they will extricate themselves from bad marriages, bad jobs, and other types of harmful circumstances. But they have to be willing to let go of their fears and to face change as a positive event.

If you're an Adaptive Supportive, you may lose sight of the following: No other human being—not your parents, spouse, siblings, best friends, political leader, or clergy—has the right to tell you who you are. No one has the right to limit your choices in life and diminish your individuality. If you put too much stock in other people's definition of who you are, you may begin to believe them and even become dependent on their approval and feedback. After a while you can find yourself needing someone else to "rubber-stamp" everything you do.

The definition of the real self comes from within. It's up to you to recognize who you are and to take responsibility for your own well-being. While the support and acceptance of others give life a pleasant and comfortable quality, you shouldn't let a need for security prevent you from seeking out your higher self.

Beyond that, you need to question the notion that stability and permanence are the most important qualities in life. They definitely have their place, but so does the process of change. Look at the way you are living and try to determine if it has real meaning for you. Think about the work you do, the relationships you form, and the values you express daily. Are you happy with these aspects of your life? If not, give yourself the freedom to try some new ideas and to attempt some new physical, mental, and spiritual approaches to the challenge of daily living.

Above all, recognize that the beliefs that have been handed down to you by others are not necessarily the beliefs you should accept and adhere to in life. Yes, they *may* be the right beliefs for you. Or they may be 99 percent right for you, or 75 percent, or 50 percent. The point is, beliefs are something you can accept or reject, whole or piecemeal, and it's every human's right to do so.

You don't have to be a revolutionary. Stridency and committing acts that will get you on the six-o'clock news may not be your style. Still, you can work within our society's institutions without relinquishing your power and control to those who run them. What it boils down to, in the end, is that you don't want to end up disillusioned and disappointed in your old age because you accepted someone else's prescription for living as the only possible one. There are so many ways to live. Decide what values are important to you and your family, and then define yourself according to what you truly believe.

Guardians Of Order And Stability: Adaptive Assertives

There is a small subgroup of the Adaptive Supportive energy type that shares this type's strong need to fit in with the majority but that differs from the type in that its members will take on limited leadership roles. This subgroup is the Adaptive Assertives, and it's a group that's distinguished by having some of the most fulfilled, least dysfunctional members of society. Adaptive Assertives, like their close energy cousins the Adaptive Supportives, mold themselves to society's expectations and live within the social contract they are given. The difference is that Adaptive Assertives will challenge wrongs within their immediate environment. Unlike Adaptive Supportives, who accept things just as they are, Adaptive Assertives try to correct problems within the system. In that way they have an assertive component to their natural energy.

An Adaptive Assertive might be the unionized worker who challenges corruption at the top of the union, the farmer who chooses to "go organic," the neighbor who encourages others to get involved in preventive health, or the parent who tries to improve the local school system. These people are, in a sense, leaders within their own social and work environments, although at times they are following the lead of Dynamic Assertives within those environments, or working in tandem with them. The thing that distinguishes the Adaptive Assertive orientation from that of Dynamic Assertives is that Adaptive Assertives are not interested in challenging whole systems; they're just trying to right a wrong, or to correct a flaw, within a small microcosm of a system. They remain obedient in that they don't question the big picture—the larger issues of how our world view might be improved or how society is organized. As Adaptives they do what society asks of them, whether it be joining the army, voting the party line, or keeping their front lawn trimmed to an acceptable height.

Nonetheless, Adaptive Assertives are smart, idealistic, and conscientious people. On the high side of their energy they play just as important a role in society as any other energy type. Adaptive Assertives are often willing to facilitate change on a personal scale, and their constructive efforts feed into the larger forces for change. They form bonds with other energy types to help make the world work better and more honestly. They may be more predictable than those with the Dynamic energies, but their high-side efforts are useful and positive.

In short, Adaptive Assertives are superb pragmatists. While Dynamic Assertives may be able to offer more sophisticated critiques of what's wrong with various societal paradigms, Adaptive Assertives will actually get down in the trenches to make one particular corner of society run well. They'll do the fact-gathering that's necessary to keep any enterprise running optimally. For instance, an Adaptive Assertive at a school board meeting might show up armed with specific information on which grades lack textbooks for what subjects, and where in the budget the money for these might be found.

Since they're willing and able to deal with the nitty-gritty of change in a limited, familiar sphere, Adaptive Assertives excel in supervisory positions. In this group you'll find people who aren't afraid of detail work and who can use it to effect positive results—people such as foremen, department heads, school principals, police chiefs, and engineers. All of these occupations require highly developed organizational ability, which is generally an Adaptive Assertive forte.

In Tune, On Top . . . Intolerant?

When they're living on the high side of their energy, Adaptive Assertives focus on making the best of what they have. In fact, members of this group are often the most fulfilled and happy of all the energy types. This makes sense when you consider the following: This world as we know it is basically an Adaptive's world—that is, however much the visionary Dynamics or dreamy Creatives might want to change things, at any given time, except perhaps for a short period after a revolution, the world we're living in is the status-quo world of the powers that be. It's an imperfect world that has to be adapted to. And who better to enjoy that than the Adaptive Assertive? All the Dynamics, and the Creatives, as we've said, are perpetually itching to change things; they're too idealistic to be consistently happy. As for the Adaptives, the Adaptive Supportive usually has too little control of his or her work and economic life to be really fulfilled. And the Adaptive Aggressive, although often well off economically, is by nature a constantly striving person, always seeking the next big opportunity for a power play; this predatory lifestyle doesn't make for long-term happiness either.

But the Adaptive Assertive doesn't have these roadblocks on the way to contentment. In the Adaptive Assertive you have someone who's in tune with prevailing values; someone who's generally on top of things workwise, in that he or she may have a supervisory post and thus some measure of control; and someone who's not power-hungry. So there's a greater potential for happiness in this group than in the others.

These are family-oriented and civic-minded people who attempt to do something constructive within the boundaries society has set. They seek creative outlets for their ideas, and they take pride in living an autonomous and highly principled life. When they are on the high side of their energy they will have a healthy home, a healthy family, and a healthy workplace. What's more, the world around them will be a better place for their efforts.

A lot of high-end qualities of the Adaptive Assertive are the qualities we think of as traditional, conservative virtues—"the things that made America great." Thrift, punctuality, hard work, honesty, persistence—all of these bring to mind Ben Franklin's aphorisms, and Adaptive Assertives on their high side. We can laugh at these "nerdy" attributes, but we do so at our own peril, because without them we'd have no viable workplaces, schools, or neighborhoods. We'd have no PTAs, Elks Lodges, Boy or Girl Scouts, or any of the other nonglamorous organizations that work to keep our civilization civil.

One of the adages we can probably all remember from our youth is "A stitch in time saves nine." Adaptive Assertives have taken this seriously in that they tend to be excellent at planning ahead, taking steps to forestall any potential disaster. Thus this is the group whose members hardly ever declare bankruptcy. They're good savers, family-budget makers, and buyers of insurance. You hardly ever see an Adaptive Assertive operating in a crisis mode. They don't have to—they've planned for every eventuality.

Saving for the future is one of those traditional American activities that seems to have gone out of fashion in some circles, but not with Adaptive Assertives. Others may squander everything they earn in a quest for immediate gratification, but members of this energy group are still firm believers in the virtue of systematically saving for their children's education, their own retirement, or that proverbial rainy day. So Adaptive Assertives aid the national economy by being this country's "master savers." And they're "master buyers" as well, in that they pride themselves on being educated consumers who research the market before making purchases so they can get high quality at the best price. They eschew both schlocky goods at rock-bottom prices and the extravagant. In their shopping habits, as in much else in Adaptive Assertives' lives, moderation is the preferred mode.

If you're trying to think of Adaptive Assertives you know, and none stands out in your mind, that may actually be a result of another of this group's attributes: They don't stand out. Members of this energy group are basically humble, nonflashy people who have no desire to call attention to themselves. They tend to dress and house themselves conservatively, and are happy to live calmly according to their principles, letting others create the noise, crises, and drama of life.

But the quiet quality of this group does not mean they are pushovers. Adaptive Assertives are idealistic people who value order and justice and who will work to clean up an environment where order and justice seem lacking. So on their high side, Adaptive Assertives serve as the conscience of a particular environment—the watch dogs who want to keep it honest and make it all it should be. They are very connected to their communities—where they often live their entire lives—and have a natural inclination to protect their own neighborhoods. They are the ones who say to others, "We have to deal with this problem. It's our neighborhood, it's our jobs, it's our community—let's keep it healthy." In this respect they serve as role models for others by showing them that change is a worthy and achievable goal.

On the down side, a facet of this group that can be problematic is that Adaptive Assertives are not particularly tolerant. This is a highly functional group—good at coping with reality, working hard, feeling reasonably contented with what they have, and planning for a rainy day. So they sometimes have trouble understanding why others can't always operate in the same way and achieve the same things they have. "Why can't they work hard like I did?" they'll ask about the poor, or "What do they want, anyway?" they'll ask about a group with a political grievance they can't quite comprehend.

The trouble is that Adaptive Assertives, while good with detail, are not all that practiced in their imagination skills. So they sometimes have trouble imagining how someone could have grown up in different circumstances than they did, with different gifts or liabilities, or even with totally different values. Some of these suppositions are beyond their ken, and so an Adaptive Assertive on his down side is capable of dismissing individuals, or even whole groups of people, as "lazy," "weird," or even "no damn good."

"Let's Do It Right!"

One of the most distinguishing characteristics of Adaptive Assertives is that they believe in doing things correctly. They don't just want to get a job done—they want to get it done right. This energy type is responsible for upholding the quality and dependability of many American products; in fact, where they've been permitted to, Adaptive Assertives have helped stem industrial degeneration in this country by taking enormous pride in the quality of their work. They approach their jobs with professionalism, and they can be especially effective as supervisors or foremen who pass their high standards on to others in the company, specifically the Adaptive Supportives who are working just beneath them.

Better Homes and Gardens

The Adaptive Assertive's strong desire to do things the right way is also reflected in his or her home environment. Their homes tend to be sensibly decorated, sparkling clean, and organized to the hilt. These are the people who have a place for everything, and everything is in its place. What's more, everything works, and if it doesn't, it's repaired immediately. There's a meticulous quality to the Adaptive Assertive's approach to life, and it shows.

Take a top-to-bottom, inside-and-out tour of the Adaptive Assertive's house and you see order everywhere: In the attic, old suitcases are piled in size-place order. So are old magazines, with chronological order entering in here as well. In the bedrooms, mattresses are rotated on a schedule, so that no part gets unduly worn. There are wall thermometers in each bedroom as an accuracy check for the thermostat thermometers (and if one of the wall thermometers was wrongly calibrated so it reads a couple of degrees too low, if you took that one off the wall you would see this fact penciled neatly on the back). In the bathrooms, toothpaste tubes are rolled up from the bottom and towels (color-coordinated with the tile) are stacked on a shelf with the folded edges all facing out.

The kitchen? Hospitals could look to it as a model of antisepsis. And note that there's nothing random about the placement of magnets on the refrigerator. In the living room—well, you may not be allowed to sit in it, but if you were, you wouldn't see or inhale a speck of dust. The dining room (it *was* dined in once!) could pass the white-glove test too. In the basement, well-cared-for tools are all hung up on hooks—*labeled* hooks. Outside, the flower garden is a perfect rainbow of color surrounded by a knockout lawn; in fact, the whole yard is a showplace, and that includes the doghouse—even the inside! And the yard, like the house, is kept up daily, even hourly. Soon after it snows, each flake is dutifully transferred from where it doesn't belong to where it's permitted, and ditto for the errant leaves of fall. You could make fun of neatnik Adaptive Assertives ad infinitum, but on the other hand, they're responsible for a lot of the beauty and stability found in neighborhoods all across this country.

By the way, concerning the Adaptive Assertive's prompt repairing of what's broken, he (or she) often will not have to wait for the repairman, because he can fix it himself. This group has a high percentage of superb, intuitive mechanics who can figure out how to fix almost anything. What's more, Adaptive Assertives often enjoy helping others, to the extent that they'll gladly tackle neighbors' minor household emergencies—gratis.

I had an uncle who exemplified this. Whenever he found out that a neighbor or relative had something that had broken down in or around that person's house, he made it a point to fix it. And he didn't make a big deal about this either. He simply showed up at the person's house as soon as he could fit it into his schedule and, without fanfare, fixed the thing. He didn't need any helpers—he seemed to like working alone—and he would never accept money or any other payment for his efforts. To those relatives with no mechanical ability, this Adaptive Assertive uncle was a godsend!

And one might say that he was a godsend in another sense. You see, it was this same uncle who, if you were homebound, would keep you supplied, weekly, and for the rest of your life, with a copy of the minister's latest sermon. And he certainly wouldn't accept payment for that service either. Payment would have been beside the point anyway, the point being that my uncle just wanted to keep things in order, to keep things humming.

Loyal to the End—With Some Strings Attached

Adaptive Assertives generally do not come across as warm people, but they can be loving to their family members. In fact, family life is very important to the Adaptive Assertives. They tend to center their lives around these relationships, socializing with siblings, cousins, aunts, and uncles, for example, more often than with coworkers or others outside the family.

An Adaptive Assertive can be a good friend to a select group of people. They don't tend to form a lot of friendships, and in many cases they have the same friends throughout their entire lives. Once they bond with certain people, they remain true to those relationships. An Adaptive Assertive would never betray a friendship; like their Adaptive Supportive counterparts, they are exceptionally loyal people.

The drawback is that Adaptive Assertives generally expect others to behave in a prescribed fashion. They have been conditioned to accept society's manners and morals, and they expect others to adhere to those same standards. That doesn't leave a lot of room for individuality and warmth in their relationships. However, Adaptive Assertives can form lifelong and loving relationships with those who share their beliefs.

Many Adaptive Assertives also develop relationships through their civic activities. They are likely to be Scout leaders, for example, or to serve as elders in their churches. They are conscientious people who will perform volunteer work for organizations that help the homebound or elderly in their communities. While there is the tendency of Adaptive Assertives to come across as too opinionated or intolerant, if others can accept these idiosyncrasies, they will benefit from the checks and balances that Adaptive Assertives provide in their immediate environments.

Energy Combinations

An Adaptive Assertive and an Adaptive Supportive, sharing similar energies and attitudes as they do, can form a solid relationship, as can two Adaptive Assertives. In the latter case, an interesting situation sometimes develops: With an Adaptive Assertive couple you get a very stable, ordered, mutually supportive unit in which doing things right becomes such an art form that, after a while, the rest of humanity begins to look wrong to the couple. They can develop an "us against the world" mindset, and their union can evolve into something quite insular and intolerant. But their house always looks great—and they're happy together!

A coupling with a drastically lower chance of mutual satisfaction would be an Adaptive Assertive and a Creative Assertive. These two don't tend to attract each other, but if they did get together, it's not hard to imagine the troublesome scenario that would follow. The Creative would shortly come to feel stifled by all the Adaptive Assertive's rules, which would probably run the gamut from not putting your feet on the coffee table to the necessity of earning a living. As for the Adaptive Assertive, she or he would soon be disgusted by the Creative's erratic schedule, moods, housekeeping, etc. No, these two, paired, would not be happy campers!

Personal Growth—Within Limits

There are two main factors that put a damper on personal growth for Adaptive Assertives. One is that, as the energy group experiencing the most life satisfaction, Adaptive Assertives don't feel the impetus to change as much as others might. This is understandable: If you're happy with life, you don't want to upset the applecart unnecessarily. Of course, you don't want to remain totally stagnant either, and Adaptive Assertives on their high side are willing to grow intellectually and spiritually. For example, they might stay abreast of issues relating to preventive health and use the information to make constructive changes in their lives, such as supporting organic farmers in their local communities, growing some of their own food in the backyard, taking vitamins, or adding an air purifier to their homes. The other main factor working against growth in this energy group is the Adaptive Assertive's tremendous need for order and security in life. Given this aspect of their energy, their growth patterns tend to be circular, covering the same ground upon which they have always felt familiar. In essence, Adaptive Assertives stay within the social and work systems that define their lives, rather than reaching out to experience something totally new or connecting with the larger contexts in life.

If you're an Adaptive Assertive, then change at a broader level is not going to come naturally. But you might want to consider this: It's fine to focus on correcting the wrongs within your own circles. After all, these are problems that others may overlook because they are not affected by them. However, it pays to at least occasionally look beyond the inner workings of your particular milieu to examine the very nature of a system itself. In addition to having minor, localized flaws that need fine-tuning, the systems you have come to accept may have larger-scale limitations that need to be addressed. By learning to question these systems you could promote your own personal growth, as well as further enhance the important role you play in society's progression toward constructive change.

Adaptive Aggressives—
The Facilitators

❖

You can call them opportunists. They are. But you can also say that Adaptive Aggressives are resourceful, socially aware people with a keen sense of where their interests lie. They are goal-oriented, long-term planners who are drawn to people they believe have the power or capacity to help them reach their goals. Bottom line, they are survivors. As professionals, they may be top-management advisers, lawyers, sales and marketing people, actors and actresses, office managers, or lieutenants in the military.

You can call them climbers. They are. But you can say, too, that Adaptive Assertives are bright people who bring vitality, joy, and a sense of openness and healthy acquisitiveness to life. They know what they want and they go out and get it, and this aggressive go-getter spirit can be a refreshing thing—provided it's not cloaked in deception. If an Adaptive Aggressive is upfront about his (or her) ambition, and if he maintains a general standard of honesty, it can be an exhilarating experience to be around him. In fact, this is the wildest and most exciting energy type—bar none. Yes, the Dynamic Aggressive shares the strong drive of the Adaptive Aggressive, but in the Dynamic the drive is more focused; it tends to be tailored to a specific goal. The Adaptive Aggressive, on the other hand, is more restless and all over the place with his drive. He'll try anything!

Adaptive Aggressives often seek power and status, but they are not dynamic creators themselves. Thus, on their down side, they may lack confidence in their own abilities and turn to other people for focus and ideas. They become attuned to what others need or enjoy and try to make themselves indispensable to these people by fulfilling their every desire. Adaptive Aggressives have an ever-present need to be accepted; thus they may behave like emotional chameleons by adopting the beliefs and ideas of the person they identify with at the moment.

In many cases Adaptive Aggressives are driven people who have not been appreciated for themselves. They lack self-assurance and a sense of grounding in their own individuality, perhaps because they learned early on to become what others wanted. Their emotions go up, down, and all around, depending on how secure they feel in the situation of the moment. Despite this emotional volatility, though, they try to present themselves in a dignified and controlled manner.

Adaptive Aggressives can be so hypersensitive to criticism that they cannot bear to consider their own shortcomings. On their down side, in fact, they generally are not interested in improving themselves, other than to upgrade their external circumstances. Nor do they have a capacity for self-observation—they are too outwardly focused. They may appear to have a strong ego, but what they actually have is a strong persona.

Adaptive Aggressives' attachments are often based on neediness, and because others are instrumental in making them feel significant, members of this energy group tend to blame others when they don't feel good about themselves. This can be frustrating for everyone involved. Also, the personal lives of those with this life energy are often cluttered and chaotic because they hang on to their emotions, their past, and their pain. But they disguise this pain because they believe they must hide their vulnerability.

When other people interact with an Adaptive Aggressive, they must use all their senses and their intuition to determine what the Adaptive Aggressive is feeling and how he or she is responding to them. Is the response honest? Or is it less than honest? Adaptive Aggressives may believe for the moment that they are being sincere, but if any group can fool a lie detector it is this one because they have an adeptness at self-deception as well as at deceiving others. Sometimes their deceit consists not so much of out-and-out lying as it does of lying by omission, or of exaggeration or rationalization. This group has a great ability to rationalize, and it is one they make full use of. Of course, others eventually realize that the Adaptive Aggressive is playing fast and loose with the facts. Hopefully this realization comes before too much harm has been done.

An Adaptive Aggressive on the down side does not develop an internal set of values that remains stable across all situations. Their integrity is linked to the momentary standards of the person or situation to which they have attached themselves. Thus they tend to be unpredictable and skittish. They will end something very quickly if they are betrayed. In fact, they may even expect to be betrayed, because they do not trust others easily. At the same time, they may fear losing what they have if they believe it is the best they can do for the moment. These kinds of strategic considerations are always on their minds.

In fact, strategy and planning are key to this energy group, with other people playing an instrumental role in their plans. Whether this role is a witting or an unwitting one depends— as so much does for this group—on the circumstances. In other words, sometimes Adaptive Aggressives will let you in on their plans, and sometimes they won't. If they believe that informing you will help them, they will let you in on the plan. If they think you might resent it, they won't; they are masters of the hidden agenda. In any event, they are savvy people who see all that is around them. They can see the big picture and develop short-and long-term goals within its framework.

Adaptive Aggressives take advantage of every opportunity, and not only that—they make opportunities happen. That's why salespeople are often Adaptive Aggressives: This type has the chutzpah to walk into a place and get someone interested in their product or service. On their up side they are energetic and highly effective in the sales field, but on the down side they may go for the cheap approach. If this tactic fails, they tend to make excuses for themselves.

While occupationally Adaptive Aggressives may be good as salespeople, in life they sometimes seem more like shoppers—comparison shoppers. That is to say, Adaptive Aggressives are constantly comparing what they have to what they see around them, be it in the personal or the professional area. Then they'll shop around for the better opportunity. Why are they always on the lookout for something better? It's usually because they're unhappy, insecure in themselves. The irony is that to other people, Adaptive Aggressives often appear to have a secure, even cushy, environment. But for them it's always only temporary.

Adaptive Aggressives tend to be clandestine because they sense their weaknesses may be exposed and they'll be "found out." On their down side, then, they may lie, cheat, manipulate, and execute all manner of power plays to pit people against each other. The goal of these low-side machinations is a hidden but desperate urge to protect their image, as well as what they have, and they're not likely to feel remorse when operating in this mode.

Adaptive Aggressives are shrewd socially in that they're familiar with the social scene and know how to use it, and they've mastered enough etiquette to be able to maneuver smoothly through various situations. Also, you almost never see an Adaptive Aggressive who's not dressed properly. Whatever the occasion, they've got the image down. For instance, if they're in the office they'll be dressed to precisely the level of formality the boss favors; if they're working out they'll have on whatever exercise wear is currently in vogue—not for them the old shorts and T-shirt that just happen to be in the drawer. For a weekend at someone's country retreat they'll be sporting just the right mix of the casual and the costly. Others at the retreat may use the weekend to become at one with nature, but it can look as if the Adaptive Aggressive is more at one with the fashion ads!

Because they are concerned with appearances, Adaptive Aggressives give the impression that they have control over their energy. But there's a frenetic quality to that energy, unlike that of other people who combine a high energy level with a certain calmness. The Adaptive Aggressive's energy tends to be turbulent. In a serene setting, such as that country retreat, the Adaptive Aggressive's inability to relax really shows up. She will sit for a moment, start to fidget, read one page of a book, put the book down, turn on the radio, walk around the room for a while. Then she might go into the other room, pick up the phone but have no one to call, watch a movie, get something to eat, walk around the grounds, but be spooked by the quiet. People in this energy group are not ones to appreciate quiet; in fact, they're sometimes scared by it. Returning to her room, the Adaptive Aggressive might try to nap, give up on that idea, turn on the TV, consult her schedule of trains back to the city.

Even in ordinary circumstances, Adaptive Aggressives always seem to have a surplus of energy. When you're in a room with them, you can never forget that they're there because they're tapping their feet, or pacing, or even saying things to themselves under their breath. Adaptive Aggressives sometimes have a bull-in-a-china shop quality to them that can make them uncomfortable to be around—unless you're up for a prolonged, intense energy jolt.

If you are, then it's another story. An Adaptive Aggressive can motivate you as no one else can. A Dynamic Aggressive or Assertive may inspire you, but an Adaptive Aggressive can get you chomping at the bit and primed for action; it's as if they have a surplus of adrenaline flow that—if you're receptive—somehow transfers itself to you. Members of this group make great athletic coaches for this reason.

One reason Adaptive Aggressives are often restless and troubled is that their sense of self is so fluid. They depend in an ongoing way on interaction with externals to keep them from feeling unsettling emotions. When they stop moving, planning, and scheming, they are frightened by the emptiness and insecurity they feel. These feelings drive them onward, toward the next goal. And when that one is reached, then there's the next; they're like the ever-swimming shark, unable to stop.

When frustrated, Adaptive Aggressives tend to react impulsively. They blame their frustration on others, and they may live in a state of turmoil that embroils those around them. Neither do they handle stress well. In a crisis situation, Adaptive Aggressives tend to panic. As a prisoner of war, for example, an Adaptive Aggressive might fold immediately and volunteer information about others in his group.

The Adaptive Aggressive woman is an emotional chameleon; she can adapt to any person or environment. You like Italian food? She does, too. You like the opera? She's an old opera buff. You'd like to go to France? Best country in the world for her. No matter what your needs or desires, this type of woman will adapt to them and reflect those needs herself. (It should be noted that up to at least the 1960s, young women were trained—by teen and women's magazines, and by the prevailing wisdom—to be exactly these sort of mental and emotional mirrors of their dates' and mates' frames of mind. For instance, to be popular with boys, girls were supposed to find out what their dates were interested in and then get interested in it themselves—or pretend to be; that would do, too. So there's no doubt that some of today's Adaptive Aggressive women are the products of pervasive social conditioning a few decades back.)

Many Adaptive Aggressive women have a hidden agenda. In other words, they adapt themselves to you for a time, all the while getting what they can from you until it benefits them to move on. Perhaps they can no longer obtain what they need from you, they think they are going to be exposed, or someone better comes along. And if a man should discover that an Adaptive Aggressive woman does not belong in his life, she will no doubt make him pay for having been involved with her at all.

The Adaptive Aggressive woman can be exciting, and even scary. Think of the character played by Glenn Close in *Fatal Attraction*. That's that Adaptive Aggressive woman on her down side. On the up side, an Adaptive Aggressive woman would have enjoyed that same experience without degenerating to the point of vindictiveness. In fact, the Adaptive Aggressive woman is generally controlled, self-assured, independent, and methodical on the high side of her energy. She's a great person to work with because she's not afraid to assert herself and take charge. She has more confidence than any of the other energy types when it comes to dealing with people. She will get a job done right.

Likewise, Adaptive Aggressive men have strong personalities, and, on the surface at least, they are committed to their beliefs. They are determined, organized, no-nonsense people. They can bring order to a disorganized environment, fix something that is not working, and offer good ideas on how to resolve a problem. As a result, they make excellent management advisers, office managers, and sales and marketing people. But on the down side, there may be no virtue they hold sacred. Thus the Adaptive Aggressive male can become self-interested, manipulative, and conniving.

These men can survive anywhere due to their adaptive nature. Put them in any environment, positive or negative, and they will adjust to its conditions by mirroring the needs and desires of the people around them. Take Oliver North, a perfect example of an Adaptive Aggressive on his down side. North did what he believed was right because he honored the authority of his superiors. He adapted to the situation in which he found himself and the problem he was presented with. Nor did he betray the people behind him when the situation was exposed. In fact, others betrayed him. Like any Adaptive Aggressive, North was dismayed when the people he protected made a scapegoat of him.

Ronald Reagan was a Dynamic Assertive on the down side. But he surrounded himself with Adaptive Aggressives such as Attorney General Meese, and others who could hide his limitations, and serve as the brains, mouth, and conscience behind the president's actions. We should remember that a Dynamic who holds public office will almost always have strong Adaptive Aggressives behind him. These behind-the-scenes people pull the strings, and they are the ones we must identify and watch.

Hitler, for example, was a shrewd, clever, and powerful man, but he was not intelligent. He, too, supported himself with strong and intelligent people such as Joseph Goebbels, who had several Ph.D.s. Even institutions such as the Catholic Church have leaders who are powerful, clever, and ruthless. Pope Leo X was not smart, but he surrounded himself with insiders who could serve as his voice.

Many actors and actresses are Adaptive Aggressives who can excite others with their ability to take on any emotion and mimic any attitude. That adaptability is a unique part of their energy, and, used in the show business arena, it's a positive thing, a far cry from the schemings and manipulations that characterize some Adaptive Aggressives' use of their energy.

In Charge of Their Energy—or Ruled By It?

When operating on the high end, Adaptive Aggressives will get in charge of their energy so they don't burn out and resort to using other people. In this phase they are exciting, supportive, and spontaneous. They take a constructive approach to anything they do. On the down side, they do burn out and use themselves up, as well as others. There is a wide range between these two extremes, and an Adaptive Aggressive's position along this spectrum will depend on his or her conditioning and the influence of other people in his or her life. The Adaptive Aggressive needs to take these other factors into account and then choose to bring out the higher side. If he or she does not make that choice, the higher side may not emerge on its own.

While Adaptive Aggressives often get ahead by using a relationship as a vehicle for their own growth, in and of itself that approach is not necessarily negative. Where it does become problematic is if they are on their low end, where a lack of balance can cause them to be ruthless. Then they may use other people to their own advantage, and they will continually look for the next opportunity. As soon as they identify a better situation or relationship than what they currently have, they may disengage and move on.

Indeed, the Adaptive Aggressive can be quite dangerous on the down side. They are aware of the world in which they live, and they tend to align themselves with questionable causes or even radical and harmful ones. Thus they may carry out deeds that serve their own interests but undermine everyone else's. At their lowest level they cannot be trusted for a second. They may betray others even as they are taking something from them.

Adaptive Aggressives on the low end include many of the M.B.A.s who enter banking, government, and industry with purely opportunistic goals in mind. They generally work for a Dynamic person, and they will be loyal to that Dynamic and do his or her work as long as they get promotions and have their backsides protected. If something they work on succeeds, Adaptive Aggressives will take credit for it. If it fails, they may avoid taking responsibility.

Many Adaptive Aggressives, though quite capable people, do not carry projects through to completion on their down side. They start all kinds of projects that just seem to evaporate. I often think of them as "emotional magicians" who create a lot of illusions in their lives. Like all good illusionists, they can be entertaining and exciting, but much of what they do amounts to distracting motion. The potential of a project or idea excites them, but finishing it may require more emotional stability, determination, and focus than they have.

Adaptive Aggressives also have a difficult time expressing their emotions and revealing their true selves. Eventually their high level of self-criticism will be turned outward and applied to other people and to their environment. Indeed, they often try to change their environment because they find it dissatisfying. And if things do not go well, the Adaptive Aggressive, more than any other energy type, will cut and run. They will run out of a marriage, a relationship, or a job. Many Adaptive Aggressives repeat this pattern over and over again and fail to learn from the experience.

Open to the New—and to Now

But for every negative there's a positive, and that certainly holds true for this group. When they're in charge of their energy, one of the Adaptive Aggressives' positive qualities is that they are open to new ideas. If something excites them, they can go into the moment with openness and verve. They take advantage of the moment the way a football player sees an opening in the field and runs for a touchdown. On the up side, these openings in life will always appeal to the Adaptive Aggressive. And they will use their higher energies to plan for the future and determine how to get things done. They are smart and capable people who can calculate long-term plans. In this respect, then, their ability to scheme is a positive quality that allows them to formulate effective plans.

What's more, nobody is more attentive to details and to immediate follow-up than the Adaptive Aggressive; nobody organizes better. Without Adaptive Aggressives on a work team, the process of achieving an important goal can be chaotic, or even break down.

Adaptive Aggressives also have a great deal of flexibility and spontaneity, both of which compensate for any lack of creativity they may have. After all, what good are great ideas that sit around to gather dust and never get executed? The Adaptive Aggressive gets involved and makes sure things actually work. They're expert facilitators—and as such they serve a vital function.

When Adaptive Aggressives keep their energy high, they are not Machiavellis running around trying to take over the world or cheat their way to success. They are effective, can-do contributors to all the activities of life. They are exciting people to be with. They are flexible, in the moment, spontaneous, fluid, and fun. The other energies need that excitement. In truth, we are drawn to people who represent action, who do something worth reading about and considering. Witness the popularity of magazines and tabloids that continually show us people who have done something exciting.

Want to Make It Happen?
Hire an Adaptive Aggressive!

In the world of work, each of the life energy types has something essential to contribute. Typically the Dynamic Aggressives are the macromanagers, the ones who create and direct large organizational frameworks. Dynamic Assertives have input here, too, although they're less concerned with the directorial aspect of management, and more with the ideological. Once systems are outlined within these frameworks, Creative Assertives develop and refine the actual mechanics; then their plans are given to Adaptive Aggressives to see that they're implemented.

So it's the Adaptive Aggressives who actually make things happen. Masters of detail, they can set systems in motion, and if they're not always there for the long haul, the Adaptive Assertives—those organizational wizards who work just beneath them—are. Then, of course, there are the Adaptive Supportives, who contribute physically to the system with their hard work.

Concerning Adaptive Aggressives not sticking around for the long haul, this group tends to job-hop like crazy. They, like many others, make career choices based on what they believe will make them happy. But they rarely end up feeling happy or fulfilled with the work, and so they jump from one thing to another. Also, they tend to deny that they have failed at anything.

On the high end, Adaptive Aggressives do not like competition. Much like Creative Assertives in this respect, they don't think other people have the right to judge them. Adaptive Aggressives do not believe that their insights, skills, and creativity should be pitted against those of another, because they don't see themselves as being the same as anyone else. Also, they don't want to risk losing and being shown up. Therefore they generally don't want to play the game unless they write the rules.

Still, achievement is very important to the Adaptive Aggressive. They believe that the more successful they are, the more other people will appreciate them. As a result they tend to exaggerate everything they do and will try to make themselves indispensable. This orientation toward achievement can make them quite effective in the workplace, especially when, on the high end, they follow through on details. Generally, though, Adaptive Aggressives are responsible only to the degree that they feel appreciated for their efforts. And, they prefer to be responsible to a more powerful person. Then they really get the job done.

An Adaptive Aggressive is great at reading a crisis situation quickly and coming up with solutions. If someone presents a business problem to an Adaptive Aggressive, he or she will offer a dozen viable ways to resolve it. The other person will be drawn by these abilities. The catch: While on the up side, an Adaptive Aggressive helps another person with the intention of staying around for a while; on the down side, they help, but with the idea that doing so will get them to the next place they want to be.

Unfortunately, they do not always balance the ethical and moral implications of responsibility with the practical aspects. When they do value the moral implications of their actions, they can be conscientious, valuable contributors to an enterprise. But if they are operating from their lower energy, Adaptive Aggressives may start a lot of projects but rarely bring any to completion. They take shortcuts and look for instantaneous gratification, rather than execute a job from beginning to end. If something better comes along, they leave. Or they feel slighted, and leave.

Nevertheless, for facilitating short-term goals—no matter how difficult—the Adaptive Aggressive is unparalleled. In fact, members of this group relish a challenge, and their willingness to confront difficulties head-on, rather than shrink from them, is one of their virtues. If something hard needs doing now, an Adaptive Aggressive is your best bet for getting it done.

A friend familiar with my views on the natural life energy groups emphasized this point in a conversation we had recently.

"Gary," she said, "I get the impression that you're not too crazy about Adaptive Aggressives because they can be exploitive. But there's another aspect to them—they are, in a sense, the most helpful group. They can be real life-savers, simply because they'll do things that no one else will do."

She went on to tell me about an experience she had years ago but that she still remembers vividly. It was her first day as a college freshman. The dorms were crowded that year. Settling into her room, she was disconcerted to find that although her two roommates had claimed desks, there was no third desk in the room for her. As a creative writer who liked to write on a hard surface, she felt that she was starting her higher education on a bad note.

But talking to the RA—the residential assistant who supposedly managed her hall—was no help. This person claimed that there was a furniture shortage and that no more student desks were available at the moment. All the RA had to offer was the prospect of filling out forms and waiting. The upstairs RA had the same story, and my friend suspected that although these people professed to care that she was starting her college career without a desk, her problem was not really a priority for them. She began to get discouraged about college even before her first class.

Yet the day was saved. What happened was that two girls who roomed next door got wind of the situation. These young women, whom my friend later got to know, were, she reports, classic Adaptive Aggressives. For instance, on that first day, although they hadn't been on campus much longer than she had, they had already scoped out the whole place, and they seemed to know a million people. They were loud, pushy, all-over-the place types who would do anything.

And they proceeded to do just that.

First they immediately grasped the problem, and the fact that something had to be done before classes started. Then they told my friend that they'd seen where there was an unused desk. "Come on," they said to her, "let's go and get it. With three of us, we should be able to drag it to your room."

The desk was in an area that they were not authorized to go into. "Won't we get into trouble?" my friend asked. "This desk looks different from everyone else's. Besides, aren't I supposed to fill out a furniture request form and route it through the administration?"

These considerations meant nothing to the Adaptive Aggressive young women. "Don't be silly!" they said. "You need a desk, there's one here, and you're getting it!"

The problem was solved.

My friend reported that although she did later get to know the two helpful students next door, they never became friends. "I was a quiet Creative, they were obnoxious Adaptive Aggressives, and we didn't have much in common. But here's the important thing," she continued. "I needed something done. They, and nobody else, were the ones who could get the job done, and I'll always remember those two for that." She also says that thinking about that incident helps her see how people of each life energy type, no matter how alien or annoying that energy might seem to different types, can work to support the well-being of others.

And on their up side, Adaptive Aggressives *are* supportive. They can do a great job as part of a work team that includes creative people, since they have the capacity to follow through on a good idea and handle all the details. They can also take someone's work and present it to the public. The Adaptive Aggressive generally likes the limelight and enjoys interfacing with others, while the Creative may prefer to work behind the scenes.

The Conditioned Aggressive

By the way, there is an interesting "dual energy" phenomenon that we see with some people who are Adaptive Aggressives and Dynamic Aggressives in the workplace. These people, while aggressive and authoritative at work, are passive and obedient at home. They seem to have succeeded at mastering two energies. But the natural energy is always the one that does not make a person feel conflicted. In some cases the dominant role these Aggressives play at work will be their real energy. They remain passive at home, even though they hate the role, because they were conditioned to be Adaptive Supportives.

More often, however, the role a person plays at home represents his or her real energy. We tend to reveal our true selves in personal relationships because it is in these that we are most vulnerable. Generally, then, people who are Adaptive Supportives at home truly are that way. They present their conditioned, Aggressive self at work to achieve certain goals, even if they must be insensitive to others. If they were to be submissive at work, they would not get raises and promotions. If they did not get raises and promotions, their partner at home (who may be a true Dynamic!) would not be satisfied with the relationship. Thus a person will play out his or her conditioned self to sustain the relationship of the true self.

Exciting—or Exploitive—Relationships?

Relationships are important to Adaptive Aggressives, on the down side because they use relationships as tools. This is the energy group whose favored means of coping is to distract themselves with visions of future glory, and other people become the means for achieving goals related to these visions. So where others might derive spiritual nourishment from relationships, Adaptive Aggressives nourish themselves with the fads and addictions offered by society, using relationships as means to this end.

Their specialty is attaching themselves to powerful people. And they're good at this because they can be appealingly exciting. They are adventurous, energetic, and able to take on the energy of another person at any time. This unique ability can lead other people to believe that an Adaptive Aggressive is the perfect person for them. This is especially the case with powerful or influential people who, because of their lifestyles, are often short on friends. Along comes someone who seems like the answer to a prayer. What they like, the Adaptive Aggressive likes. The apparent similarities are enticing. The other person may think, "God, this is really a great person. We're so much alike." Perhaps. But the similarities may be an illusion. And the Adaptive Aggressive may in fact be manipulating the relationship because he or she has an ulterior motive.

Whether you're a power broker or not, a relationship with an Adaptive Aggressive can be a complicated and tricky thing because they bring a lot of expectations and emotional baggage into it. But they won't show you that at the outset. So it's as if, initially, they come into your life with a little suitcase of emotions. And then once they feel that they've got you, the doorbell rings, you go to the door, and there are twenty-seven tractor-trailer-loads of emotions they want to bring in!

Many Adaptive Aggressives do not have close friendships. They are afraid to trust people or let people really get to know them. Thus they can be quite lonely. Compounding their interpersonal problems is their inability to take criticism well. It makes them feel too unworthy, and it often mirrors what they've been telling themselves all along. In general they anticipate negativity from others and don't want to risk being brought down from good feelings.

Members of this energy group can have a "here today, gone tomorrow" air that makes other people not even bother to keep their telephone number. They always seem to be halfway out the door, and this lack of stability is another factor preventing Adaptive Aggressives from forming strong friendships. They are too unpredictable and skittish to establish a sense of permanence. But all their activity is something of a cover-up for identity problems.

These same identity problems can trouble an Adaptive Aggressive's relationship with his or her children. They tend to pressure their children to achieve what they have not. The child becomes an extension of the parent's ego, which is not a healthy situation for either of them.

Actually, problems begin in many Adaptive Aggressive-run families before the achievement stage, with infancy. Adaptive Aggressive parents bore easily, so they don't have the inner resources to change their usual mental rhythms to relate to a baby for any length of time. They're the type who say, "I can't get into this diaper-changing stage, but once the kid starts to talk, it'll be interesting, so I'll get involved." Then, when the child starts to talk, it's interesting, all right—for about five minutes. The Adaptive Aggressive does not have a long attention span or much patience, and the toddler stage, like all other phases of childhood, requires a great deal of patience. In addition, Adaptive Aggressives may be too preoccupied with their own professional interests to give their children much time.

They are good at providing their children with material things; in fact, they're highly responsible in this regard. But they may not be able to meet children's needs for large blocks of parental time and for unconditional love.

Have We Got an Adaptive Aggressive for You!

A more positive facet of Adaptive Aggressives in relationships is that they're great partners for just plain having fun with. They're spontaneous, they like adventure, and they're full of raw energy. Not everyone appreciates these attributes. But for those who do, an Adaptive Aggressive on his or her high side can be a perfect partner.

Who can best pair with an Adaptive Aggressive? A Dynamic Aggressive or a Dynamic Assertive. They're the ones most likely to have the energy level, smarts, and backbone necessary to tangle with this type. And these Dynamics are attracted by Adaptive Aggressives because they're usually looking for someone who agrees with them, who compliments them, who's willing to do what they like to do, and, if work is part of the equation, who can help implement their ideas and plans. Adaptive Aggressives fit the bill in these ways. What's more, while most people are intimidated by the two fast-moving Dynamic energies, Adaptive Aggressives are not. That's a big plus from the point of view of the Dynamic who is tired of being shied away from. Dynamic Aggressives and Assertives can be volatile, demanding, and even insulting to their intimates and work partners, but Adaptive Aggressives can take whatever's dished out. They're tough. And so if they can keep their exploitive tendencies in check, they can make good matches for the two most demanding Dynamic types.

If collaborative work is part of the relationship picture, Adaptive Aggressives can serve as effective lieutenants for these Dynamics. On their high side they'll remain loyal to their Dynamic counterparts through adversity. Of course, their low-side potential for disloyalty and betrayal is always a danger.

Consider Elvis Presley, a classic Dynamic Assertive who often surrounded himself with Adaptive Aggressives. Like many Dynamic Assertives, Elvis wanted people around who would understand him, agree with him, and be willing to do what he liked to do. But he ended up being exploited to the hilt. His "friends" betrayed his confidence by writing books that revealed every little thing they knew about him.

While the Dynamic Aggressive and Assertive may sometimes be up to the challenge of a relationship with an Adaptive Aggressive, a Dynamic Supportive has a harder time of it. Consider an Adaptive Aggressive woman who marries a Dynamic Supportive man. She may think she can motivate her more mellow husband to help her achieve certain material ambitions. But when this unrealistic scenario doesn't work out, it's all downhill after that.

Interestingly, the Dynamic Supportive man may not realize this until the bitter end. The Adaptive Aggressive is the type who will leave her mate and only then tell him all the things he "did wrong" over the years, or all the things she couldn't stand about him. She never brought these things up at the time, because then there was still some benefit that could be squeezed out of the person. But the whole story finally comes out in the end, which is one of the reasons that breaking up with an Adaptive Aggressive is hard to do. The other one is that they will generally seek a large settlement for their trouble. And even if you're talking about a parting of the ways of friends and not about a romantic relationship breakup, this can be the case. Sometimes it seems as if you practically need a written pre-friendship agreement before you get involved with an Adaptive Aggressive!

Spirituality Not a Priority

Spiritual growth is not a priority for Adaptive Aggressives. Instead, they seek intellectual growth to acquire new skills, and perhaps emotional growth to help them better adapt. They are also interested in physical development, and will often take pride in their bodies.

Adaptive Aggressives have a lot of peak experiences because they are more willing than other energy types to try new things. One of the reasons they are exciting people on the up side is that they will do things that other people would never even consider. They welcome new experiences, which, in a world peopled mostly by frightened, let's-stick-to-what-we-know types, is like a breath of fresh air. On the down side, however, they may have peak experiences that are not necessarily constructive for themselves and others.

Sometimes Adaptive Aggressives take a stab at spiritual enlightenment, but they do so more in form than in essence. For instance, they may treat spiritual events as yet another opportunity to maneuver themselves into someone else's life. Go to any New Age retreat, for example, and many of the people there will be Adaptive Aggressives. But they never surrender to the experience because they need to be in control at all times. They're the ones who meditate with their eyes open, the ones who are supposed to be in a deep sleep but are thinking all the while. To grow, you have to let go, and they generally can't.

The Adaptive Aggressive may be involved in personal improvement, but the effort is likely to fit into their utilitarian scheme of things in some way. Reading is not an idle intellectual adventure for them; it's a get-ahead thing. An Adaptive Aggressive might be the type of person who litters the coffee table with art books, philosophy books, and New Yorker magazines, while hidden underneath they have copies of People. Their true interest lies with techniques for getting ahead, making deals, dressing for success, picking up men, (or women), etc. They're always looking for an advantage and a way to better their circumstances.

Can You Move Toward Trust?

If you're an Adaptive Aggressive, it doesn't mean you are doomed to be a chronic user, or a loner. You can have a balanced work life and mutually fulfilling relationships if you try. But there are a couple of issues you'll have to work through first.

To begin with, you have a particular energy—one that's very strong—and you should honor it. But you can refine and channel it to get along more harmoniously in the world. You can learn to harness your power and control your energy, in order to construct positive relationships and achievements. Your energy should be constant, like the electricity that supplies a light bulb. If it's like the electricity that causes lightning, it will be spectacular and exciting, but also spastic, undependable, and potentially harmful.

Think about your life. Do you continually start and stop projects due to the spastic quality of your energy? Do you feel powerless and trapped when you find yourself in relationships that require commitment and stability? Do you feel angry when you can no longer control everything around you? If so, begin to recognize that these are excuses not to relate to others. They are problems you need to work on.

Your energy must be harnessed and developed to its highest level so it can be applied in a positive way. Learn to accept being alone as a constructive state, rather than dwelling on the negative feelings that come from loneliness. Move away from being manipulative and predatory, and you will be freer to exhibit your sharing and caring qualities.

Learn to identify environments that suit your energy. You have as much potential as any other energy type—perhaps more—to be happy with your energy. But you may be so caught up in searching for something that you fail to look at what you already have. Or you may come across a healthy environment for yourself but pass it right by in your haste. Look for situations that satisfy the needs of your energy type.

Ideally, you need to be acknowledged for your special skills and attributes, to cooperate rather than compete with other people, and to avoid the harsh judgment of others.

Adaptive Aggressives tend to look outward. That's okay up to a point; we all need feedback to see how we're functioning. But if a person is to grow, he or she must begin to turn inward. So stop looking to others all the time to validate and improve your life. You may be in a terrible bind because you don't trust others, yet you depend on other people for so much. As a result you may feel resentful when you don't find satisfaction in the things other people bring to your life.

Concentrate on appreciating yourself. Learn to be less harsh on yourself and to trust your own competence. You must learn to love someone affectionately rather than for the qualities that serve your needs or allow you to live vicariously. The extreme swings in your feelings, from idealizing others to being overly negative, can drive other people away. Like many Adaptive Aggressives, you will get fed up with the things you do to ingratiate yourself to others, and end up feeling enraged.

Adaptive Aggressives, in particular, have the potential to grow and become more genuine if they form relationships with people who treat them with kindness and regard. But you must overcome some difficult obstacles to establish such relationships. Most important, ask yourself, "Can I work on becoming more trusting, and more able to experience others as benign and caring?"

If the answer is no, you may continue to manipulate and mistreat people, and they will not tolerate such treatment for long.

But if you've answered yes, you'll have taken the first step toward making the most of your exciting, powerful, and potentially fulfilling life energy.

Conclusion

What We Can Learn
From One Another

After reading about the seven natural life energy types you probably have some idea about which type best describes you. To test your idea and review the concepts in the foregoing chapters, you can take the quizzes at the end of this book. They will help you determine which type you are, although keep in mind that people's life energy identities are not always clear-cut; you may display attributes from two or three predominant types. But whatever the case, you might at this point be asking the following question: If I am a particular NLE type (or types), does that mean that I must necessarily and always display a particular pattern of behavior?

The answer is, of course, no. As a member of a particular energy group, you may *tend* to display a certain pattern, but that's not at all the same as saying that you're destined to act in a certain way. We are, after all, unique individuals and possessors of free will.

It is with this idea of the personal freedom that we each

---

possess that I conclude this book with the following thought: Each natural life energy has something of value about it that members of any other energy group can emulate. This is not to say that, for instance, an Adaptive Supportive can or should decide to turn himself into a Dynamic Aggressive. But it is to say that there is at least one characteristically Dynamic Aggressive trait that an Adaptive Supportive, or anyone else, might try now and then to incorporate into his or her life.

So let's start here, with Dynamic Aggressives. What is there about the Dynamic Aggressive energy that might serve as a model for anyone? We know that this group's defining quality is that they exhibit a tremendous drive to get to the top, and, in truth, we don't want the rest of the world emulating this; it would be too much of an unnatural strain for most people, not to mention the fact that it would result in unparalleled bloodshed. But there *is* something about Dynamic Aggressives that people of all energy types could emulate: their affinity for hard work. A member of any energy group could benefit from injecting a little more of the work ethic into his or her life—at particular times, anyway. So when these times come up, a Dynamic Aggressive could be an appropriate inspiration for anyone.

Likewise, not everyone could or should go around spouting opinions on how to change the world, as is the wont of Dynamic Assertives. But there is something about Dynamic Assertives that others might want to observe and learn from. Specifically, Dynamic Assertives depend on multiple, as opposed to single, interpersonal relationships. They are the ones who best understand that no one individual can fill all a person's relationship needs, and even that relationships themselves cannot fill all our emotional and intellectual needs. That's why Dynamic Assertives tend to have a variety of people coming into and going out of their lives, and sometimes to have low-intimacy withdrawal periods.

The way Dynamic Assertives live in this regard is somewhat unconventional, and no one is saying that everyone should follow suit. But by at least observing and thinking about the Dynamic Assertives' way, perhaps those individuals of other energy types who are too clingy and relationship-dependent can change their perspective into a more realistic one.

What does the Dynamic Supportive have to show us? Most of us are not, after all, constitutionally cut out to become nurturing helpers in the Dynamic Supportive mode. But we can all try to emulate the group's warmth and friendliness. Sure, if we all tried this, our imitative efforts would be a superficial thing (and maybe the whole world would begin to seem like Southern California!). Still, communicating in a more pleasant way might be beneficial anyway.

We can't all be Picassos or Shakespeares, and there's no use trying, but there is a trait of Creative Assertives that anyone can try to develop. Creatives have associative minds. It's the way they create—they look at a thing and, instead of connecting that thing with what it's usually associated with, they let their mind wander all over the place to create new associations. And any person can do mental exercises to develop a loose, wandering, associative mind, like the Creative's. This may be difficult at first, but it's doable by anyone and probably helpful for everyone in that it would increase people's problem-solving skills.

What can we learn from Adaptive Supportives? Probably not how to become millionaires; this is not their forte. Nor is innovative thinking. But a hallmark of this group is devotion to family values—meant in all the positive ways. This is the group that stresses family in their social lives and in their loyalties, and in today's rootless, transient society, standing by one's kin is a virtue that should be encouraged whenever possible.

As for Adaptive Assertives, one of the things this conscientious group can demonstrate for us is the virtue of being well-organized. Whatever energy you have and whatever work you do, being neat and organized will help you optimize your life.

Turning to our last energy group, while some Adaptive Aggressives might be able to offer us seminars on how to backstab your way to the top, this is not the area in which we should emulate them. But we could all look to their openness to opportunity.

It's sad, but some of us don't even concede the existence of opportunity. And while others may wait for opportunity to knock, the Adaptive Aggressive is the one who's got the door wide open and is ready to sprint out and meet opportunity halfway down the block! This is a great spirit to have. After all, how many times do you hear excuses as people fail to grasp good things that come their way?

"Oh, I don't have the energy for that."

"Oh, that would be too much trouble."

"It would never work out."

"They won't like me."

"I couldn't."

These are defeatist attitudes that you don't find Adaptive Aggressives hobbling themselves with. We could all learn from them in that.

Finally, whatever your NLE type, and whatever you choose to learn from those living out different energies, one thing is certain. If you are living out your own on the high side, with respect for your own unique gifts, you will be teaching others even as you learn from them.

Appendix: Test Yourself— Which Type Are You?

❖

The following series of quizzes is intended to help you determine your predominant natural life energy type, or types. Go to any sections you think might apply to you—there may be as many as three or four—and answer the True-False questions in them. Be honest; answer *true* only if a statement seems highly applicable to you. If a statement represents only something you *wish* were true, or something you think others would like to see in you, answer *false*.

In general, answering *true* to six or more out of the eight questions in a quiz means that you are that type. But since every individual is unique and has a different constellation of attributes and attitudes, you may not fit into any NLE pattern that definitively. Therefore, look to whichever quiz yields the highest number of *trues*. This is your predominant energy.

Am I a Dynamic Aggressive?

1. Ever since childhood, I've always seemed to want more out of life than my peers did.
2. I can work harder than most people, and I enjoy doing so.
3. I spend much less time than others do on what I consider pointless leisure pursuits, such as TV-and movie-watching; novel-reading; and card-, computer-, or board-game playing.
4. I find myself getting frustrated because most people operate at a slower pace than I do.
5. I could never be really happy working for someone else.
6. I don't have much time or patience for long family gatherings, such as a whole afternoon spent celebrating Thanksgiving.
7. Managing a big job and having underlings carry out the detail work is my ideal kind of endeavor.
8. I'm more intelligent than most people, and others almost always recognize this.

Am I a Dynamic Assertive?

1. I enjoy thinking about large issues, such as how society is organized politically.
2. The idea of a lifelong and exclusive intimate partner doesn't seem desirable or realistic for me.
3. Being alone does not scare me; in fact, I do some of my best thinking when I'm alone.
4. I find myself getting frustrated because most people's worldview is so limited.
5. I have a drive to express my ideas and influence the thinking of others.
6. I have no trouble getting people to listen to me and grasp what I'm saying.
7. The makeup of my social circle is constantly changing.
8. I can't fathom the idea of holding one job for decades.

Am I a Dynamic Supportive?

1. I get asked for help a lot, and have a hard time saying no.
2. When I meet a person I'll give that individual the benefit of the doubt; in other words, I'll like him until he gives me a reason not to.
3. I procrastinate a lot.
4. People usually like me.
5. I'm happiest interacting with people and aiding them in some way.
6. It sometimes takes an outside force to get me motivated because I tend to be satisfied with what I have.
7. People tell me I have a great sense of humor.
8. I'm good at smoothing over others' conflicts and helping to mediate them.

Am I a Creative Assertive?

1. When I'm in a new situation, such as a new job setting or relationship, I spend a lot of time comparing it to analogous situations I've been in previously.
2. I can sometimes work creatively at full throttle for hours on end and not notice the passage of time.
3. I'll periodically go through extremely low-energy periods during which I have to remind myself that it's only a phase.
4. I find myself getting frustrated because most people are not on my mental wavelength.
5. Working by myself is no problem; in fact, I prefer it.
6. At times, ideas just "come to me," and if I can't put them down then and there—on paper, canvas, etc.—I'll be uncomfortable until I can.
7. Throughout my life there's been a pattern of people calling me one or more of the following: "temperamental," "moody," "sad," "flighty," "different"; and I never really felt like I was "one of the boys," or girls.
8. I find competition distasteful.

Am I an Adaptive Supportive?

1. I believe that respect for authority is one of the cornerstones of good character.
2. A lifelong relationship with a romantic partner is one of my goals.
3. My extended family is the most important part of my social life.
4. Directing a big job and supervising a lot of underlings is my idea of a headache.
5. Holding one job for decades would be okay with me if the conditions were good and the boss was nice.
6. Trying to lengthen your life by eating the "right" foods doesn't make much sense to me because when your time's up, your time's up.
7. I believe that blood is thicker than water and that it's more important to be loyal to your relatives than to your friends.
8. I prefer to work at a job a set number of hours each day and then have the rest of the twenty-four hours for relaxation.

Am I an Adaptive Assertive?

1. I feel I'm good at supervising a small group of people, and I enjoy doing so.
2. I believe that divorce is to be strongly avoided whenever possible.
3. When it comes to spending and saving habits, I take pride in being more thrifty and less foolish than most people.
4. I generally believe that if individuals behave outside the norms of society, they should be prepared to pay the price.
5. My home is more organized and cleaner than most people's in my neighborhood.
6. I enjoy the feeling of my life going along at an even pace like a well-oiled machine; too many stops and starts and ups and downs would really upset me.
7. I understand that detail work is what ultimately gets a job done, and I have the gumption and know-how to tackle details.
8. I would never dress in a flashy, bohemian, or otherwise attention-getting way.

Am I an Adaptive Aggressive?

1. When I first enter a new environment, such as a workplace or a school, I make it a point to become acquainted with as many people as possible.
2. I rarely seek quiet.
3. My vacations are always highly structured; several days of just sitting in one place and vegetating would drive me crazy.
4. Networking as a career and life tool is something that comes naturally to me.
5. When tackling a problem or task, I'm usually less defeatist than others.
6. I like associating with influential people and am not intimidated by them.
7. I'm happiest moving and doing, as opposed to sitting and thinking.
8. I thrive on setting goals for myself and then figuring out how to reach them; I can't imagine just drifting through life without a plan.

Be Kind to Yourself

Explorations into Self-Empowerment

Accentuating the positive and eliminating the negative, the program that Gary Null offers in this book begins with self-exploration and ends in self-empowerment. Once you have discovered who you are, really—once you have realized the source and force of your natural life energy—you can put it creatively and profitably to use; for energy lies at the heart and in every part of the process that yields achievement.

To achieve, then, energy needs to be freed of the restraints that inhibit spiritual growth, dull a sense of well-being, and lower self-esteem. The pages that follow demonstrate how to break down the emotional roadblocks and overcome any shadowy hazards on your highway to good health, security, success, and happiness.

Contents

Introduction

❖

How can you best be kind to yourself? Although it's a simple question, finding the answer isn't always so simple. It's too important a question to be answered by other people because their solutions may not be right for you. For instance, certain parts of the recovery movement advocate delving into your past in order to understand the traumas and problems that have contributed to your present difficulties in mastering life. But delving into the past is only a tiny beginning step. If you wallow in thoughts of past problems and abuses, and blame others for your present problems, you'll be stuck in your past forever.

So becoming mired in the past and in blame is not being kind to yourself. You have to go beyond blame if you want to live up to your potential. That's what this book is about—going beyond blame, and beyond the past—and moving squarely into the present to explore how you want to live, and how you can actually empower yourself to reach your own goals.

Many of the sections in this book begin with a question that you can ask yourself as a way of exploring your thoughts and priorities. There are, of course, no right answers. And while I have offered answers of my own throughout the book, you certainly don't have to accept these. In fact, if you question and reject any of my answers, you will be acting in the same ever-questioning, ever-critical spirit in which I wrote this book.

I believe that one should always be asking questions. I remember asking myself some of the most important, and saddest, questions I've ever pondered, on the night of my thirtieth high school reunion. This event is something I keep coming back to in my mind because it made such an impression on me. It wasn't just the fact that most of my former classmates seemed to have physically neglected themselves to such an extent that they now seemed like people who had joined my grandparents' generation. Sure, as a health advocate, that bothered me a lot. But it was much more than that. It was that my former classmates were all so defeated-looking. There was unhappiness in so many of their eyes. And when I asked them about their lives, I heard many unhappy tales—of divorces, tragedies, and, over and over again, alcoholism.

Why? I asked myself. Why were these people so beaten down by life? Why were so many of their faces unsmiling?

One idea seemed to lighten their expressions. A bright aspect of many of their lives seemed to be the thought of retiring. It was as if after twenty-five years of work they were now nearing the end of a grueling obstacle course, and would soon be able to relax and enjoy collecting their pensions. Yes, retirement in the near future was one thing that my former classmates seemed eager to talk about—retirement, and the good times we had had in high school. So those were the highlights for them: the past—school days, and the future—retirement. What was missing was joy in the present.

This is, I believe, a major factor in the problems in our society. We're not taught to value the present. The prevailing belief system tells us to educate ourselves for, to work for, and to generally orient our thinking toward, the future. Prevailing belief systems being the powerful forces that they are, this is what we do. What gets lost in the process is the present, and whole lives can go by without the present ever being given its due. That's what I was seeing in those faces at the reunion.

This book, then, is dedicated to our finding fulfillment and success in our lives right now—and to doing so using no one else's notions of success but our own.

By the way, here's my own personal notion of success. It consists of three parts:

1. Knowing who you really are;
2. Spending each day doing what you really should be doing, based upon your knowledge of who you are; and
3. Doing so with joy and love in your heart, so that those you come in contact with feel the effects of your fulfillment.

What's your personal idea of success? In answering this question, it may help to actually write your thoughts down. In any event, as we brainstorm together, please remember the goal.

Be kind to yourself.

Be Kind to Yourself

Getting Rid of Negative Influences in Your Life

Growth has to begin somewhere. Start by exploring both the constructive and the destructive aspects of your nature. First you must deal with the negative. By dealing with what doesn't work in your life, you're going to know what excuses not to fall back on. You will know why you are not doing the things you've dreamed of doing. You will know why you stay with people who don't support and love you. It's a simple matter of deciding which direction you want to put your energies into—positive or negative. Once you understand the consequences of your negative qualities, you could say: "Hold on—do I really want to feel this way or go down this path again? I've been here so many times and I know that what I'm about to say or do or feel is not going to change things. I'd rather choose a positive option when dealing with a negative situation which hopefully would help me resolve this constant repetition of old patterns of behavior." Once I have decided that I can make a positive change, then it merely takes the courage to give it a try.

Breaking destructive patterns is the gateway to getting on with your life. Positive input only becomes significant after you deal with the limiting negative factors. Sure, confronting the negative will make you uncomfortable, but the discomfort is necessary. Change never occurs without it.

Once you understand your negative characteristics, you can claim your real self by saying, "Hold on, I don't buy into this anymore." Once you resolve these issues you will be able to reclaim the dreams of your youth and enact them as an adult. For every problem, you will be able to find a positive solution.

Do You Get Unconditional Support From Your Friends and Family?

Think about the people in your life. How do you feel about them? Do they care about you? Are they supportive and giving or are they takers? What do they want from you?

Fold a piece of paper in half and record your feelings about each person in a double-entry journal. On one side record your positive responses, on the other side the negative ones. You'll probably have mixed feelings about many people: in these cases write on both sides of the page.

This exercise will help you clarify some of your feelings. You may find that some people expect you to serve their hidden agendas.

Once you define your feelings about these people, you will know which relationships need more nurturing and which ones require more honest communication. If you find there are some people you feel comfortable with part of the time, ask yourself whether the benefits of being with them outweigh the detriments. Are there certain activities you can enjoy together? This will allow you to plan your time accordingly.

Be honest about who supports you and whether that support is conditional or unconditional. Then you will know who is healthy for you.

What Are You Willing to Accept From Others?

Be very clear about where you draw the line with others; otherwise, people will overstep your boundaries. Let people know when they are making you feel uncomfortable and that their behavior is unacceptable to you.

One evening last week, for example, someone came to my home unannounced. He said, "I just thought you'd be in," to which I responded, "I'm glad you did. It's good to see you. By the way, I'm so busy lately, you might want to call next time, so you don't waste a trip if I'm not here." It was a thoughtful and polite way to remind him to call first.

If you don't set boundaries, you're saying that any area of your life is free and open for people to explore. Then you have no sanctuary. Every human being needs a sanctuary, a place on earth that is exclusively and uniquely his or her own. Sure it's good to be spontaneous at times—to call someone at an unexpected hour—and sometimes it's just plain necessary to do so—but you should always consider other people's boundaries, and their need for sanctuary as well.

One of the most important sanctuaries is the emotional and intellectual sanctity of yourself. When people say your ideas and feelings are all wrong and start to correct them, they're dishonoring you intellectually and emotionally. That's an emotional assault, a serious offense.

What Do You Expect From Others?

Do people in your life know what you expect from them? Tell them right up front. Either they can meet your expectations or they can't. If they can't, then end the relationship. There's nothing worse than someone saying they can do something when they can't. It creates unrealistic expectations and results in anger and fear of failure.

I look for honesty in my friendships; it's a first priority. I won't allow anyone into my life who lies to me; in fact, I don't believe in second chances once a person has lost my trust. If you give someone a second chance, before long they'll be asking for a third chance, a fourth chance, and a hundredth chance. From what I've seen in my life, I'd say being dishonest is always a pattern of behavior, not just a onetime thing. It's a character flaw that keeps coming up, although sometimes people become clever enough not to get caught.

Unless you tell your friends what you need from them, you'll have ambiguities and contradictions in your relationships. Honest, open communication is essential. If you have trouble expressing your real needs, think about what's holding you back. Are you afraid to lay out your real needs because you worry that no one will honor them? Well, in some cases you're right: they won't, or can't. But it's better to modify and explain your feelings than to engage in a superficial, meaningless relationship.

Remember, if you're not clear from day one about what you want from a relationship and what someone can give you, much of what you share in that relationship will be built upon false expectations. If it ends, there will be unnecessary blame and recrimination. Who needs that? Just be honest right up front. And be patient. No one can be all things to you, or anyone, all the time.

Do You Stop Yourself From Attaining Basic Assets?

Consider the following assets. Do you have negative habits that prevent you from attaining them? You'll find that it helps to actually write these down.

Happiness

Write about the habits you have that keep you from being happy. Perhaps you tend to worry, or you have specific fears. You procrastinate, get angry, suppress your feelings, or compare yourself to others, assuming that other people have something you don't. If only I had their looks, wealth, mate, children, or house, you think, then I'd be happy.

I was running with a man who told me he didn't think we were going very fast. He was comparing our speed to that of some other runners who had just passed us by. I pointed out to him that those guys were bolting at a four-minute pace and must be world-class athletes. We were going at a five-minute pace and doing very well. We weren't as good, but then again, we weren't twenty-two. Don't compare yourself to someone or something you're not.

Health

Write about habits that undermine your health. These might include drinking, being lazy, not exercising enough, thinking negative thoughts, not getting enough sleep, overeating, and worrying.

Fulfillment

What do you do that prevents you from being fulfilled? Look at these possibilities: needing to make a career change, but keeping yourself back, not working up to your potential, never having enough money, procrastinating, being dishonest with yourself, making excuses, having no confidence, lacking focus, not trying for fear of failure, denying yourself the things you want, and giving up.

Respect

What do you do that prevents you from being respected? Perhaps you don't respect yourself because your self-esteem is low, you avoid necessary confrontations, you dishonor other people, or you gossip.

I never gossip. If I have something to say, I say it to a person's face. Anyone who talks to you about someone will talk about you. It's a destructive activity that many people engage in. They see someone looking happy, but instead of being happy for that person, they make some kind of snide remark. I won't do that; it dishonors not only the person I'm talking about, but myself as well.

Love

What do you do to prevent yourself from being loved? Unless you love yourself, you'll be unable to project love to others and to receive love. You also need to be vulnerable and to be able to take risks. It's difficult to be lovable if you're not open, because no one knows what you're really feeling. When you hold your emotions inside, people can only guess your feelings toward them. Perhaps you're afraid to be honest for fear of rejection, or because you're out of touch with how you really feel.

Financial Security

What do you do that prevents you from being financially secure? Perhaps you're afraid to take risks because you're afraid of success.

People who are truly financially secure aren't motivated by money, nor are they afraid of losing what they have. People who are afraid of losing money never seem to have enough.

No matter how much they have, they continue to work like crazy to acquire more. That shows insecurity. You see this in immigrants who work themselves to death even after they've acquired more than enough money. They never let their children forget how hard they work and how much they suffer. As a result, their children feel guilty about anything their parents give them.

You need to be happy with who you are and what you do. You find security when you adjust your lifestyle so that you're happy with what you're doing regardless of the amount of money attached to it. Of course, you need to accept that your lifestyle is going to be commensurate with what you're doing. For example, if you want to work for charity, your lifestyle will not incorporate fancy cars and lavish furnishings. If you realize that you're getting something else that's more important to you, accepting a simpler lifestyle won't make you unhappy.

When I wrote the first book in this Mastering Life series, *Change Your Life Now*, I didn't seek my regular publisher, Random House. Instead, I chose a publisher with a background in transformational books. My earnings for this book didn't compare to my usual earnings, but the circumstances were different. Random House publishes books on nutrition, but this book was about helping people change their lives. This was particularly important to me because I had just come to understand that people need to learn to change their beliefs before they can change their diets. I'd been doing it wrong for all these years. I'd been writing about nutrition, thinking that people were getting healthier, when they weren't. They needed to change their attitudes first. Then they could change their eating habits. Otherwise, they weren't going to stick to the right diet.

The point is that although I was paid less, I felt that this was the most important book I'd done. I gladly accepted the terms because it was what I needed to do. I'm not measuring my book, or my self-esteem, by my income. That would be dangerous. I'd start basing decisions on money and end up betraying myself in the process.

How Do You Control Others and How Do Others Control You?

Think of the chase, the capture, and the conquest. After you conquer something or someone, do you begin to lose interest? Look at all the things you thought were important. You put a great deal of time and energy into those projects. Afterward, was what you did no longer important? If so, then control was what you were after.

Or perhaps you've been in this situation. You were the object of someone's affection. As long you were being pursued, the person had an interest in you. But the situation changed as soon as you said, "I'm yours." Suddenly the interest was gone. You were just another trophy. Again, control was the issue.

Do you try to control people? Do you assume that you have the right to? I see this in parents who try to dominate their children instead of respecting them as individuals. Children need to know that they count. Even when children say things that make no sense, a parent needs to respect their right to say them. Too often you hear comments such as, "That's stupid," "You're wrong," "Don't embarrass me." Such remarks teach children to stop being honest. They become afraid of expressing anything, because their parents might judge what they say as being unworthy. They would rather say nothing than risk feeling the pain and discomfort of their parents' rejection.

That starts a pattern of holding back that continues on into adulthood. People refrain from sharing positive, constructive insights. They relate to authority figures as if they were their parents. They follow their boss's dictates unquestioningly as if their own opinion counted for nothing. They search out partners who control everything they do.

When someone controls you, your life is no longer your own. It belongs to someone else. Someone else is building his or her own ego by controlling you. The person never cares about your dreams or treats you as an equal. The person is never there to support you.

Think of how different it would be if you were with people who supported you unconditionally. You'd think, maybe I could really run that marathon, or change my career. Of course sometimes the people in your life *would* really support you if you were honest with them about what you really want to do and be. If you're not honest, you're never going to know.

The people who really care about you for who you are have got to give you the freedom to be who you are. If that means letting go of some control, then they've got to let go of that control. That's why you have to look at who controls you.

Where in Your Life Do You Feel Empty?

Look, for example, at the following areas of your life:

Empty Friend

Are you an empty friend? Here's how I define the empty friend. He (or she) is the person who always needs something from you. That's the only reason he calls. An empty friend calls and says, "How are you doing, Bob? What's up? It's been three years but it feels like we were just talking yesterday. You're not using that house up on the lake, are you?"

True friends aren't users. They enjoy being with you and they honor who you are. They never criticize or betray you. They defend you when someone else attacks you and they never talk about you behind your back.

If you don't have integrity within a friendship, then what's the point? It's better to let go of that relationship and find another friend. There are no shortages of good people out there. Look for people with good hearts, people who can laugh and who are fun to be with.

about the kind of friend you are. Are you able to
ople for who they are? If you can't, you shouldn't be
n. Don't be with someone whom you constantly crit-

Empty Lover

The difference between an empty lover and a real lover is that
the latter will always take part of the responsibility for the
relationship. The empty lover never does; if something goes
wrong, he or she blames you, perhaps calling you a user. When
the relationship is working they never complain about your
using them.

An empty lover tries to make you feel worthless for wanting
to end a relationship that is no longer working. The person
doesn't accept that there's a time in a relationship when each
person has a right to say good-bye. An empty lover sees the
relationship as an investment, and tries to make you feel as if
no one else will want you if you end it.

If someone tries to make you feel bad about yourself, just
say, "Wrong. I'm not going to feel bad about me." The next
time someone tries to put you down, simply refuse to allow
that energy in. Then their reality doesn't become yours.

It takes two clashing egos to fight. They can't put you down
by telling you how much they enjoyed the time spent together.
They're not going to say, "I'm sorry we're not going to spend
any more time together but the time we did spend was good."
You don't often hear anyone say that, but how much healthier
that would be!

Empty Patient

Are you an empty patient? I know people who see holistic doctors and then get very angry or disappointed because the doctor
is not meeting their needs. They say the doctor gives them too

little time or doesn't treat them because they don't have enough money to pay for the treatment they need. Or they say the doctor doesn't believe their symptoms are real. Yes, these may all be legitimate complaints, especially considering that some "holistic" doctors are holistic in name only.

However, I also see people ignore the insight and advice their doctor gives them. They never become holistic patients. No treatment ever works for them. They keep going from doctor to doctor.

The empty patient never does anything for himself. When I ask these people why they don't use what they know, they give excuses: "I don't know what to do." "I'm not a doctor." "I don't know what my body needs." Yet they never seem to start educating themselves about what they need to know.

Empty Worker

Empty workers resent people who work harder because it shows how little they do by comparison. These people work on automatic. They're at their job just to collect a paycheck. They don't care about what they're doing. They never take responsibility for anything they do and they never give constructive suggestions about how to make the job better.

An awful lot of people in this country are empty workers. I watched people strike at a plant in my hometown. My uncle worked at the plant and I talked to him about it. I said, "You're making a certain income. It's enough to cover your basic needs. I know you want more but there is a price war on with a foreign importer. The importer is subsidized by his government, allowing him to cut prices by twenty-five percent. If your company cuts its price by twenty-five percent it cuts itself out of the business and you're out of a job. Would you rather have a job where you can maintain your standard of living or would you rather go on strike and cause your company to go bankrupt? Then you'll have no job. You will lose your home and a lot more."

I was amazed that these people hadn't thought of that. They were only concerned with having more and milking their company for all they could get. They didn't care about making production more efficient. Six members of my uncle's family were working at a job that required only one person. They were causing their company unnecessary expense. They admitted they could have found other jobs.

Perhaps you've really got to be in business for yourself to appreciate what I'm saying. When you are responsible, you care about making your product or service better and more efficient. Then you're *not* an empty worker, but a caring one.

Starting Now

❖

Most of us have something in common: We get caught up in our dreams of yesterday. This leads us to think in certainties when practically nothing in our world today is certain. For example, real estate is no longer the investment it once was. In the 1950s you could buy real estate and expect to retire in twenty years. Jobs guaranteed security for life and promised to meet the rise in living expenses. Marriage and relationships used to be more certain too, to the extent that you could often get away with taking people for granted.

When and How Do You Change?

Positive change won't happen without your input; nothing positive just happens by itself. At some point in your life someone has probably told you that things will get better. Think about what that means. Do things get better on their own? If you don't actively construct a program that allows you to move from one place to another, you'll never reach your goal. You must have a program and you must be the architect of that program. No one else can make changes for you. You can have support from other people, but making the change is your responsibility.

Change usually happens over a period of time, not all at once. When I help people train for a marathon, I teach new skills in increments. Only when the new runner has mastered one portion of the training do we take them forward. Otherwise they will burn out.

Compare your journey of self-appreciation to the old tradition of apprenticeship. An apprenticeship can take years and years. You can't expect to instantaneously get in touch with your real self at a weekend workshop.

When should you start making a change? My suggestion is right now. Making preventive changes in your diet and lifestyle, for instance, is better than waiting until after the diagnosis of a disease. Then you have some life-threatening problem to face and are more likely to respond out of fear, and to follow some outside authority's dictates of what is right for you, rather than your own inner motivation.

Are You Changing to Please Others?

Most people look for direction outside of themselves and neglect to look within. Right now there are over five million Americans involved in cult practices. Most are not in Moonie groups or something that obvious. Rather, people embrace things that on the outside seem reasonable—The One Heart Movement, The One Mind Movement, The One World Movement. But ultimately these are still cult practices. They preach about how life really is and how it should be. They point out all the things in your life that don't work and show you that by doing things their way, everything in your life will work. People who engage in such practices are giving someone else the responsibility of making their own lives work and are ultimately disempowering themselves in the process.

You will never be able to sustain changes that another person makes for you. All you will do is be obedient to that other person's program. You will be eating certain foods, chanting, meditating, doing service in the community to show that authority figure what a good, obedient person you are. Finally you will have changed by discarding all the features that make you unique. You will no longer be you. You'll have become the person that the authority figure won't get angry with.

Ultimately, change, to be meaningful and sustainable, must come from within. When you do something, ask yourself whether you're doing it because you want to. Are you honoring something inside? Or are you doing it to be recognized by some father figure, mother figure, or religious figure who is validating your existence?

In What Ways Do We Disguise Our Real Self?

Do you disguise your true nature? Why hide something that's naturally you? Are you insecure or ashamed about who you really are? Are you afraid of rejection? Do you feel inadequate?

Our society makes us feel as though we must achieve something in order to be acceptable. You feel that you are not acceptable just as you are. You try to react to everything people say. You think if you don't conform, people are not going to like you. I'd better give them what they want, you think. There's less hassle. After all, you get rewarded if you give them what they want, and you get punished if you don't. The problem is, without honesty there is nothing natural in what you're doing or how you're feeling. Your life is then based upon the artificial, and the artificial has no bottom, no base.

When you're dishonest in your work, you will overcompensate and try to get the emotion you want from your friends and family. But that doesn't work. You're still in a bottomless pit. You can't be one thing to one person and something else to another. When we project different images to different people it can create enormous confusion.

Being honest makes you vulnerable. Conversely, only when you are vulnerable are you honest. When you are vulnerable, you're open. When you're open you're expressing what is natural with a sense of self-balance. In other words, you're acknowledging who you are. You're sharing true intimacy.

Intimacy means you're expressing what you really feel. You're laying it out. A person can accept or reject it. But they must also respect that you have a sanctity within which you alone make the decisions. You alone decide who comes into your sanctuary and shares the self. And if others are going to share the self, you make sure that they share the self as you have expressed it, not as they would manipulate it. The result is that you have allowed yourself to be vulnerable without changing what you're being vulnerable about in order to meet the needs of other people.

That's the desired result, anyway. What sometimes happens is that when someone knows you're being vulnerable and open and honest, they take advantage. They try changing you. You have given them access; you've said, here's what I am. Here's what I feel. But then they say, oh good; now let me set you straight. Suddenly you realize, hold on, that's offensive.

And it is. No one should offend you when you have opened yourself up to them. You have the right to say, "I shared my real inner self with you. If it's not good enough as it is, I'll have to say good-bye."

If you don't resolve this issue—either feel completely comfortable or walk away from the situation—you're going to be hurt.

Vulnerability allows you to be as free and flexible as possible. It gives you movement, fluidity, a full range of intellectual and creative expression.

Without vulnerability you are closed, rigid, fearful of being discovered for your inner passions. When you're not vulnerable you can't move. You're stuck. You get stuck in a job, stuck in a relationship, stuck in a career, stuck in a place. You may try to defend the merits of being stuck rather than open yourself up to move on. You may spend more time defending the ego than you do in realizing that there is nothing to defend in being open.

You never have to defend vulnerability. You never have to defend the true and honest self.

Compassion, sensitivity, and openness come when a person feels comfortable with who he (or she) is, and when he is willing to give the quality of that energy to another human being. But remember—it serves no purpose to give the quality of your inner being to people who either abuse it or deny its virtue. Give your gift to one of the many deserving people in this world who would honor that gift and do something positive with it.

To know yourself requires knowing what you're not. I think it's very important that you determine what you are not! Frequently to understand what you are is to acknowledge what you are not.

For instance, if I am not a liar then I'm honest. If I'm not a thief, then I can be trusted. You might find it helpful to make an entry in your journal for each thing that you are not. It then becomes easy to generate a list of what you are.

When You Remove Your Masks, Whom Do You See?

Everyone has a mask. Some people wear many. They spend their lives perfecting their images. Most people want to look a certain way, talk a certain way, be a certain way, cultivate a certain presentability and a certain acceptability. Usually the image is not the inner person but altogether different.

Why do we do this? Perhaps it's because as children, we learn to act a certain way in order to be accepted. At home we adapt to our parents' needs and in school we work to please our teachers. For every positive lesson, twenty more are negative and limiting. We learn that we are not smart, not right, not good, and that we will be punished for being ourselves. We change to appease the adult world. It's a survival mechanism.

Then one day, many years have passed, and we've forgotten who we really are. The mask becomes like a virus in a cell; it thinks it is part of us. So how do you change this situation?

Begin by looking at what doesn't feel right. Ask yourself whether you are wearing a mask to hide an essential part of you. Only during the process of being honest and open can you begin to change. You can begin to see who you really are beneath the mask.

Write about the masks you wear in life. Is there a particular one that you usually wear? What is it meant to protect? Remove the mask and listen to the person underneath. What do you hear? Do you hear the same perspective or a different one? Are you an obedient person or a challenging one? A dynamic person or a passive one? Do you hear a person who wants to join something, or a person who wants to lead the way?

Asking yourself the next question will help you explore some of the reasons you might mask your feelings.

What Causes You Discomfort?

Many things in your life can cause discomfort. These are just a few to consider.

Change

Change takes you to unfamiliar territory, and that can be unpredictable and scary. When you're in a new situation, there are no guidelines to follow and you don't know what will happen next. Your old masks may not work for you there.

Change is a necessary prerequisite for growth. But most people will only allow change into their life when they are so dissatisfied with their circumstances that they can no longer bear life as it is. Seldom do people change just to try something new and different. That means that some things in your life will change, but an awful lot won't. And often, it's what you don't change that is counterproductive to your growth.

Stress

You need not fear stress. Stress-provoking situations can be used to your advantage. You can challenge yourself and become stronger for facing stress. Ignoring it, on the other hand, will only cause you more *dis*tress and make you weaker. When I get into a cab that's not air-conditioned on a hot summer's day, I have a choice. I can either worry about becoming clammy and sticky or I can relax, roll down the window, and enjoy the breeze hitting my face. You have choices as to how you will handle a stressful situation.

Most stress comes from inappropriate reactions. You can keep from becoming stressed by getting into the habit of watching yourself for overreaction. If your accountant says you owe this or that tax, you can blow up at her as if it's her fault or you can simply deal with the situation. When I get audited, the first thing I say to the accountant is, "Worst-case scenario, how much will I owe?" Then I write out a check and say, "If it turns out that I don't have to pay that amount, you'll return the balance." I go on with life. After all, it's only a piece of paper. It's nothing until I make it into something.

Telling the Truth

Telling the truth can be uncomfortable. It can startle people because they're not used to hearing it, and it puts you in the position of dealing with their reactions. Therefore, upon reflection, you may find that you're rarely, if ever, completely honest with anyone.

Start being honest, in a sensitive way with no intention of hurting anyone, and just expressing what's inside. Right away people will know where you stand. It's better, I feel, to be right up front with people so that they can accept or reject you based on who you really are. Otherwise, you're playing the game of trying to get acceptance for what you don't really mean.

Make a list of values that are important to you. Be honest about what they are, how you feel, what you want, the real you.

Recall situations in which you have been dishonest with someone. Ask yourself the reason. Did you want the person's approval? Know that your happiness does not depend upon another person's accepting you. Know too that you are really doing yourself a disservice by lying to people.

You can say anything when it is in the spirit of love. Not only will you help others that way, you will be true to yourself as well.

Failure

When you experience a failure, what do you see and how do you feel? Failure can be perceived positively or negatively.

When you experience a failure you may interpret it as you being a failure. You may equate what you accomplish with who you are. Failing, then, becomes a judgment against your self-esteem, an affront to your ego. This misperception goes back to childhood, when you were made to feel uncomfortable or unacceptable for doing something wrong. Perhaps your parents reprimanded you for getting a C on your report card when your brother got an A. Suddenly, you were no longer good enough just as you were. You felt you had to succeed to be loved and accepted.

Ironically, once you're in this mindset, no matter how successful you become, you never feel that you're good enough.

Look at the actions of businesspeople dealing in millions and billions of dollars who never find contentment no matter how much money they have. They play with other people's money, caring only about how much they can profit themselves. Look at what we went through in the eighties, when billions of dollars were made and lost and lives were devastated. According to an article in *Spectrum* magazine, five million lives were displaced in the 1980s by leverage takeover buys. Even middle-class Americans who didn't play a part in the game were harmed in the process. Think of the legacy left by these Wall Street manipulators. We haven't even felt the full effects of it yet. How many of those people were living with a fear of failure?

Fear of failure can stop you from trying again. A lot of people never try to do anything a second time because the first time they tried it, it didn't work. Failure to them becomes a way of justifying that they should never have tried in the first place. It then justifies what they suspected all along: "Gee, I can't be a writer." "I can't run a marathon." "I can't work in another career." That attitude keeps people in the same old predicaments.

And it's not a realistic attitude. Hardly anyone does a thing right the first time. Most people do things consistently wrong, repeatedly failing for a long time before they succeed. When you look at Fred Astaire flawlessly dancing, what you see is the finished, edited product of a year's effort to make a film. What you don't see are all the mistakes, in the hundreds of outtakes, that led up to that point of perfection. Likewise, when you see a martial artist demonstrating tai chi or karate, you don't see all the practice it took to get that person to his or her level of mastery.

The best way to perceive failure is as something that didn't work. This just means that you need to do something different the next time. Then, failure never becomes something that limits you or takes you to a dead end. It becomes something that strengthens you, helping you to see what doesn't work. This is a healthy way of looking at failure.

Be willing to learn from your errors. Learn like a child learns. Children fall down, get back up, and try again. They don't expect to walk the first time they try. They don't let their falling affect their self-esteem. That's an attitude adults should adopt as well.

Fear

Most fears are the result of imagination. You imagine a situation, worrying about what might happen *if.* . . . You think, "I would change my job, but what if I don't find another one, or what if I do find another one and it doesn't work out?" You start seeing all the negative possibilities instead of the positive ones.

Unfortunately, many people don't know how to respond positively to fear. They may develop obsessions for anything from food and alcohol to sex. They may blame their problems on the lack of a loving relationship. They may think, if only I had someone to love, everything else in my life would fall into place. People have many ways of disempowering themselves in the face of fear, rather than confronting what's bothering them.

The only way to deal with fear is to face it. Once you confront what you are afraid of, you can start looking at all the possibilities and preparing yourself for change. You can focus on gathering the tools you need to get the job done. The fear often vanishes in the process.

Name one thing you would like to change in your life but feel fearful about confronting. How do you circumvent the issue? List the negative and positive consequences of changing. Then list what you can do to minimize the negative and prepare for the change you want. Repeat this exercise every week. At the end of the year you will have changed ten to twenty negatives into positives.

Loneliness

When you feel lonely, you generally feel sorry for yourself. Sometimes you're just a victim of the unquestioned assumption that aloneness equals loneliness, when in fact aloneness can be a wonderful opportunity for introspection and growth. Sometimes you decide that you can't feel lonely if you belong, so you might become a joiner to evade feelings of isolation. Joining something is not necessarily a bad thing to do, but you have to look at your reasons for doing it. Are you joining a group only because you don't have a life without it? Or are you bringing something positive to what you do?

There are other areas to explore when you're looking at sources of discomfort; these include feelings of guilt, pain, and disappointment.

What Limiting Patterns Do You Engage In?

Do an honest self-evaluation. Each week look at one area of your life to see if you can improve it. Notice any habits that limit your ability to grow, perceive, communicate, share, feel, and be honest with yourself and others. For instance, do you keep your appointments, or do you tend to break them? Do you organize your day to get in what you want to do, or do you just meander through the day? Do you overorganize? One way to never get anything done is to overplan. We do not appreciate that constant planning can take us away from the process of change. Some people constantly plan for what never gets accomplished; all they do is engage in the procrastination game.

Another important question to ask yourself: Do you have the patience to listen to others with care, or are you always simply waiting for them to shut up so you can talk?

List the patterns that you perceive as being self-limiting.

Then work on changing them. By doing that, you will be able to grow.

Being Wrong

How do you know what's wrong? Is your idea of wrong based on what someone taught you? And do you find that much of what you were taught is accurate based on your own experience?

Look at sexism. How much male behavior is based on the conditioned belief that women are sexual objects for conquest? I would say most of it; it's a big part of human male behavior. Yet we know it is wrong to use someone purely as a sexual object and not to see her as a human being.

On the other side of the coin, many women are taught that they are nothing without men and that their primary goal should be to make themselves indispensable to men, doing things for a man that he could easily do for himself. This is common behavior, and it's disempowering, to say the least.

Most people are trained to be obedient and never challenge authority. Even when they see a gross injustice, they learn to keep their mouths shut. Everybody in our society, with some rare exceptions, is taught to obey authority. Is that a behavior to be questioned? Is it wrong to speak out against authority when you see injustices done?

And what about education? How many curricula in this country are designed to help a child explore his or her own needs in a constructive way? On the contrary, students are conditioned to passively accept what they are being taught and never challenge the instructor. Is it wrong to have your own ideas when they disagree with the teacher's? Is it wrong for a teacher to teach a curriculum that differs from the course his superiors have set? Whom do you threaten when you want to grow beyond some of the limitations, biases, and prejudices in the educational structure? When I was in school studying nutrition, I repeatedly tried to question the teachers when they said sugar was good. It wasn't long before I was told that I would be thrown out of class if I opened my mouth again.

Explore your own beliefs of right and wrong. Do your beliefs disempower you and others? If so, look at where those beliefs come from, and begin to challenge them.

Feeling Inadequate

What in your past leads you to believe that you or other people are inadequate? Particularly, what role does society play in contributing to that notion? Let me give you an example. In this country, fewer Native American children go on to higher education than in any other demographic group. Yet, when is the last time you heard anything about the problems of the Native Americans and their educational system?

The fact is that our war against Native Americans has continued into this century. In this century, Native American children were not only forced to learn English; they were actively discouraged from engaging in their own cultural practices. They were not even allowed to practice their native rituals. When they would start their rituals, helicopters from the American Forestry Service and the Bureau of Indian Affairs would come in and disrupt them. Their practices were considered heathen.

Native Americans couldn't own land off the reservations—which was a good way of keeping them there. Long after everyone else had the right to vote, the Native American did not.

The stereotypes still persist. I know of a Native American woman who auditioned for a role in a movie. Although she was educated and intelligent, she was asked to act as if she were stupid. She didn't fit the image people had of Indians, she was told. The woman refused to act dumb just to fit a stereotype.

Other cultures are also excluded from power and made to feel inferior. Have we ever had a Hispanic Supreme Court justice? How often do you see Hispanics featured in major motion pictures, or in a television series in a real-life situation? Usually Hispanics are portrayed as pimps or gang members. You see only the worst stereotype, and by portraying only this biased picture we make a group feel inadequate.

Another way people are made to feel inadequate is through age discrimination. This is especially true for women. Often in our society, women over thirty or forty stop revealing their age because they are afraid of being judged for it. Older people have been made to feel inadequate and no longer an essential part of society. We try to dispose of them instead of seeking out their intellectual and emotional wisdom and learning from their lifetimes of experience. Sadly, excluding our aging population is a loss to everyone, young and old.

But then, such losses are inevitable considering our society's superficial point of view. We notice a person's looks, build, age. What happens when a person doesn't have those things anymore? Is he or she suddenly less of a person? We set standards for perfection that nobody can meet.

You can have wonderful relationships with people of any age if they are based on equality. Some of my best friends are people in their eighties and nineties. I became friends with them when they were in their seventies and eighties. And what did I share with them? Everything. I didn't focus on our differences; I looked at what we could share equally.

Being Judgmental

Being judgmental is a way of defending your self-esteem, because if you put people down, you feel better about yourself. But this is a terrible way of feeling good about yourself.

What if people are being unfairly judgmental about you? I find it's best to choose a loving reaction. I can take a step back and say, "You don't like me? That's alright. You don't know me. If the time ever comes when you want to know me, maybe you'll think differently. But you can go ahead and have your feelings. I'm not going to have any anger in return." That kind of response is going to make a person think.

Obsessing

You obsess when you become constantly preoccupied with unresolved conflicts. For example, you are spurned by a loved one. You feel rejected because someone you love will not reciprocate. This causes you to become preoccupied with thoughts about why the person is not returning your love. What's wrong with the person for not seeing how wonderful you are? Or what's wrong with you that is making you unacceptable to that person?

You must accept that if someone does not want you in his or her life, that's the person's choice. You need to move on. There is no shortage of nice people who will enjoy and accept you for who you are without all the extra effort.

Obsessive behavior is obviously unhealthy. Once you become obsessed, it's hard to see anything from a balanced perspective. When you see yourself obsessing over someone or something, you should seek professional help.

Blaming

Many people find it easier to blame than to think. What if you don't blame but just accept certain things being the way they are? For example, if you're a parent of a teenager who doesn't keep his room neat, plays loud music, rushes through meals, and leaves dirty clothes all over the place, your first response might be, "What's wrong with this person?"

But perhaps it would be better to stop and think, is it possible that this person's perceptions, though different from mine, are justified? Maybe he is at a time in life when it's okay to be messy and disorganized and to have multiple interests all competing for his attention. Maybe it's all right for your teenage daughter to be inconsiderate toward others in her immediate environment. This is generally something people grow out of once they become responsible for themselves and others.

Consider the behavior of the person you are blaming. Is their behavior really the issue, or are you making it an issue to avoid dealing with your own pain?

Are you the kind of blamer who tends to criticize virtually everything and never feels good about anything? For example, you go away to a resort in the middle of winter, where you have the opportunity to sit in the sun and relax for a few days. Instead, you're concerned about the size of your room or the waiter who gave you poor service. You blame someone or something for your inability to relax and be happy. You take your pattern of blaming with you wherever you go. No matter how good something is, you find a way to make it less enjoyable.

Are you the kind of blamer who blows everything out of proportion? For example, you're a homemaker who cleans so much that the moment someone comes in and makes even the slightest mess, your day is ruined.

If you are a blamer, you should seek help to understand the cause of your blaming. You should also try to get some feedback from the people you've been accusing about how they see you. Usually these people will keep their thoughts to themselves because you like to be in control and to have the final word. But if you are open to feedback and ask for help, people will generally offer you an honest picture of yourself. Then you will start to see how your actions affect others. This is not to assume that you should see yourself only as others see you; rather, you should use it as a reference point, keeping in mind that everyone's perceptions are different. Your sense of humor, funny to you, may seem cruel and insensitive to others. The question is, is it cruel? Or were you simply looking at something from a different perspective? Clearly, we cannot please everyone, but it would be wise to be aware of how others perceive you so that you can modify your actions and be more sensitive. This does not mean that your jokes are not funny—but they might not be funny to everybody.

Begin Your Own Twelve-Step Program

You must take action to actually start improving your life. After examining old patterns of behavior that limit you, you can take steps to obliterate those patterns by adding one new thing to your life each month. You create your own one-year, twelve-step program. (Of course you can work faster or slower as needed, and you can tailor the program to meet your needs. The key is to start by assessing what you need to make your life work.)

Gradually change all areas of your life. Don't trick yourself by changing only one aspect. That's creating imbalance; a perfect example of this is when a person works nonstop at his or her career but neglects other important areas of life, such as personal relationships. People who do this are still looking for approval, and not dealing with real needs in a way that will ultimately lead to greater happiness for themselves as human beings.

Here are some steps you can take to become more whole. There are twelve of them, in keeping with the idea of a twelve-step program.

Include Sacrifice and Service in Your Life

This comes from within. What do you give back to the world? You cannot serve others if you think the world is there just for your taking. John Wayne said in a 1971 interview that he believed we were fair with the Indians. They weren't using the land, so we took it to make use of it. The underlying premise was basically that if one group is stronger, smarter, and wealthier than another, it's okay for them to take the other's land, assume ownership, and displace the other group from their homes. That mentality is the opposite of service and sacrifice.

For me, Rachel Carson exemplifies the idea of sacrifice and service. She said back in 1960 that we can't keep abusing the environment without repercussions. She cautioned us about the finite amount of abuse that anything can take; she took a lot of abuse herself for performing the great service to mankind of warning us about DDT, our disappearing bird life, and our responsibility to the planet. Sacrifice and service take great courage in our society.

Every movement in this country starts with one person's efforts. One individual can make a great difference. Ask yourself what difference you can make. What do you have to offer? Become an expert in one area and share what you've learned. Your life can be an example to others.

Set Your Goals—Then Get Going

Once you've set a goal for yourself, don't let apprehension impede your progress. Your negative expectations can overwhelm you. It's never good to concentrate on your problems; focus instead on what you want to achieve.

When I've got to get a job done, whether it's making a documentary, writing a book, or presenting a workshop, I don't let my expectations of the project limit me. If I started thinking that I need to come up with $300,000 before I can make a documentary, and worry about finding a camera crew and getting it on the air, I'd never make it happen. Similarly, if you want to write a book but spend all your free moments worrying about finding time to write, you'll never get it done.

Instead, I forego any expectations I might have and simply start to make my documentary or write my book. When selecting a documentary to produce, I try to find one that will be relevant to the most people. For example, with one like "A More Natural Approach to Treating and Preventing Cancer," it may take me a year of research before I begin filming—I have to interview patients who have been successfully treated, doctors who have gone beyond the limitations of the orthodox treatments, and therapists such as herbalists and homeopaths who play an essential role in prevention and treatment. But during every step in the process I continue to reshape and remodel what will become the final product. In the interim I send out letters explaining the documentary as if it were complete to see which noncommercial stations in the United States would find it of interest. By the time filming is completed I know how many will air it, and which video rental and sales catalogs will offer it to the public. It's not a difficult process.

Evaluate the Possibilities For Your New Self Every Day

When you get up in the morning and look at yourself in the mirror, be happy with what you see. Know that you are growing and learning. Be pleased with the progress you've already made.

Then do something different. Every single day do at least one new thing. Say something positive and encouraging to someone you meet. Dress or cook in a novel way. It can be anything. The important thing is to change something each day.

Relinquish An Old Pattern

Give up one pattern of behavior that no longer serves you, such as always talking over someone, never allowing them to finish a statement—it shows disrespect for the person as well as lack of interest in what they're saying. Instead, try to listen fully to what someone says before responding. When you see that pattern emerging, don't allow it back into your life. Do something more constructive instead. Reaffirm the new behavior, which will in time become a new pattern that helps your life work.

Create Or Join Support Teams

Anytime you need help in your life, you can find people willing to support you. Many fine people in this country have gone through crises, survived them, and are now stronger for it. Sharing what they've been through helps you and strengthens them as well.

Have a Daily Conversation with Your Old and New Selves and Write a Headline

This is an activity I engage in each evening for a half hour before going to bed. First I consider how I would have lived that day if I were not growing. Then I look at the way I actually handled my day. I write a headline for myself, based on my day. Today, for example, I went out of my way to help a senior citizen. I went to a soup kitchen and spent an hour helping to serve meals to homeless individuals. I helped the environment by cutting out a couple of articles from an environmental magazine, making 50 copies, and distributing them through my office in the hopes of raising the consciousness of others. And I honored my body by only feeding it good, healthy food.

As the architect of your day, what would you like to say about what happened? Perhaps you will write something like, "I forgave my parents today for the abuses of a lifetime." Once you write a headline, you reaffirm the new way you are living. This helps you continue the process of change.

Write a different headline for each day. At the end of a year you'll have 365 headlines describing how you changed your life.

Burn the Negative Bridges Behind You

The symbolism behind the idea of burning bridges is that you acknowledge your movement from a comfort zone. You are allowing yourself to move forward and get on with your life.

When you resist the idea of moving ahead you choose to re-cross the same old bridges. It seems simpler because you know the outcome. People respond to you in a familiar fashion, and you get your way.

Although it seems easier on the surface, that approach to life has serious shortcomings. If you follow the old patterns of be-havior, you stay stuck in the same old problems. You turn to food, drugs, or alcohol as an outlet, or to negative people for advice. You repeat destructive actions.

Once you realize that you can't get back in a door that's closed forever, you reaffirm life every day. You don't devote time and attention to old patterns of thinking and behaving. Instead of feeling frustrated and blaming yourself and others for your life's failings, you now recognize that this is a different day and you need to live a different way. The only way to do that is to realize that yesterday's bridge is burnt, and to affirm that today you are waking up with a new focus that is going to make the day productive and positive.

Then you simply disallow that the old bridge is useful. You turn away from the old system and choose to honor life in-stead. Even if it's rough, you're going to leave your comfort zone and feel the discomfort of uncertainty. You're going to stretch your mind, body, and spirit to learn new patterns of behavior, new ways of relating, new ways of listening, and new ways of doing things. You're going to go over a new bridge.

Realize That Reality is Better Than Fantasy

Most people dream of doing things but never actually do them. They may make an attempt to start something new, but stop themselves short of actualizing it. They dream about finding a new job or starting their own business, but never do anything about it. They remain where they are, and continue to live in frustration. Perhaps their work environment is very toxic and they're breathing in unhealthy chemicals. Maybe their job provides no challenge or fulfillment. Instead of changing that, they just fantasize about working someplace else.

Maybe they're in a relationship that is more harmful than supportive. Although they're unhappy, they do nothing to change their situation. They fantasize about ideal relationships with people they've never met, even when making love.

At some point you need to say, "It's my life, let me live it. Let me be honest about what I need to make my life more fulfilling." That's the hard first step, but it's worth it because when you actually start making changes, those changes can be so profound and exhilarating!

Keep Everything In Perspective

Don't blow things out of proportion. Question your perceptions of the world and know there are other ways of looking at things. If you want a really humbling experience, spend some time on an Indian reservation. See people who are trying to survive with almost nothing, who are still trying to find life and meaning in the midst of almost total deprivation.

Look at our own culture's values and compare them to those of the Indians and other cultures around the globe that value Mother Earth. We dishonor the earth and use it to serve our needs without giving back to it, but not all cultures approach life that way. The Indians lived making only imperceptible changes to their environment, while we have radically changed the earth. We assumed we had the right because we had the might.

Question what you see, and know that there are different ways of viewing the world. Then you're not in conflict with others, and you can pull back and see life in a larger perspective. Things won't get blown out of proportion. Have you ever wondered how the world would be different if you had never been born? What difference have you made? Native Americans have long realized that there was a deeper meaning and purpose to life. That, in turn, shaped their perception. They never killed more buffalo than they needed to eat and to clothe themselves. They would not deforest an area just to have a better view. The idea of random exploitation of people or environments was alien to them. In our culture, however, many people are trying to assess the significance of their lives. Everyone has something to share that's positive and meaningful and lasting. Think of the doctors who know they've saved lives: the draftspersons who, because of their labor and ideals and pride in their work, have created products and services that have allowed untold numbers of people to enjoy a better and safer quality of life. When you begin to look at all the conflicts you engage in, ask, "Could I change my perceptions to see these conflicts from a different perspective? Would it change my response as well as the outcome?" By doing this, we see that so much of our reality can be altered in a positive way by changing our perceptions and looking at the larger context in which we live and coexist with each other and with nature.

Share Your New Power

When you're learning and growing, share the positive changes you're seeing. Sharing is an essential part of communicating and belonging. It helps you grow.

Connect to Your Higher Self

Know you are not alone but in the company of a silent spiritual witness. You are accompanied by a consciousness that is higher than your conscious self. That awareness will connect you to a deeper, more essential meaning of life, which will help you to have more compassion, sensitivity, and honor. You will feel less lonely and afraid.

You won't be afraid of making sacrifices when you feel they are necessary. Look at Gandhi and Martin Luther King, for example. They were very strong-willed people, but I do not believe that they could have accomplished what they did in life if they weren't spiritual. Acknowledge your spiritual side and manifest it.

Face One Fear Each Week

List your fears and then select one to overcome. Work on conquering that fear all week. Every single day of that week, face and confront that fear. It may be fear of fighting an injustice, improving your communication skills, or facing the fear of rejection, for example. No matter what you fear, it's better to fail and learn from your mistakes than not to try at all. So put yourself out there.

When you put all of this into action you have a twelve-step program to begin making your life the way you want it to be. The changes are no longer just in your head. You're starting to actualize them.

Reaching for Excellence

❖

Most of us do not accept ourselves. We spend a lot of time and energy disguising who and what we are. We make ourselves into something that's uncomfortable and artificial. We set ourselves at odds with our beliefs and then we feel we must justify the imbalance. We feel we won't be safe until we have disguised our motives, intents, and agendas to make it seem as if we are someone else. We feel that if people know who we really are, they won't accept us.

We become dishonest in our communication, and many problems result from that. Expressing fears and uncertainties is not generally admissible in our society. Showing we're afraid of something means—in our society—that we are not to be trusted. If we communicate that we aren't sure we can do a job, we won't be allowed to do it. So we have to cover up our uncertainty and appear certain, even if that's not how we feel. We've been taught to think that such a cover-up is right. But is it?

A lot of people today are sick and stressed because their actions don't reflect their feelings. This book strives to show you that many of your most closely held beliefs cause you to be imbalanced in many ways. By correcting this imbalance you can have happiness and a life that is uniquely your own—your own brand of excellence.

A lot of people wouldn't be stressed out if they realized that play is as essential as work. People have been made to feel guilty if they play, especially if they have responsibilities that are not always being met. But how many of your responsibilities are artificial? An example of artificial responsibility might include continuing to do all the cooking and cleaning up of meals when other members of the family could very easily chip in and help; or doing all the laundry, cleaning the entire house, and doing outside maintenance (gardening, cutting grass). Are these responsibilities being properly shared? In a social context, you might be the person in your Jaycees or Kiwanis Club who is always expected to do more—the person who "gets the job done." In time, people expect you to do things they very easily could help with. The whole idea of being a part of any organization or cooperative effort is to *share* responsibility. For example, would you feel guilty if you got to work on time, instead of an hour early, and left on time, instead of one half hour to one hour late?

I believe that life is for work, but not for work done only to attain things you don't need, like a color television set, a big wardrobe, a fancy car, anything fancy. I really don't want to be rich. I want a life. So while everyone else I knew was making a big income, I was making a life. I took time off to go to a Native American reservation and study their culture. I spent six years in Harlem working as a scholar and writing the first book on the psychological and social impact of African-Americans in Hollywood. I spent time writing a book called *Black Geniuses: The History of the Afro-American Experience in Inventing*. I learned about life and people. These were things I did because they were a part of living life and learning about life. They weren't mainly about making a living.

It's amazing what happens when you don't think you have to knock yourself out to make a living, when you're not going overboard on the money or success angles. You become almost like a child—in a good way. Do you ever notice that a child will play with something without the need to control it? A child doesn't have to win; she or he just likes playing. Children learn from playing.

As adults, though, most of us don't do something unless we win. We ask: What's in it for me? What am I going to get for it? How much am I going to make? Suddenly, when you make all of your time worth something, you don't want to do anything unless it has financial merit. Thus there is no time to just hang out. The people today who are dying of heart attacks are the people who have that "I need to have it in order to feel good" attitude. If you don't realize you have to make a life, not just a living, then all you will do is make a living. No matter how much of a living you make, it will never be enough to make you happy. The more you make, the more you'll spend.

Let's take a look at some ways we can rebalance ourselves. Then we can have a focus that comes from within, and reach for the kind of human excellence that transcends the limits of monetary, material, and ego-gratification considerations.

On a Scale of 1 to 10, How Do You Rate Yourself?

Look at the following areas. How do you rate yourself as these?

Adventurer

Are you bored with your life? When was the last time you did something really adventurous? It's important to be able to take risks from which you can learn, challenge yourself, and grow.

To become adventurous, you may have to break through fears, illusions, inhibitions, and expectations that can stop you. The most important thing to learn, by far, is how to give up old knowledge that is no longer relevant. I wrote a book once containing the most important information I knew at that point in my life. Four years later I wrote another book that completely contradicted the first. So I simply bought up and destroyed the remaining copies of the first. I had to let go of my old beliefs to reshape my thoughts.

When you replace old thoughts with something new and more apropos, you encourage the adventurer in you.

Parent

A parent is someone who does more than provide a place to stay and food on the table. A really good parent is also a friend, someone a child can trust and with whom a child can share his innermost thoughts, someone who won't betray the child or put him down.

A good parent encourages communication. One of the best things parents can do is to ask their children, "What could we do differently to help you? Could we be more patient and understanding? Could we give you more time or be less critical? Could we develop a friendship by doing more to respect you?"

A parent also has to be able to accept criticism. Most parents are not good at this. Being in a position of power and authority, parents tend to insist on doing things their way, making their children feel powerless in the process. As a result, children learn not to speak up for themselves. They fear retaliation, overreaction, and overdiscipline. A lot of parents make the same mistakes over and over and never know it because there is never any feedback.

Parents and children need to be able to share thoughts in a safety zone. Before there is any reaction, before there is any condemning or ego-defending, children should be able to simply speak their minds freely. A parent can say, "Go ahead and tell me what you think. Tell me whether you feel what I'm doing is right or wrong. I'm not going to react to it; I'm just going to listen." Then parents can take that time just to listen and be open.

Let's say a child confronts a parent with something like this: "Mom, it's my room. You've got the whole house to keep organized and clean. I want my room to be my room. It's the only place I have that I can call my own. Let me be as messy as I want." If the mother were to react without thinking, she might say, "No, it's not your room. It's our house." That makes the child feel like a boarder in the parent's house. If the parent thought it through first, she would have time to consider her child's viewpoint and respond differently. She could then say, "I understand that you need your own space. I've been so concerned with keeping the house in order that I've been neglecting your needs." By taking a step back, you give yourself the opportunity to understand your child a lot more and to foster better communication and cooperation.

Friend

Explore your friendships. Ask your friends why they want you in their lives. Ask yourself what you like about the friendships. What do you gain from them? What would you like to be different? Are there things that annoy you about your friendships? As an example, let's say one of the things that bothers you is that every time you go out with your friends, you go where they want to go—whether to a movie, dinner, or whatever—and they rarely ask what your interests are, the assumption being their decision is good enough for both. Or you may have a friend who talks about what a great time they had the night before with some of their friends, but who never invites you—and never realizes that always talking about the good time they had with other friends can make you feel left out. If it bothers you, you've got to bring it up.

Lover

I'm not talking about sexual love alone. I'm asking whether you are open to expressing and sharing the joy and inner harmony of life. Or do you see love as being exclusive? Do you say, "I love you only, and I love no one else?"

We like to think that love, like everything else, is limited. But I've found that, on the contrary, there are no shortages. Although we think that everything is in short supply, really there is no limit on most things, especially love.

Why is love made to be exclusive? Why do you think you can only love one type of person? Why not love everyone? Think of the consequences of that. If we had been taught to love all people, could we have tolerated over two million Vietnamese civilians being killed, incinerated, and bombed out of this world, or any of the seemingly endless brutal conflicts that permeate our daily lives? I think not. Life would have been seen as too precious.

Teacher

We all have something to share. Think of all the lessons you have to teach others. Think of all the joy and love you can receive by giving unconditionally to others. If you honor your time instead of wasting it, you can share with people the things that you value in your life. If you had more time to get outside your home and enjoy nature, you could, for example, take your camera and indulge in some weekend nature photography. By inviting your friends, you can accomplish three things: spend more quality time with your friends, do something creative, and appreciate what it means to organize your time so that you have more time for activities you value. Another good example is attending a cultural event: most people enjoy crafts fairs, and although they don't take up much time, by freeing an extra two hours a week, you give yourself the advantage of the company and the event.

Doer

The key is not just to do things but to do things that honor real goals, real needs, and real balance. If most of what you do meets artificial goals (buy, address, and mail the perfect Halloween card to everyone you know) then you're not doing. You're filling your days to avoid doing.

I've never understood facing a problem with a problem. Negative thoughts, or projections of vengeance or anger, can't resolve anything. Yes, expressing anger is a natural reaction, but it should be directed toward allowing something to change. If I have a problem, I actively search for solutions, looking at all the possible answers I can come up with. I ask other positive people for their input as well. This is different from wanting sympathy. I want to be with someone who will help me out of my situation, someone who can make me laugh, who can put my predicament in a completely new light. Positive solutions help resolve problems.

Creator

Most people believe they aren't creative. But that's just not true. Most adults have simply forgotten how to engage in creative pursuits.

When you engage in a craft, such as weaving, painting, sculpting, or woodworking, you derive a great deal of psychological benefit. And there are thousands of classes across the country that will teach you arts and crafts. There are centers where you can learn everything from flower arranging to rebuilding car engines to remodeling homes. You can save a lot of money making things you want and doing repairs yourself. The purpose of this exercise is not merely to distract you from something that would keep you busy. We have enough busyness in our lives as it is. Rather, this provides us an opportunity to match the needs of the inner self to something in the external self, that can give us greater inner peace and harmony by expressing the joys of our outer life.

Most cultures pass down skills from generation to generation. Traditionally, this has been a part of our culture as well. When I was growing up, my father would fix just about anything. He would repair the car, paint the house, and lay cement block. This was a part of what parents taught children.

Many Americans see repairs as a laborious, tedious waste of time. After all, didn't we want to be successful partly so we wouldn't have to do unglamorous chores like cleaning, repairing, or maintenance ourselves? However, there's another way of looking at these jobs. In fact, one of the reasons I bought a farm—on which I toil away many of my weekends—was to actively engage in maintenance, repairs, and improvements. It is a great stress reducer; and things like planting flowers, raking leaves, or repairing a roof are all relaxing exercises. Someone from another culture—China, perhaps, or India or Japan—would find these chores to be meditative. We have mistakenly adopted the idea that only so-called productive work, work that earns us an income and enhances our career or our public position, is worthy of our time and attention. It seems Americans have forgotten how to do for themselves. Many baby boomers, particularly in the 1980s, figured that they made enough money not to have to do things on their own. They stopped being creative and put all their energy into making more money. Specialized services proliferated for people who had the disposable income to pay for them.

Now, in the nineties, a lot of that disposable income is gone, so people are having to relearn a lot of old lessons. In the process, people are noticing how economically, as well as psychologically, beneficial it is to do things for themselves.

What skills would you like to develop? What do you need to do to get started? Be creative and learn to do whatever it is you want to do.

Humanist

Quite simply, being a humanist means that you are willing to take responsibility for how your actions impact others. In effect, you're living up to higher spiritual values. Spiritual values are not necessarily associated with any religion. They simply involve being kind and ethical, i.e., not cheating, stealing, lying, committing adultery, or betraying people. These are concepts every religion recognizes, and they take you to a point where you're honoring the best that you are.

Do You Take on the Feelings of Others?

Don't take on other people's negative feelings. Many of us are taught to believe that in order to honor our family we must take on their guilt. How many times have you gotten calls—used as control mechanisms—intended to make you feel guilty? All you have to do is say, "Hey, I understand you're not having a good day, but I am. Good-bye." That's what I do. I won't listen to anybody else's negative comments, and I don't care who it is. My family never calls me to complain because they know I'll hang up on them. When the negative people in your life realize they can't manipulate you, they'll stop trying.

Imagine doing just the opposite, calling people to feel good and make them feel good. That would be creative and constructive.

How Do You Rate Yourself At Being?

We're always *doing* something, but never thinking about ourselves simply as *beings*. What I love about visiting other cultures is seeing people who feel they don't have to do anything to be. They can just hang out. Have you ever gone to Venice, California? Its culture is based on people who are easy to be with. But we like to make fun of them, implying that these people don't have an intellect or a life. We call them flaky just because they're having fun. But they're good at being.

I've noticed this in other countries as well. The people in Trinidad, Barbados, Venezuela, and Argentina, for example, despite their differences in class and work ethic, all have something in common. They're very comfortable hanging out and being. They don't base feeling good on having something. Even people owning almost nothing have the capacity to enjoy life.

I had a wonderful time visiting some families in Jamaica. They were very poor, but never allowed a lack of money to get in the way of their enjoying their lives. They never used poverty as an excuse to be abusive or neglectful parents. They never dishonored their lives. I think of one woman, in particular, who had a large, wonderful family. Even though they had little materially, they had a great sense of the spirit of life and never felt diminished by what they didn't have.

In our culture, we believe the lack of money causes all our problems. We think it's the reason relationships are unfulfilled. One day we'll have enough money to restore our relationships. How foolish, though, to believe that money is more important than the essence of a relationship and what you have to share. You can be just as happy poor as rich. You can start a relationship with absolutely nothing in the beginning and end up with boundless joy just by being together. Just feel the love and grace of being with another person you feel honored to be with.

When material things become all-important, you displace the importance of being together. Now you have things and debt.

And the pressure of trying to meet the debt can cause you to lose the relationship.

How Are You Unique?

List your unique qualities. Are you able to express them or are you afraid for other people to see you as different? When you're concerned about what other people think, you edit yourself. You don't express what is naturally inside. You think, "I would allow this to come out but they're not going to like it or they might think I'm strange." Look at the average middle-class American, for example, who keeps everything within very narrow confines. Nothing is done that will in any way betray the person's middle-class ethic. What results is a very boring life.

I find the most interesting part of being with a person is his or her uniqueness. When you remember someone as being fun to be with, it is his or her unique qualities that you think of. Honor your own unique qualities. Make them important, overcoming your fear of allowing them to emerge. That will rebalance you.

Of course when you start being who you really are, some people may reject you. You have to accept that, and remember that the most important thing is that you not reject yourself. It's your life. Outside of certain common standards set by society, there's a lot of room to be unique, fun, creative, and constructive. Why not use that room?

Do You Envision What You Really Want?

Look carefully at what you want to change. See it in your mind. Imagine your ideal body, for example. If you were to look in the mirror, what would you like to see? (And dismiss all those images that television and magazines bombard us with. Those aren't real.) Once you know how you want to look, it's easier to find the patience and persistence to make it happen.

This holds true for all areas of your life. How do you envision your career? What do you want your home to look like? Where do you want to live? See it first to make it happen.

Three years ago a couple sat in my audience in a lecture on changing your life. She was an accountant and he was an artist. They couldn't afford living in New York nor could they see their ideals being met there. I spoke with them about what they wanted their home to look like. They shared their image and from that I suggested they consider moving to Colorado, Arizona, or New Mexico.

They wondered how to get started and I advised them to start by realizing how much they could do on their own. They didn't need to rely on any other expert because there were enough books about housebuilding to teach them what they needed to know.

They spent nine months traveling and finally found five acres of land in Arizona. It was magnificent land, and not expensive because it was not near anything. Then they started reading about how to build.

They built a 7000-square-foot home with a greenhouse in it and circulating water. It was a most unique house. They spent less than $100,000 on their home; today it's worth $900,000, but they have no intention of selling it because that's where they love being. That's what they envisioned.

When you begin something, visualize what it will look like when finished. There's no shortcut to making it happen. It takes time, effort, and mastery. But it's a wonderful feeling to put time and energy into what you really want and to feel good about doing it. It's better to have a life in which you make sacrifices for your happiness than to have things and not have happiness because those things you attain have nothing to do with meeting your real needs.

When You Go on Vacation Do You Work or Relax?

Most people forget what a vacation is for. A vacation is to separate your mind and body from your everyday environment. Wherever you go—mountain climbing, trail hiking, fishing, to the beach, or to an amusement park—you should be going to relax, to have fun, and to energize. If you do that you'll have a whole new sense of self-awareness when you come back.

Don't take your work problems with you on vacation, and don't take them home over the weekend. They'll interfere with the quality of your relationships with friends, family, and yourself.

Identify Your Filters

What mechanisms have you devised to filter out things you don't want to know about or deal with? Identify them. You've got to be aware of what's going on and you've got to deal with it.

Perhaps the first thing you need to do is to eliminate the filter of procrastination. Identify that part of you that says: put it aside, hide it, disguise it, avoid it, deny it.

Yesterday, after broadcasting my show, I immediately started setting up for the next day's show so that I'd be ready to go right on the air. It gives me peace of mind knowing that I'm set up and ready to go. And why not? It only takes a few moments to set up, label tapes, and file them away.

Yet I'll go into friends' houses and find they've got their desks stacked with stuff. Books are on the floor, paper is all over the table and the other furniture. You know what I'd do in that case? I'd take everything and first sort it. Put bills and necessary papers in a pile, and throw the rest in the waste-basket. Obviously they don't need all of this stuff. Otherwise they would have dealt with it.

Here's a suggestion. Stop procrastinating. Start cleaning up one room. Take everything in the room that you no longer feel is essential to your happiness and either throw it away or give it away. Each day clean another room. Keep only what is essential. Look through your closets. You'll probably find many clothes you no longer use because you wear the same clothes over and over. Take all the things you don't wear and give them away to someone who will wear them. Give them to the Salvation Army. Better still, give them to someone on the street who needs clothes. When you stop using things with joy you lose respect for them; they just accumulate. Giving away things you don't want is a good way of feeling good about getting rid of stuff that's no longer important.

Also look at relationships you've neglected. Make a list of all the people you haven't communicated with lately whom you still would like to remain in your life, and write them a letter. Tell them why they're still important to you. I let my friends know that they are my friends, and why.

I don't believe we should ever take anyone or anything for granted. Think how many times you've done things for people who have never said thank you. Some people expect you to do certain things for them over and over. You've done it before, they assume, so you'll do it again. They forget to honor the fact that you didn't have to help them.

Stop doing things for people who have lost respect for you, because that's wasting your time and imbalancing your life.

It's better for you to give that time and energy to someone who will appreciate the gift. Plus it will make people who have taken you for granted appreciate the loss.

Do You Complete Projects?

Prove to yourself that you can complete things by involving yourself in a single project that will be important for your growth. Be sure to specify a goal and a reasonable timetable, and then take the steps necessary to complete it. For example, if I'm writing a book I plan in stages. There's a research phase, an interviewing phase, transcription, writing, and editing. I keep track of each phase of every project on a board in my office. At any given moment I can tell you exactly where I am on any project. I never procrastinate. Every single day I work on one of my projects.

People ask me how I've written 50 books, 165 television shows, 45 documentaries, and 500 articles, and prepared 1000 workshops as well. I am able to do all these things because I don't allow myself to become distracted. If I start something, I finish it. I honor my word and don't make excuses for not getting the job done.

Sometimes, to complete a project, you have to master a new skill. Don't be intimidated by this. Mastering a skill may have less to do with being extremely gifted than with being relaxed in the pursuit of yourself. When you pursue yourself you're honoring your special gifts, whatever they are. You're exploring and developing your talents instead of letting uncertainties bury them.

Perhaps you would like to write a book but think, "I don't know if I can write." Well, no one starts off as a writer. I didn't come out of the womb writing. I didn't even study journalism in school. Instead, I asked a literary agent if I could work for her for free full-time. In return, she set aside three hours a week to critique my work. In the five years I worked for her I didn't earn anything, but I was able to become part of an extremely intellectually stimulating environment, which was an incomparable reward in itself. Plus each Saturday the agent would set aside some hours to go over my work. That's how I learned.

I had to be willing to give up all that time at no pay in order to learn something about mastering a skill.

Are You Open to Change?

Most of us identify with the things we have accumulated, but these things can be easily lost. What would happen if you didn't have your possessions anymore? Has it ever occurred to you, when you see news stories of people running from bombed-out towns they've lived in all their lives, with absolutely nothing except for the clothes on their backs, that these people have got to start all over again? What would you do if you had to start over from scratch? Would you try to build the same kind of life, or would you do things differently?

If you don't think much of yourself and your ability to adapt to change, then you believe that you're not worth anything without your possessions. Your accumulations become like a ball and chain and you never get far.

When you are too attached—to things, places, or ideas—you give yourself a lot of excuses for not changing. You think you can't move because you've always lived in one place, or you can't leave a job because you've worked there for twenty years. People justify not changing by saying things like, "I've got emphysema, I got cancer, I'm stressed out, but I've got to stay at my job. In four more years, I'll get my pension. Then I can go to Florida." They have an "I've got to be taken care of" mentality.

They never think of changing by creating a job and an environment that's health-promoting. Too much conditioning and too many expectations from others get in the way.

What Standards of Excellence Do You Strive For?

Without striving for excellence and achieving mastery in at least one area of life, you will be mediocre in all things. This will lower your sense of self-esteem.

Conversely, you need to value yourself before you can concentrate your energy on purposeful goals. Attaining excellence, therefore, is a growth experience. If you want to take consumerist or environmental action in order to help people, for example, you can't just arbitrarily do it. You have to first prepare yourself by broadening your knowledge. Growth is not instantaneous but a gradual striving toward excellence.

Developing excellence requires change. When people want to become excellent New York City marathon runners they have to put all their energy into it. To do that they have to eliminate a lot of unhealthy habits and imbalances. If they train correctly, in six months their lives will change. They'll be able to take on challenging projects and issues, and to confront things in their lives that they never would have thought of approaching before running the marathon. The courage and strength the marathon gives them will allow them to do almost anything.

I'm suggesting you start to create excellence in one area of your life. Begin by asking, at what do I want to excel? That will provide a focus. Write on a piece of paper: Area of Excellence. Under that write down one thing at which you are going to excel, one area in which you are going to be the best you can be. Bring your focus and energy to achieving mastery in that one area of your life. Once that's achieved, focus on another area. And then on another. This way you can continue to grow.

Are Your Goals Realistic and Obtainable?

Of course you have to create realistic goals, ones that are reasonable and attainable. It's pointless to create goals that you're never going to be able to achieve.

Your goals should help you get into balance. Goals requiring excessive energy usually create imbalance; you're focusing so much energy into one area that you're neglecting other important spheres of your life. In order to create more income, for instance, you may end up imbalancing yourself nutritionally, emotionally, spiritually, intellectually, or physically.

In the process of achieving your goal, you should be able to replace negative qualities with more positive ones. If your goal is to have a healthy body, for example, take everything unhealthy out of the refrigerator and throw it away. That's step one. Then you have to take the second step—restocking the refrigerator with healthful foods. You're replacing the negative with the positive.

Set a goal for yourself of enhancing your relationships with yourself and others. Each night when you come home, instead of turning on the television or radio, set aside time for creating, for friends, for play, and for meaningful interaction with your family. You're replacing unwanted habits with more positive ones, and as a result you're creating a healthier life.

What is Your Legacy?

A legacy is a contribution you make to the world, something that shows you have made a difference. I believe that every human being has both the opportunity and the right to leave a legacy. Leaving a legacy doesn't mean you need to do outstanding things that the general public has to know about. You can leave a legacy in small ways. When you touch people with kindness and joy, for example, you are leaving a legacy.

Think of people who have touched your life. It's not necessarily the outstanding achievements you remember, as much as who the person is or was. Gandhi isn't remembered for being a particularly good politician. But the way he lived his life motivated a lot of people to change theirs.

Even the poorest person living in Selma, Alabama, or living in a rice field in Thailand, can leave a legacy, because a legacy is not necessarily based upon materialism or wealth or education. It's often based upon what's in your heart. We have a rather distorted view of the components of success. For instance, we will look at success most often as what an individual has achieved: the accumulation of wealth, power, and control, and the public's acknowledgment of that. Generally a person becomes wealthy and can change his or her standard of living. Frequently the person has been able to achieve this success and still maintain all of his or her principles. Other individuals, however, may be successful without increasing their power, control, or position and without receiving public acknowledgment. For example, they may be very healthy because they eat foods they feel will prevent disease. They may have a very fit body because they have a disciplined, focused-exercise regimen. They may have happy and healthy children, hence they have success as a parent. They may have matched their inner needs to their exterior work and therefore enjoy going to work each day. Greed and money may not be a part of their lives because they have learned not to focus on what others have, and therefore have no motivation for envy, greed, and jealousy. So in essence, they may have very successful lives. The point is that true success comes from honoring what is important to you and measuring value through your own standards, instead of an artificially created social norm.

Start thinking about what you would like to be remembered for.

Do You Honor Your Real Needs?

No two people have the same needs. Therefore, no one but you can know what your needs are. No one has the right to tell you what those needs should be. They are *your* needs.

I once had a relationship with a woman who gave me an ultimatum. Either I honor her needs or I honor my own. Our needs were different and I chose to look to my own and she became angry. That's what happens sometimes; you're not always going to please people.

I suggest you make your needs come first. Otherwise you will become imbalanced and frustrated at putting someone else's needs ahead of your own. Of course taking care of others is necessary at times, but if the other person denies your needs, and if you get into a self-denying pattern of behavior, you forget what your own needs are, and can eventually lose your sense of identity.

Begin by asking what your needs are. What do you need as a human being to feel good about yourself and to be fulfilled? Write these things down. Honor the real self rather than an artificial one; this is crucial to your well-being and happiness.

How Do You Keep Yourself Balanced?

What do you do to maintain your equilibrium in the following areas?

Intellectually

Set aside time for intellectual growth every day. Challenge your existing thoughts and knowledge. Be willing to give up ideas that can be replaced by something more relevant and vital. This will help you to grow, solve problems, and become more self-sufficient.

I suggest buying five nonfiction books, each about a different subject. Choose books that take you where you have never been before to help expand your insight. You'll start to think differently and to open yourself up to new ways of looking at life. If you read about Native Americans, for instance, you'll learn about another culture's perception of nature as sacred, and you'll contrast that to European thought. This will give you a whole new perspective on environmental issues.

Each day spend one hour reading one of the books. At the end of approximately three months you will have learned something new in five different areas.

Also, set aside time to learn through adult education courses. That's another way you'll be learning something new that interests you, and stretching yourself intellectually.

Environmentally

There are over twenty magazines written in lay language that inform you about environmental issues and explain how they are directly related to your health. You may have radon being emitted from your basement. You may have asbestos, formaldehyde, and bacteria in your air. Your home has the potential of being an incredibly toxic place but you won't know it unless you read up on it. Reading will help you learn how to recognize problems and know what to do about them.

Read any one of 300 books written about the environment, and subscribe to five or six magazines. That will make you aware of what is going on, how it affects you, and what you can do to help create a healthier world.

Then involve yourself in a cause that will improve the environment. Perhaps after reading you'll feel motivated, for instance, to join a local group fighting incineration. Do something to connect yourself to your world.

Physically

To improve your body, give yourself some short-term and long-term goals. Your short-term goal might be to lose a pound a week. You might want to run or walk a mile or more regularly. That will help you lose the weight, as well as increase your endurance. You might decide to go to a gym three days a week. Make a point of staying on this program.

A long-term goal might be to run or racewalk in six months. You might want to train so that a year from now you can complete a marathon.

You can also help yourself physically through detoxifying and rebalancing with good nutrition. You can rid yourself of the candida in your gut, for example, by drinking fresh raw juices, and by taking vitamin C, caprylic acid, garlic, biotin, and acidophilus cultures each day.

If you are still eating meat, you may decide you are ready to become vegetarian. You can make the change gradually by switching from meat-eating five days the first week to three days the second week. The next week you will eat meat twice and the week after that once. Then you will have no meat. Do the same for chicken and fish.

You'll start to replace the beef, chicken, and fish with more grains, beans, seeds, nuts, fruit, and juices. You'll start to take vitamins you haven't had before, such as quercetin, vitamin E, and B complex.

I balance the physical by ingesting only those foods that build health. There's never confusion about whether or not I should have sugar, meat, alcohol, caffeine, or refined carbohydrates. If foods don't honor my body, I don't eat or drink them.

In the process of seeking physical balance you can cook the most delicious recipes and interesting dishes. Your body will appreciate the creativity.

Emotionally

Are you able to express your feelings freely or do you find that you edit, change, and distort your feelings for fear that others won't accept them? If you hold back anger instead of expressing it constructively, you will only end up displacing it. It will become cancer, constipation, high blood pressure, or some other bodily ailment. If you feel some passionate feeling (and anger is part of that passion), learn to express it in a nondestructive way. People may accept or reject you for it, but you'll be doing it solely for yourself.

Choose to be with those people who support your emotional needs. If I want to be comfortable acting silly and crazy, for example, I'll be with someone who will accept this kind of behavior, not with someone who will tell me to grow up and act mature.

Spiritually

To be spiritual is to see life through a greater perspective. You realize you are part of something spiritual, whatever you want to call it—God, Goddess, universal consciousness. When you honor the spiritual self you come to realize that you are in this world to make a difference. You act in a way that respects life and you are conscious of your actions. You don't spend your time complaining, bad-mouthing, stabbing people in the back, or trying to get something for nothing.

You never intentionally hurt people and you don't act from hidden agendas; these actions would not be spiritual. Everything you do should honor the spiritual side of life.

It's easy to see how people can be negative, bitter, condescending, vile, and destructive when they are not conscious of the spirit. When you're not, everything else becomes meaningless and you have no balance. Many times I have tried helping people on a spiritual level who were not willing to help themselves spiritually or emotionally, and it was all for nothing.

How will your life be different now that you are aware of the silent witness to everything you think, say, or do? How will you do things differently?

Define the True and False Parts of Yourself

Your life is either working or not working based upon how in touch you are with yourself and your real needs. Recently, I spoke with a woman who was out of work. She told me that instead of running out and finding any job in her field of hospital administration, which is what she would have done only a year or six months ago, she was taking the opportunity of having time to match her real self with a job that meets her inner needs.

The job she chooses may not be in hospital administration. She realized that her experience in that field taught her that she is more interested in working with people than with statistics and budgets. As a result she will expand her options. Making important changes requires knowing the truth about who you are. If this woman didn't have a sense of who she is, she would just take the first job to come along.

In looking at who you are, don't get too caught up in trying to figure out where you went wrong. There won't ever be enough therapists to help you resolve what went wrong in your background. The current fad, for instance, is to blame dysfunction on sexual abuse. Just about everyone in America has now been sexually abused, it seems. That's why their lives don't work. They're sure of it. They've heard it on *Oprah*.

The truth becomes grossly exaggerated. Of course there are abuses, but everyone shouldn't be using that as an excuse to put off having a life. You're either completely dysfunctional, in which case you should be in Bellevue, or you're functional, in which case you should give up living in the past and have a life now. If we're afraid of actualizing, we use our background as an excuse. Our parents become the reasons for our limiting our lives. That's a cop-out.

Get in touch with your real identity by looking at what works and what doesn't work in your life. Are you in a job that you really don't like? Are you in relationships that don't meet your needs? Let go of the beliefs that keep you from being yourself. Start looking for ways you can actualize your real identity. And remember not to overlook any part of your life that works; rather, appreciate it, honor it, and focus on it. Don't replace that.

What Fits and What Doesn't?

When you're in the right place, in the right job, and with the right people, you feel as though everything fits. You feel comfortable and natural. There's a rhythm to life and you feel that you're in the flow of things.

You know when things don't feel right. When relationships don't work, for example, it's not because one person is to blame. No one has to be wrong. It may just be that two people don't fit together. You can have a good job but it may not be the right job for you. You don't have to blame the job.

An attorney friend of mine was always feeling hyper, critical, negative, bitter, and cynical, until he changed his circumstances. Now he's practicing law, but a completely different type of law. He left New York and now lives in Seattle, in an environment that fits his needs. He's become a completely different human being.

Think back about the people and places you've most enjoyed. What made you feel so naturally good? Where do you feel you belong? Where you feel the best is where you should be. Start preparing yourself to be there instead of sitting around and yearning for that place. It takes time, but you can begin to prepare yourself now for where you really want to be and what you really want to do.

Gary Null

Describe and Define Conflicting Realities in Your Life

Figure out where your life is out of balance. Only then can you rebalance it. Be honest. It's easy to deceive yourself. You get so used to your life being a certain way that you begin to believe you don't know how to change. You start to believe you can't when you can.

Ask yourself who in your life is trying to define your reality by keeping you exactly the way you are. People tend to want to keep you from changing when they want to maintain the power structure of a relationship. In the process, they try to keep you away from your path. You've got to recognize this and stop it. Then you'll be able to choose a more fulfilling and rebalanced life.

Finding Happiness

❖

People constantly seek happiness from some external panacea but they never quite grasp it. They have moments of joy, but are not able to sustain it. In the absence of happiness, everything becomes an issue. Your energy, instead of being spent on the enjoyment of life, is spent on meaningless chores.

How much time and energy do you spend on things that aren't significant? Do you make insignificant tasks significant because you're looking for something that's missing? What's really lacking is the honoring of the inner self. The questions in this chapter are designed to help you understand what prevents you from finding happiness. If you sort through all the obvious problems and deal with them one at a time, you'll slowly come to grips with the reasons for your unhappiness.

How Do You Justify or Resolve Pain From Your Past?

Look for ways in which your past conditioning might limit your happiness. For example, you might crave physical affection, just a pat on the back or a hug from a friend, but you don't allow yourself to give or receive it because you were taught not to seek or initiate physical displays of emotion. Perhaps you're a man, and you were led to believe that it was necessary to project a masculine, stoic image all the time. Now you're denying yourself an experience you need because you were taught it was wrong. This can be especially isolating.

You can limit yourself in more subtle ways as well. Perhaps you would like to share your feelings with someone, but you prevent yourself from doing so because you fear rejection. You may avoid closeness because you trusted someone in the past and were hurt. Perhaps you confided in a friend who later used what you said against you. That experience may have taught you to guard yourself.

Maybe you learned to deny yourself happiness by living your father's or mother's dreams, instead of your own. Perhaps you're a man who wanted to be a musician but your parents wanted you to become a doctor. They scolded you and made you feel unmasculine for your interest in music. As a result you learned to put on a façade by acting very masculine and over-achieving in business, sports, or some other area. You repressed the genuine, sensitive side of your nature because you feared it would be used against you. And you may still be holding on to pain from the past.

Stifling your true self might keep you from getting hurt again, but it also prevents you from experiencing real joy. You lose sight of inner qualities that make you special. You seek approval from the world by acting cool, dressing a certain way, or buying fancy cars. You're looking for happiness outside of yourself, but that kind of happiness can only be momentary.

Being unhappy is emotionally toxic. You've got to eliminate the toxins before you can rebuild your health. Only then can you change. You don't rebuild your health by bringing in something new without eliminating the old.

Many people in our society don't understand this. The style is to be super-hip and try something new—a new twelve-step program, a new self-help group. Everybody wants to take a shortcut to the new without first resolving the old. But nothing changes that way. You just plaster another layer on top of an already overburdened psyche and push the real you further down.

First examine your current patterns of behavior. Ask yourself where they come from. How are they getting in the way of your happiness? What real needs are you denying yourself? How can you let go of old patterns that keep your life from working? What first step can you take to validate who you really are?

What Have You Relinquished to Gain a Better Standard of Living?

Most people buy the American dream. They believe that happiness is external and they want materialistic success. Thus they organize their daily lives around making money and tend to spend more than they have on things they don't really need. But concentrating on what money can buy often creates an insatiable desire for bigger and more expensive things. Whole relationships can be centered around the attainment of tangible things, such as cars, houses, more money. Many couples make these things the focus of their being together; they believe they are being responsible and showing loyalty by giving things to their partner. One wonders what would happen to the relationship without the things? Would the people involved no longer have a basis for being together?

I've lost many friends over the years who felt they needed to upgrade their lifestyles once they started making a little money. They directed all of their creative energies toward this purpose and, in the process, gave up valuable time and energy. They stopped having time for themselves or their friends, time to take trips, time to read, study, and engage in hobbies. They gave it all up to work long hours for a "better" standard of living.

People are terrified of the idea of lowering their standard of living. Couples feel miserable because they can't buy a house. This is really peculiar to my way of thinking because not owning a home means greater freedom from debt. When you receive your paycheck at the end of the week it's yours to save or to spend on more important things. And the purchase of a vacation home is another questionable thing, from my point of view. Rather than buy a house in the country that you feel obligated to go to every week, you could travel first-class and visit places you've always wanted to see.

I frequently counsel people who can't figure out why they're unhappy after attaining all the trappings of material success. The problem is they've lost touch with the essence of who they are, as well as with the ability to really relate to others. Most of their conversations, for example, are about how well or how poorly they are doing, in a material sense. And they never ask how you are.

As a child growing up in a small town in the South, I remember watching the old men sitting around and whittling away. They wouldn't carve anything in particular and they wouldn't say fifteen words in a day. There was a sense of contentment, though, a feeling of camaraderie. They had an idea of what life was about, why they were alive, and what they wanted to do with their lives. They were doing it. They knew how to just *be*. The key is to appreciate being alive.

Today this scene is hard to find in our society. Most people rush frenetically from task to task. They communicate superficially and then wonder why nobody understands their essential needs.

Think of all the things that you consider essential. Are they really? Do you look at what you don't have and think that acquiring those things will make you happy? Does thinking about the things you don't have cause you stress? Have you acquired a "successful" lifestyle and given up a happier way of life?

What Generates Happiness?

What is happiness? Health? Love? Good friends? A nice place to live? Creative expression? Freedom? Inner peace? All these things are important. Who creates them, and where do they come from? You do, and they come from inside.

You are happiest when you are living up to your own expectations. Living according to other people's expectations limits you. If peer pressure dictates that I must have a family to be happy, then without a family I should be unhappy. Accordingly, if I don't have a love in my life, then I will be unhappy.

Why is it, then, that as a single male I'm so happy? The reason is I live according to my own ideals. I know what is essential to my own happiness, and it doesn't depend on other people's expectations. Happiness starts with health of mind, body, and spirit, and a sense of inner peace.

You need to restructure your life so that you have time for what is important to you. Start with the idea of freedom from obligations, of being responsible first to yourself. That gives you the freedom to be. Each day gives you only twenty-four hours. But if you use your energy to change your life, you can make those hours work for you.

In my daily life, I use my time to my advantage and only share energy with people who honor me. I'm working on a book project, for example. I met with a publisher last week but rejected his offer because I realized I would be doing a lot of work for nothing.

Later I found another, smaller publisher and decided to work with him. This person wanted to work with me and planned to help with the editing and research. When another person cooperates on a project there's a constructive effort that makes the project happen twice as fast and with half as much difficulty. He's on my side and we're working together. I chose that.

My agent reminded me that I wasn't going to make any money with this publisher, but that didn't deter me in the least. My life is not just about money. It never has been and it never will be. It's about what is going to make me happy.

Ask yourself, are you generating your own happiness or living according to the expectations of others?

How Can You Make Each Day Exciting?

Start the day by listing all the things you would like to do that day. It doesn't matter if you get to them all.

Here's what I do. No matter what, I set aside two hours a day to work out. My body counts. If I don't take care of it, it will become dysfunctional. I don't want to end up with cancer or heart disease.

I make time for my friends each day as well. They're important to me; I don't like to have a friend in name only. Therefore, I allow myself a minimum of two hours a day for my friends.

I also set aside time to pursue cultural interests. I live in a city with wonderful museums, theaters, and concerts. How in the world can I live in New York and not take advantage of these things?

Scholarship is important to me. Every day I spend six hours studying. When I study I engage my mind. The more I learn, the better able I am to teach. Find me a teacher who continues being a student, and I'll show you a good teacher.

Every day I take a walk in the park. There I am totally relaxed and not thinking about anything in particular. I'm living in the moment by just being.

Of course there must be time for work, food, doing the laundry, and all the other responsibilities I have. It all gets done without hurrying and scurrying. I make time each day for fun, for seriousness, for friends, and for the body and the mind. One of the reasons that people do not have a lot of energy—and as a result, much positive activity—when they get home from work is that they're tired. And, realistically, what are you going to do if you're tired? Eat, sit in front of the TV, then go to bed.

To gain more energy, I would suggest starting with the basics, like a thyroid test. You can test your thyroid in the morning, before you even get out of bed. Put an oral thermometer under your armpit for ten minutes each morning for three consecutive days. If your temperature is below 97.5, then you may well have an underactive thyroid. Other symptoms include intermittent depression with no apparent cause; thinning of hair and dryness of skin; and cold hands and feet.

A second possible cause of fatigue is exhaustion of adrenals, overuse of sugar and caffeine, and stress. In this case you should have a complete physical, or go to a chiropractor, who might do kinesiology testing to determine the health of your adrenals. Taking B-complex vitamins (50 milligrams twice daily for two weeks) and vitamin C (1000 milligrams five times daily) will certainly help improve overall adrenal function.

Overeating at lunch, especially if you also consume alcohol or foods that you may be sensitive to, can cause brain fatigue. One way to discover whether food sensitivities are a factor in your tiredness is to undergo a one-week rotation diet, eliminating all the foods you commonly eat and replacing them with different ones. For example, if yours is a wheat-heavy diet, replace all wheat products with rice. Switch from sodas to juice. And try to eat smaller, more frequent meals, because hypoglycemia is the most common cause of afternoon fatigue. But fatigue may also be caused by intestinal parasites (giardia, for example), and by the presence of electromagnetic radiation, such as that emitted by computer screens.

On a nonphysical level, we always know when we're excited by something: When we have something to look forward to, we have more energy, and invest our days with some project, craft, or activity that we know will keep us stimulated and enthusiastic.

What I don't do is as important as what I do. I don't waste my time. I don't spend time whining, complaining, kvetching, looking for the ideal relationship, and talking fifteen times a day on the phone about things that don't matter. I don't waste time watching television unless there is something specific that I want to see. Thus I have time to structure my life around what I want and need to do to feel healthy and fulfilled.

You may think that you don't have the time to integrate all the things you want to do into one day. Once you realize how many unnecessary responsibilities you've been taking on, you will find time to do the things that are important to you. You must not spend time doing things just because other people expect you to. For example, are you always cleaning another person's room? Do you cook for others and do their laundry? If they're over five years old, why not let them start taking care of themselves? Even youngsters can do simple tasks—making beds or sorting laundry, for instance. Doing things for other people unnecessarily takes time away from yourself. You're letting other people waste your time.

Families can waste your time the most: specifically, you need to address adult family members who like to spend time complaining. If, instead of asserting your need to be somewhere else, you assume they have the right to make demands of you, a lot of your time is going to be eaten up by negativity. Let complainers know that you don't want them wasting your time. That doesn't mean you don't love them. It means that the time you spend with them should be quality time. You don't want to argue, complain, blame, or gossip.

Until you realize how much time is wasted in a day, you cannot appreciate how much time you have. Simply eliminate all wasted time. Don't engage in gossip. Don't let people talk to you for more than a few minutes on the phone. Don't let people share negativity with you.

When you spend time with the important people in your life,

really *be* with them. Use that time constructively, not just to vent problems.

Write a positive affirmation each day about why the day counts. Every day should be exciting; there is something wrong with living only for the weekend. So make the priority you. Build the day around your needs. Make yourself count. Justify your journey.

Are You Secure in Your Identity?

People often keep themselves from rewarding careers and limit their creative expression because of what someone else has said. Perhaps one person once told you that you aren't smart enough, and you still believe it. Or maybe someone says you're an old woman and you take it to heart. You start to act and dress like you're old, not because this is the real you, but because of someone else's expectations.

Realizing you are free to grow and be who you are can reverse the self-limitation process. People from every walk of life succeed far beyond the expectations of others. You find them in every profession. And if they can do it, why can't you?

First, you need to feel secure in your identity. You need to affirm who you are and to get in touch with what you believe in. Then others won't be able to deter you from your convictions.

Have the courage to express yourself every day even if that means people are going to abandon you for it. It's better to be alone than with others who don't understand or accept you as you are.

People who live their lives as I do have been denigrated for years and years as health nuts, quack promoters, charlatans, scam artists, people who only want to manipulate the public with false ideas about eating right. There are those who have wanted us denied, dismissed, or destroyed. What if we took them seriously? We would never be able to stand up for our principles and live healthy, productive lives.

Do you allow yourself to be the target of other people's insensitive statements? Do you internalize what people say and keep yourself from following your dreams and goals, and from reaching your potential? If so, it's time to affirm where you want to go in life and who you want to be. If you allow others to see who you really are you will attract like-minded, positive people. Believe in yourself, persevere, and you will succeed.

How Much of Your Real Self Do You Share?

Relationships are a lot more exciting when you let the real you out. Work on that. Let who's really in there out. Forget about your image. Forget about what you've manicured. Forget about what you've let people believe is the real you. Let people see what you're really about. Let the real you come out. As an example: Let's say you have an interest in sports, but because your friends have a certain image of you, you haven't made time to participate—even though you really want to be active, not a spectator. Well, tell your friends that you're getting involved in some sport, be it basketball, volleyball, softball, skiing, skating, or whatever, and ask them to participate with you—then schedule it. Another example might be that you've always been perceived as a jock, but you have a romantic, sensitive side that you've hidden from others: reading poetry, perhaps, or writing.

Do You Appreciate Beauty in Yourself, in Others, and in Life Each Day?

Seek out the beauty in life. Notice what is good and beautiful in yourself, in others, and in life. You let beauty into your life by acknowledging the beauty that exists all around you. Otherwise, you only see ugliness, which justifies your feeling cynical. It's your choice. Why not allow the beauty in?

What Do You Do in Excess?

Excesses of anything are signs of imbalance. Identify extremes and start to decrease or eliminate them. The following behaviors, when excessive, can lead to disharmony of body, mind, and spirit.

Worrying

Nothing constructive comes from worrying; you just get sick doing it. When you worry you waste time agonizing over things that probably won't happen, although when you actively imagine a worst-case scenario over and over again, you may actually contribute to its occurrence.

Look for solutions to your situations instead of worrying about them. You can avoid ten hours of worry by spending ten minutes looking for a possible answer. Simply think: This situation doesn't feel good. I'm going to find a way to change it.

Working

Our society values excessive work and discounts the idea of living to enjoy life. A friend of mine used to be a successful investment banker but one day gave that up to become a gardener. He gave up an enormous salary, which greatly upset his family.

I once took a trip with this friend. Everybody I met through my friend on that trip treated him like a bum, even though he is a gentle, kind, and loving man. He doesn't overwork but when he does work he's a wonderful and patient gardener. He may sit for hours before deciding where he wants to plant something, but everything he plants grows. He's designed and built beautiful meditation gardens.

Let us remember what life and happiness are about.

Fantasizing

Fantasizing unrealistically wastes valuable time and energy. It is easy to fall into the trap of believing you will never find a better way of life, and using fantasies to escape the drudgery of life instead of eliminating your dissatisfaction with your days.

On the other hand, it's good to fantasize about something reasonable and obtainable. Daydreaming allows you to extend yourself and to reach for more than you currently have. Realistic fantasies help you to grow, to have a more interesting life, and to feel good about yourself.

Replaying Past Experiences

Replaying past experiences over and over again is counterproductive. You have a life today; you don't need to live in the past. To make your life important, don't dwell on yesterday's memories. This keeps you stuck in a time warp and prevents you from living more fully now.

One thing you can do to make your life happen now is to create a project for yourself. Engage in something you've never done before and take responsibility for its completion. This means that you are going to have to stretch yourself intellectually, creatively, and emotionally, with discipline and focus. Whatever the project, give some time and attention to it each day. When it's complete, accept whatever it is as successful. The habit of creating something new every day allows you to rejuvenate and to acknowledge your powers in the present. Thus every day has meaning.

People ask me why I create documentaries, write books, and engage in multiple other projects. I love the passion of living in the moment. Once I finish a project, however, it's part of yesterday, and I'm on to the next project.

Notice your thoughts. Do they tend to drift into the past or stay in the present? What projects are you involved in currently? What can you start doing that you've only thought about up until now?

Making Wrong Choices

Do you make wrong choices over and over? You start to know in advance that you're going to regret your decision but you make it anyway because of fear or denial. Perhaps you want to go out dancing but repeatedly turn down a friend's offer. Later that night you eat a quart of ice cream out of frustration and anger with yourself.

Nothing happens unless you make it happen. To start making right choices for yourself, begin by letting go of old behaviors that no longer work for you. Take a chance in life. How many times, for example, have you heard someone say, "Things will get better." Things only get better when you pursue a course of action to allow things to get better. In one case, a man I know had a dysfunctional relationship with his daughter. They bickered constantly, and the daughter grew up to react strongly against her father, who was hypercritical: nothing she did ever seemed to be good enough. The daughter did all the rebellious things she could—keeping their home messy, inviting men she knew her father would find unacceptable, even going so far as to sell some drugs while in college. Clearly she was reacting in a negative, self-destructive way. I suggested that one of the problems was that for as long as I knew him, his daughter had to compete for affection with the other women in his life—and the women always seemed to come first. Therefore, when a meeting was held to help them reconcile the wrong choices they both had made, I suggested they spend their weekends together. Both agreed it was a good idea. The very next weekend, he told me he was going to spend the afternoon with his daughter but his evening with his girlfriend. I said, "Start making the right choices. Spend the day and the evening with your daughter. Take her to dinner and a play, not your girlfriend. The girlfriend will be there after your daughter is gone." His first reaction was to deny it would make a difference to his daughter. I said, "What do you expect? You have been excluding her for so long, she will probably say nothing, but she will feel rejected and not see you as a new person willing to grow. Why not be with her alone so she doesn't feel competition?" Finally the message broke through. He was able to let go of an old behavior that is no longer working for him.

Let go of old expectations. They only limit you. In my running club on Sunday mornings, I tell people to focus their minds on what they want to do and to allow their bodies to go to where they feel good and comfortable. Sooner or later they always go further and faster than they ever thought they could.

Depending on Relationships

Can you enjoy life without someone else, or do you depend on relationships to make you feel happy? Do you live through someone else? Are you overly concerned with how others feel about you? In other words, are you holding others responsible for how you feel about yourself? Or are you able to honor your individual needs and still find positive things to share with another person? Achieving that kind of balance exemplifies a healthy relationship.

Taking on too Much Responsibility

Being excessively responsible shows that you don't feel acceptable for who you are; you have to prove you are acceptable by the things you do. If you're excessively responsible, you might be the type of person who does everything for everybody—walks their dogs, does their laundry, takes care of their children, and so on. People start to take advantage of you; they think they can always count on you for everything. In the process, you may forget to be responsible for yourself and you will forget how to enjoy life.

Of course there are appropriate responsibilities. You need to be responsible to society and unselfish in the pursuit of life. You must do things that will help others in some way. Giving time and service to those in need is an important part of honoring the spiritual side of our nature.

Searching

I strongly believe we should spend time searching—but not excessive time. Many people are always searching and the irony is they don't even know what they're searching for—they're just engaged in a constant search. I don't believe Ivan Boesky or Michael Milkin knew what they were really looking for. They each had a billion dollars—enough for lifetimes of spending—but couldn't stop their yearning for more even if what they were doing was illegal.

There's a time when we have to ask ourselves, where is our journey taking us? What are we looking for? Perhaps we need to look inside instead, to come to grips with who we are.

Regretting

Many people ponder, "If only . . . if only . . . if only." For example, how many people regret not becoming an athlete? Instead they're weekend warriors who hang out at bars and root for teams. Not that it's wrong to root for a team and to have fun with sports. It's fun to have your heroes and favorites. That's normal. But not when it's excessive.

People who feel they've never won anything, because they've never tried anything, tend to live through movie heroes—Arnold Schwarzenegger, Sylvester Stallone, Clint Eastwood. These heroes are always loners facing insurmountable odds and winning; while sitting in the theater, audience members feel like a hero vicariously, but when the lights go up it's easy to feel a deflated sense of self.

There's a better way of dealing with regret at having lost opportunities than watching movie heroes. It's called taking action now.

Have You Experienced Unconditional Love?

Being able to love someone unconditionally is a direct result of whether or not you received that kind of love from your parents and other significant people in your life.

Children need the freedom to fail. This teaches them to take chances in life, and, more importantly, that they are acceptable for who they are, and not judged according to what they can do. I came home from school once with a B on my report card. My mother looked at it and asked me, "What didn't you like about your teacher?" I said I was just bored with the class and she let it go at that. I wasn't made to feel bad about it.

Parents can manipulate children into believing the children owe them A's with such comments as, "If you don't get A's you're not going to get into the right school and you won't get ahead in this world. We're working ourselves to death so that you can go to Princeton or Harvard but we can't do this without your help. You're not respecting what your mother and I are doing to get you through this."

Suddenly the child feels terrible. He or she has been made to feel as if he's betrayed his parents, and that he's a selfish, no-good person. Putting these unnecessary responsibilities on a child tells him or her that succeeding—not happiness—is the priority.

Parents need to ask themselves, are we just as positive and encouraging when our children get F's as opposed to A's? Good parents are.

What Does Your Life Revolve Around?

Answering this question will help you determine whether your life is focused or aimless. Ask yourself, does your life revolve around work? Relationships? Obsessing? Food? Play? Future happiness? Game playing? Changing another person or some circumstance? If your life revolves around trying to control the world around you, you won't ever know what it is to be happy.

The fact is, you can't make others change the outer reality. I learned some time ago that I can't change the American Medical Association, the food industry, and the minds of the people who are undermining our health. Of course that doesn't mean I can't do something on my own to try to affect the world.

What I can do is take action. If the rich won't help the poor I can find ways to do it. I needn't be rich to help them, just kind and giving. I can't make other people stop polluting the environment, but I can stop polluting it, and set an example for others. Although I can't keep bankers and corporations from persuading people to buy things they don't need, I can respect that money, properly used, can help people. I can choose to make money only one vehicle for change in my life and not the center of it. I can buy only what I really need. I can't make other people stop complaining, but I can make sure I don't become like them. I can wake up each morning honoring life, valuing my day on the planet, and using my time to develop character.

So you see, while I can't always alter what's out there, I certainly can control what's in my heart. I can generate unconditional self-love and other inner qualities that make life worth living: the innocence, honesty, and playfulness of the child that remains in me, as well as unconditional love, kindness, acceptance, patience, and reverence. Then there is no need for unhappiness.

Finding Security

❖

Our society reveres high-level achievers. But rarely do we ask, what is the purpose of achieving all that? What are you trying to prove? What's missing in your life for you to devote so much of your time to this success chase? Why do you always need more?

During the 1980s a large portion of the baby boom generation was engaged in doing as much with their education and careers and lifestyles as they could. But they never stopped to think whether life had a purpose outside of attaining things. They never realized that they were covering up an insecurity.

The symptoms were there—the workaholism, the cocaine use, the spending that got people into debt—but no one saw the signs. Society welcomed these high-level achievers, and the baby boomers themselves didn't think anything was wrong with their approach to life. People who are succeeding at whatever they are doing generally don't see themselves as dysfunctional. To the contrary, they congratulate themselves on taking every opportunity that comes their way.

What legacy have these people left? Today, every major corporation in America—including IBM, AT&T, chemical companies, and pharmaceutical companies—is eliminating thousands and thousands of jobs. People are now beginning to save money and not buy things they don't need. People are learning some hard lessons. They're trimming down.

The people who lost their homes, went into bankruptcy, and became loaded down with excessive debt are very insecure people. A lot of them have gone into recovery programs such as self-help and 12-step programs and therapy, to understand why they didn't take time for themselves, their families, and their physical, emotional, and spiritual health. They're analyzing why they spent all their time making money.

They were substituting money for self-esteem. It made them feel secure. It made them feel that they *were* somebody. But it doesn't work that way—not in the long run.

Guess who really had self-esteem. Guess who wasn't insecure. Guess who wasn't spending money they didn't have on things they didn't need just to prove they were okay. The people who we thought were the losers, the people we thought weren't hip and stylish, weren't the shakers and breakers of the world—our Depression-era families, our aging moms and dads. When the boom hit they didn't sell their homes to get new homes. They were happy with the homes they had. Yet many were insecure because of the eleven years of the Great Depression. But they became more stable from those years, appreciated everything they had because of what they endured.

As a result, these people own their own mortgage-free homes today. They're able to live off modest incomes and have money in the bank. They can enjoy their lives and spend quality time with one another.

A lot of the baby boomers with their MBAs, after all is said and done, have less financial stability than their parents. It goes to show that money is just a substitute for the security people feel they need. When security is lacking, money is spent to fill the void. When security is there, money is not used to prove anything. It's seen in a different, more utilitarian, perspective.

How Did You Entertain Yourself Before You Had Money?

A friend of mine confided in me that he wasn't happy because he was broke. "What used to make you happy before you had money?" I asked. We spoke awhile and I realized that it wasn't the lack of money that was making him unhappy; it was his mindset. I reminded him that if you don't have money to entertain yourself, you've still got you.

Think about the enjoyable times you've had without money. What did you do? Perhaps you engaged in hobbies or spent time reading. Sixty percent of all Americans never read a book after high school. Thirty percent read only one book a year. They stop reading because they don't have to; they forget how enjoyable reading is.

Without money, you may have spent more time with friends or family. Maybe you traveled and played. Most people need more time for play.

List ways to enjoy life without money.

How Does a Lack of Security Affect You?

Notice how a lack of security affects the following areas of your life:

Relationships

When you lack security within yourself, your relationships suffer. You feel victimized, depressed, and fearful. Somehow, you think you're not worthy, and that comes across to others.

You may place more emphasis on material success and your image than on people. Being yourself and relating honestly is not good enough. You brag about your children: "My son is a doctor." You ask friends, "How much did your engagement ring cost?" or "How much did that car set you back?" You judge people by how much they have and what they can do for you. You talk about money all the time. You think, "I shouldn't be happy and playing. I should be earning more money to have more security."

Where You Live

A lot of people refrain from moving to a new locale because they want to maintain a certain lifestyle and stay connected to the people they know. Giving that up provokes anxiety. It means readjusting their self-image.

It becomes especially difficult to lower one's standard of living. Today, because of the economic situation, we have more people going from middle class to lower middle class than ever before, but downscaling is not easy to do if you identify yourself with how you live.

Scheduling

When you feel secure you schedule your time differently than you do when you feel insecure.

When you feel secure, you plan time for personal growth. You make time for play, relating, introspection, meditation or prayer, joy, and friendship. You organize your day around what is essential to your happiness.

When you feel insecure you will generally devote each day to earning money. The trouble appears when you start giving up all your time in pursuit of the dollar and you neglect your family and friends. You don't get to see your children grow. Before you know it, they're gone. Life loses its meaning. One day you wake up and look in the mirror and you're old. You wonder where the years have gone. You regret not having used your time more wisely.

Time is a precious commodity; in fact it's priceless. So do something with your time that acknowledges its value. If you enjoy art, spend an afternoon visiting a museum. If you enjoy music, go to a concert. Make time for friends. Take your children to a puppet show. Have the confidence to live your day in a way that will enhance your life.

Freedom to Experience All Aspects of Living

When you feel insecure you cannot fully experience life. You lack confidence and are afraid to take risks.

Society encourages this risk-fearing attitude. You're supposed to maintain the status quo, to work for monetary success and never see possibilities beyond that. You are expected to become addicted to the things that money can buy and go into debt over them.

If you're like most people, you buy into this prescribed way of life because it's supposed to make you happy. Instead, though, it makes you less and less free, and the very things you thought would make you happy keep you imbalanced.

To be free, you need to go outside the boundaries of predictability and try something completely new. No one can tell you how far you're supposed to go or what you're supposed to feel. There's no feedback; you just have to experience and become the architect of your life.

Examine how completely you experience and enjoy the following areas of your life:

Sex

When you feel secure about yourself, you are free to experience your sexuality. You are willing to try things that you wouldn't otherwise try.

You are never told to have happy sex. No two people think of sex in the same way—differing perceptions are based on the messages received from parents, religious authorities, friends, teachers, and the various media. Confusion occurs when what should be a pleasurable experience between two consenting adults is tainted with fear on one side and guilt on the other: fear because what you're experiencing is condemned by parents, religion, and society, which causes shame and brings up childhood guilt because "good little boys and girls don't do that." Which in turn creates an artificial constraint—a sort of psychic chastity. How much more would you do or allow yourself to feel if you were not constrained by fear? In my experience, most people live with far less sexual pleasure than they are capable of, and sublimate their passion by reading books like *The Bridges of Madison County*, watching pornographic or explicit films, or obsessing about the exploits of Madonna and other more liberated celebrities. Whereas someone with a healthy, fulfilled sex life will be much more interested in his or her own exploits than those of other people, most repressed individuals will pay obscene amounts of money, give unlimited publicity to and keep focused attention on public, frequently exhibitionistic displays, in order to relive their sexual fantasies and pleasures.

So, after experiencing pleasure followed by guilt, what now? Should you deny the pleasure? Who could you tell? Those who will listen are more likely to listen to your stories with a feeling of envy or jealousy, and then adopt the moral high ground, perhaps admonishing you—but probably bad-mouthing you and backstabbing you. There is nothing worse than this sort of betrayal of trust. It might be better, I think sometimes, to put everything on video—call it the "No More Confidences Channel." Because everyone seems ready to betray everyone else, especially when *Hard Copy* is ready to buy the story. It makes you realize that you'd better not share anything you don't want others to know about—otherwise, chances are that everyone will know, sooner or later.

Could you imagine suddenly having the freedom to experience sex the way you want to instead of playing by the rules? You could explore and let go of all the preconditioned notions of how sex should affect you. You could stop thinking about what's right or wrong. You would no longer be limited by what your class says you can do. Instead, you would express the feelings you have without fear of condemnation.

Creativity

When you feel secure you are free to express and experience creativity. There are no limits to what you can do. Don't acknowledge limits just because you are told to. They'll keep you locked in a nonproductive mode. Decide what feels right to you. For example, I sleep two hours a night. If I were to follow the norm I'd be sleeping eight hours, even though I don't need to. I'd have less time to create. I also take certain nutrients during training for a faster recovery. If I were to listen to the advice of physicians who say that nutrition doesn't matter, I would be limiting myself as an athlete.

If you accept limits imposed on you, you lose your creativity and spontaneity. You never go beyond artificial boundaries. Ask yourself what limits keep you from being who you want to be and remove those constraints from your life. Give yourself what you need in order to be more creative.

Intellect

Intellectual freedom allows your mind to process and understand new concepts. You discard fixed notions of how things should be and start looking at things from an enlightened, expanded perspective. You are open to seeing things the way they are, and are not limited to a biased viewpoint.

I watched a television show featuring Dr. Anthony Fauci who said megavitamins have nothing to do with health. They don't help the immune system, he said, therefore they cannot help people with AIDS. I'm sure he believes that, even though it is a false statement. The problem is that, intellectually, he's not free. His beliefs are fixed. He thinks that only chemotherapy or a vaccine can stop the AIDS virus because he hasn't been open to looking at the evidence to the contrary that's been piling up.

I would offer a different perspective from that of Dr. Fauci, one based on the evidence provided by the experience of many individuals. From this I can see that antioxidants have made a great deal of difference in AIDS treatment, both in terms of delaying the onset of AIDS from HIV, and lessening the devastating effects of the illness. But in order to appreciate the value of antioxidants, you have to approach the subject using a different type of therapeutic model than the one Dr. Fauci is familiar with. And it's not unusual for a person to be down on what he's not up on.

People have a mistaken notion that as long as you have a degree—an M.D. or a Ph.D.—you automatically have intellectual insight. That is absolutely wrong. I've met people who have never been to college who possess a greater intellect than people holding advanced degrees. They're not confined to one belief; they're breaking through old paradigms and establishing new ones. And that's how we progress intellectually. That's how Einstein dissolved the notion of Newtonian physics and developed quantum physics. That's how Enrico Fermi was able to split the atom. Their intellects weren't limited by the traditional thinking of their time.

Middle-class people are not encouraged to be intellectual although society says upper-middle-class and upper-class people can be. In truth, of course, intellect has no class. Never believe that you are as smart as people have told you. Believe you are smarter.

Travel
We can travel anywhere. We can see our own city. We can see our own country. We can see the world. But I know people

living in New York City who have never seen what New York has to offer. They limit what they'll experience.

When you free your mind then you free yourself to experience any place, and you get a completely new perspective on life.

Learning About Other Beliefs

When you are free to experience other beliefs you get to learn from people with a completely different outlook on life. That will either enhance or challenge your own beliefs.

In order to be open to experience other beliefs, you have to be willing to let go of your own fixed ideas. Being closed-minded is a very dangerous thing. It causes you to become anti-cultural and nationalistic. It makes you unable to benefit from other cultures. If you visit other countries but see only the tourist attractions, you're missing the most important aspect of travel—getting to know people who lead lives different from yours.

Do You Equate Security with Being Overly Responsible?

Most people believe that if they have failed to meet their responsibilities they have failed at life. Other people look down on them and criticize them. I expected so and so, they say, and you let me down. You didn't provide. You're supposed to be this, you're supposed to be that.

Now the person feels a tremendous sense of guilt. Now he or she is motivated for the wrong reasons: guilt and fear. That drives him into desperation and frequently traumatizes him. It ties him up so he can't do anything, or it drives him to succeed in ways that are excessive. The person may become compulsive, and addicted to appearing responsible.

How many people do you know who are overly responsible?

They never know how to say no. They always take on the responsibilities of everyone else, and rarely take time out for themselves.

Are You Using Your Skills to Your Best Advantage?

A good way to find greater security and happiness is to use and develop new skills. Sometimes this means using them in creative ways. To give you an example, a graphic artist, working in a major clothing store in New York City, told me that he wanted to make a career change but that he didn't know what he wanted to do. He said that outside of graphic arts he didn't believe there was anything else he could do.

I helped him review his situation. He discovered that it wasn't his skill that was making him unhappy. He enjoyed being a graphic artist and working with computers. What was wearing him down were the schedules and deadlines. He needed to take his basic skills and use them in a completely different environment, one in which he could do what he wanted in a way that honored his time and energy.

As a result of our conversation, he started traveling around the United States to find the place in which he could best live and work. It took him three months to decide to settle in Texas. Then he investigated how he could best adapt his skills to his new environment.

Today this person works with Native Americans, helping them to preserve their history and culture in computer art designs. His is a unique and special business that combines Indian knowledge and one person's skills.

This man is as happy as he can be. When he visited me recently, he told me his business is thriving. His pleased customers tell others of his work, and people from many walks of life ask him to make their ideas into artwork.

Money is no longer his main motive for working. He loves his new environment. He sets his own schedule and has more time for himself. I asked him how much money he needs and he told me he needs just enough to get by. He said, "I'm happy being out there with people and animals. I'm happy just talking, reading, giving time to myself. I never in my whole life lived this way. I get to do something creative and in the process help other people."

Look at your skills and talents. Are you using them? And if you are, are you using them in the environment that best suits your needs?

Where Can You Get Support if Everything Else Fails?

You want to make changes but are afraid that if you fail you won't have the support you need to survive. Realize that support exists. For instance, in addition to Alcoholics Anonymous and Overeaters Anonymous many other support groups assist people with just about every addiction and dysfunction there is. The easiest way is to start reading the Yellow Pages listings for health support groups—AA, OA, GA, etc.—then also contact local hospitals that have an outpatient support group. Every hospital has several. And these groups are found not just in cities, but in small towns throughout America. Although you don't necessarily have to use outside support, you should always be aware that it is available to you. It will help you to survive and get back on your feet in a worst-case scenario.

Keeping this in mind removes some of the pressure in your day-to-day existence. You have a backup plan to fall back on if all else fails. Otherwise, you'll always be tentative about taking any steps to make change happen.

Whom Do You Emulate?

Frequently, we emulate people beyond our class. That's why we're so preoccupied with people on soap operas and "Lifestyles of the Rich and Famous." We look up to these models even when we know we will never live like them.

What does that tell us? It says that we don't want to look at our own lives. We're afraid to acknowledge our own dreams and to actualize them. We simply accept other people's idea of how we should live if we had the resources. So we often end up living vicariously.

How Does The Struggle For Security Affect You?

Striving for security prevents you from taking chances. You're never willing to do anything you're not accustomed to because that would make you feel insecure.

I remember being interviewed on a television talk show by a physician and a reporter. The physician asked me, "Gary, what would you change about the American diet?" I said I would eliminate caffeine and sugar.

People called in from all over America and asked me what was left, to which I replied, "Are the only things in your life caffeine and sugar? There's so much more to life than what you eat and drink. You've got to realize that it is necessary to let go of the negative in order to create something positive." The physician later said to me, "People are just too lazy to change. They're just not going to do it."

It's true, but it has more to do with insecurity than laziness. People feel so insecure that they won't even change the bad foods in their diet. They eat meals day after day that result in symptoms such as puffy eyes, indigestion, diarrhea, gas, and arthritic pains. But they won't give up the bad foods for a healthier diet because repeating habits they're used to makes them feel secure.

Are You Prepared To Make Your Life Simpler?

What are you willing to do to make your life simpler? Take an inventory of the different areas of your life.

Relationships

Stop fighting. Stop trying to make relationships work. It's nonsense to work on another person's psyche, to mold and readjust your partner, to make compromises. If my feet are a size ten, I'm not going to wear a size six shoe and cripple myself in the process. A relationship either works or it doesn't.

When you're with someone you know if it feels right. If it doesn't, you need to look for someone else. It's that simple. There is no scarcity of people. Our ethic says, you made your bed, now lie in it. People think that because they've become involved with someone they've got to remain in the relationship for the rest of their lives no matter how good or bad the relationship is.

What happens when you adopt this attitude? Well, you may stay together and try to find ways to distract yourself from your unhappiness. One of you becomes an alcoholic, the other becomes fat and depressed. You watch television and read the *National Enquirer*. You have an occasional affair and feel guilty about it. You're married and you feel bound by the law.

Why not feel good about being by yourself? Be free to explore life and the experiences you want. If you meet someone and it works out, fine. If it doesn't, that's fine also. No one is in the wrong. Let's stop blaming. Let's look at what's right.

There are no shortages of people to be happy with in this

world. Somewhere out there are people who complement your personality. If you make your life uncomplicated and meet someone else who is uncomplicated, you'll have the basis for a good relationship.

Possessions

In order to make your life simpler, you've got to give things up. Make a list of what you're willing to give up to make your life less complicated. What do you own that you don't really use? Why not just give away the things in your life that you're not using? Give it away, throw it away, or use it. But stop cluttering. Clutter keeps you from being free.

What Risks Have You Taken in Each Important Area of Your Life?

Your growth is directly related to the challenges you give yourself. But challenges entail risk, and change, and you may be afraid of what those changes might mean. Maybe other people's attitudes toward you will change. Maybe your attitude toward other people will change. Maybe the circumstances of your existence will change. All of these possibilities may make you feel insecure, and if they do you may avoid risks at all costs.

An example of appropriate risks: Your schedule is very predictable? So, sit down and make up a brand new schedule where every hour will be done differently. Instead of TV and radio, go for a power walk or bike ride or go rollerblading. If you don't know how, you can get lessons.

At work, if a person gossips and it's bothering you, take a risk. Sit down privately. Are they aware of the effects of gossip on everyone, and how it affects you? You have no right to ask them to change their behavior to meet your needs. You do have the right to let that person know you don't like it and you won't accept it.

Instead of working over lunch, take your full lunchtime to go out each day and try a different type of food. Sit with people you don't know to try to create new friendships.

Instead of talking to friends and family about problems, have phone-free nights when you unplug the phone. Plan your evening in advance. One night a week, enjoy some cultural event—possibly a play, folk festival, orchestra, or cabaret. Plan a night of something—bowling or billiards—something out of character—pottery or glass blowing—become a Big Brother or Big Sister one night a week. In short, take some risks. These are minor things that break old habits and routines, and in turn enlarge life-enhancing perceptions and expand your reality base. This, in time, gives you confidence to take bigger risks, including career moves, possibly selling a home you're a prisoner to because of upkeep and maintenance, and how you may really want to see other places in American but can't afford to.

What Can You Depend On?

In the world we live in, nothing is guaranteed. Human beings have trouble with this concept. The problem is, we don't like to think that something we consider permanent could be tenuous. Pink slips are handed daily to people who thought they had secure jobs. The biggest mistake most of these people have made is living beyond their means. The first thing they generally do upon being laid off is use their savings to maintain a stupid lifestyle they no longer need. Then they borrow from their friends and families and the bank. Now they're in debt.

Learning to be comfortable with less can ease much of the burden of life's stress. If you are laid off, get rid of everything and start over. Starting over is a whole new and exciting experience.

When I went to my high school reunion, many of my ex-classmates told me how their neighborhoods had changed for the worse. I asked why they didn't move and many replied that they couldn't leave because they had always lived in the same house or on the same street. It was home. They preferred to remain prisoners in their unsafe homes rather than give up the familiar.

Is any square footage worth your emotional health? It's just square footage. The energy that you have when you're there is what makes it special, and you can put out that same energy anywhere. You, and not the house, are the energy. But we give our homes a life of their own. We give them power that they shouldn't have. A house is an inanimate object that we make more powerful and controlling than it should be. We indebt ourselves to stone, brick, or wood. It's absurd when you think about it.

We need to have the willingness to let things go and say, thank you for allowing me to enjoy that when I did. Now it's time to move on.

Cultivating Resourcefulness

Did you ever think about what you should have done but didn't? Have you thought about what opportunities you missed because of something you neglected to do?

Don't beat yourself up about what you didn't do. Learn from your mistakes. The next time an opportunity arises, be willing to take some risks. And if an opportunity isn't there, go out and make it happen. That's what people who succeed do.

The majority of people want someone to make their lives work for them. In the middle class, for instance, people are waiting for someone else to make things the way they used to be. They want to live like Ozzie and Harriet and the Cleavers did. They're waiting for the politicians to give them back safe neighborhoods. They're looking for government or industry to give them a secure job so that they can have a nice backyard with flowers and swings for the kids. They're waiting for someone to intervene and make it all nice again. But that will never happen.

It's fruitless to sit around and wait for someone to come and rescue you. You have to take whatever skills and assets you have, network with others, go to groups that support and strengthen you, and make life happen. You can either make your life work or become victimized.

Finding Support

You can always find support for whatever it is you wish to do. I was talking with a man who has AIDS the other day. He said to me, "It's one thing for you to talk about eating right because you can afford to eat right, but not everyone can." I told him he was wrong. "I have not changed my standard of living in years," I said. "I live well within my financial means, but I deprive myself of nothing. I have what makes me happy. That enables me to take the extra money and work on the projects that I consider important." I went on to explain that I didn't spend a lot more money than he did on groceries. I sprout my own sprouts, which costs me about seven cents a day. This replaces more expensive and less nutritious store-bought foods.

Then I told him what he could do to eat better. "There's a house downtown that feeds about 1,600 to 1,800 persons with AIDS a month. You can get wonderful free meals made from organic food."

This man hadn't been aware of that. He was waiting for someone to come to him. But it doesn't work that way. You have to make the effort to help yourself. When you do, you will find that many wonderful connections exist. If you keep to yourself, you're not going to know about anything, and you'll remain helpless.

In almost every community in the country there are open centers. If you contact local health food stores or food co-ops, you can find a list of locations and dates of meetings. These will list dozens of self-help groups, such as the Whole Foods Project in New York City. For a person who can't afford organic food from health food stores, there are organic co-ops, and every community has organic food outreach programs—just call local health food stores. There are regular health magazines for each area of the country. There are even those specific to individual cities. They list dozens of different health care providers, orthomolecular psychiatrists, homeopaths, chiropractors, nurse midwives, herbalists, psychologists, positive transpersonal explorations, meditation, yoga, cooking classes, etc. That is merely in the area of holistic health. There are also holistic career counselors to help with career changes.

Now this man has picked up my lead and found more than enough good food for himself. His possibilities have expanded because he made one phone call.

Once you stop feeling victimized by your circumstances, you are free to make your life work. You're no longer waiting for someone to rescue you from bankruptcy, a bad neighborhood, a troubled school, or from any problems you might have. Make the breaks, and if you can't make them where you live, make them someplace else.

Bartering Skills

Yes, you do need to be resourceful to ensure a better life where you can be free to do the things you want to do and to become the person you want to become. But cultivating resourcefulness can help you in every aspect of your life. Being resourceful simply means keeping yourself open to all your options. You may want to look at what you can share with someone else. If you put your ego aside, one person's skills combined with another's create a synergy that is greater than the simple sum of the individual efforts. Get small groups together and network. That's how things happen.

Something as simple as bartering can make a difference in

your life. A friend of mine who was making $150 an hour lost his job and became sick and depressed. He was broke and couldn't find another job. He went to a food co-op and set up a computer system they needed. In exchange, he now gets organic food for free.

A lot of people don't feel comfortable with the idea of bartering. They're used to getting paid for what they do and don't know how to exchange services of equal value. You don't necessarily want to estimate the value of what you do according to its hourly worth in the consumer market. Decide, rather, on a value based upon what another person is exchanging with you, so that there is equality in the bartering. Let's say that you're a dentist and the person you're bartering with is a house cleaner. You would need to equate the service of the house cleaner with a particular aspect of what you are going to do to fix his teeth. That way you respect each other. As an example, let's say you want mercury fillings replaced with composites but you don't have the money. The dentist says the fee will be $5,000. The likelihood is that $500 is materials and $4,500 is fees to the doctor for labor. Let's say you're a school teacher and your time is worth one tenth of what the doctor's would be. So think of what you could offer someone that would establish a value for what you get. You're fluent in French so you offer the dentist French lessons in return for mercury removal. Since a French tutor makes more than a school teacher you'd charge sixty dollars per hour for tutoring—figuring it would take approximately fifty hours over a six month period to help the doctor. That's approximately one half but people in barter must adjust the value of what they're giving when giving their time. This is a human equation—it equalizes disparities between thirty dollars per hour and fifty dollars per hour so it's not a matter of working at your rate till you pay their rate—it's a common agreement that what you give of yourself is equal in effort what the other person is giving.

For example, someone wants to come to a two week health retreat which costs $2,500. The person is a dietician in a hospital and takes home $300 per week. Clearly it would take six months of part-time work to make up the difference. That wouldn't be fair; so you select an amount of time that both people consider equitable—let's say fifty hours over a six month period. This way, she could work eight hours on Saturday and a few hours one or two evenings per week—it wouldn't upset her schedule and she'd be receiving a substantial discount, but there'd be some effort on her part in return, showing goodwill. In essence, bartering has as its basis a spiritual element—the desire to share but allow each person to give what they can, and then consider that equal. Otherwise, bartering benefits the person whose services are the most expensive, and that's neither fair nor the object of the exercise. After all, the most successful people understand the importance of compassion, which is the key element in the bartering process.

You'd be surprised how well bartering can work. A friend of mine knows a man who barters his paintings. In exchange he has gotten a yacht, a car, and free dental care. He's been to Egypt where he has cruised down the Nile. This man lives off bartering. He's a smart individual who lives a very creative and carefree life filled with joy and love.

Do You Go into Debt to Impress Others?

Are you concerned about projecting a certain image? Do you buy clothes you can't afford or don't need just to be fashionable? Do you impress people with the size of your house? Do you feel you have to live in a certain neighborhood for reasons of status? Do you buy a thirty-thousand-dollar car when a thirteen-thousand-dollar vehicle is all you really need? Do you travel to where you want to go, or do you visit only fashionable places that will impress your friends?

So many people are wrapped up in maintaining an image. Recently I was working out in my health club with two people from my running group. The owner walked in and said, "We have rules in this building. Only two people in here at a time. There's also a dress code." I said, "We're wearing appropriate workout attire." (We had on shorts, tank tops, and tennis shoes.) He said, "It's a little Central Parkish. You look like you're running out there." I said, "No, we're in here working out." He said, "We like things that don't look so down there in the park." "In other words, I should wear a Calvin Klein top and Armani shorts?" "Yeah," he said, "something like that." I said, "Are you going to have fashion police come and arrest us if we don't dress right?"

When you think about where your money goes, you start to realize how many things, large and small, you do simply to project an image. Think about it: The purchase of many things in your life may have had nothing to do with making you happy.

Why not dress the way you want, live where you want, be with people you like to be with, and share in a relationship that is healthy and happy? Security isn't based on keeping the status quo and impressing those around you. True security lies in filling your waking moments with the activities that please you. When you make your choices from an inner peace, a calming effect comes over you. You are not allowing fear to lead you back into predictable, self-defeating patterns. Finally, it's your life, so try to honor it. Security comes from making appropriate changes and having the confidence to stick with them.

Honoring Your Time

❖

Most of our problems aren't the result of one error. One-time mistakes are normal and natural, and you should allow yourself and others to make them. Likewise, you shouldn't be hard on yourself if you make errors in judgment; these are necessary if you are to grow. It's the pattern of repeated mistakes that can lead you astray.

My years of counseling have shown me that most problems do not stem from whether a person is good or bad, or positive or negative. They stem from making the wrong decisions, trying to honor the wrong self. The key is to know yourself and your needs. If you don't, how can you make the right choices to honor those needs?

Describe yourself. That's the first crucial step in examining whether you honor your time.

To What Do You Give Quality Time or Attention?

You are going to be giving your life to something. The question is, to what? To what are you really dedicating your twenty-four hours each day? To a certain lifestyle? To the manifestation of ego and image? To a higher ideal? To scholarship? What are you becoming? When you're a child you can't wait until you get big enough to turn the doorknobs and wash your hands in the sink, or until you can drive a car. You look forward to what you're becoming. When you're going through high school and college you are becoming something.

Once you get out into the world, do you suddenly feel as though it's too late to become something? It's not too late. You're going to place attention on something; what will it be? Are you honoring your work, your life beyond your work, your family? Do you have to pay attention to family needs? What are their real needs versus their superficial needs? How much attention are you giving to those real needs? Or *are* you giving any attention to them?

Your Needs Versus Family Responsibilities

If yours is like many American families, everyone will be doing whatever they're going to do on their own to create their own identities, and while they'll be sharing a common space for a period of time, there won't be a whole lot of quality communication. (That's one of the reasons why grandparents in other cultures are valuable to the family. They act as the communicators for the unresolved conflicts between children and their parents. There is generally no threat from the grandparents. Rather, there's a sense of trust and patience. They're willing to forgive. They're not apt to chastise or criticize. They're looking to be the bridge.)

You've got time each day. If you don't focus attention on that time, it will be meaningless. At the end of each day, it's another day out of your life. And you will not be able to live that day again. If you're trying to do something with that time that doesn't honor the real needs of the real self, then it's wasted time. Why not put that time into focus?

This is a workbook, and, of necessity, it's advocating working in the present because, after all, you can't work in the past. So forget the past. Do not let the past dictate that you're not good enough or smart enough or lovable enough or complete enough. It's important for you to start over today. Start the game over. If this means leaving a job, leaving an area, or deciding to put time into this instead of that, then this is what you are going to do. But you are not going to change out of anxiety or haste. The whole idea is to prepare so that when you do make the change it is not superficial and you have the strength to follow through.

Recently I counseled a married couple that spend no time together. I suggested a few things they could do together each day. One suggestion was to go out and befriend a homeless person each day, talk with him or her, and give the person some food. They started going out together and found this to be one of the most rewarding parts of their day. They started seeing homeless people as human beings, not just as people they wished were in someone else's neighborhood.

How many hours a day do you waste by giving time to people who don't appreciate it? Be careful not to give your time to someone who abuses you. If all your time with someone is spent listening to him talk about himself, what's the point of being with that person? The person doesn't care about you. If you stop frittering away your time on that person and placing it where it does count, you'll be doing yourself a favor.

I'm not saying you shouldn't give time to people who are seeking your counsel. Of course you'll want to do that occasionally. But you need to cut loose the people who come back repeatedly with the same problems but never do anything with your advice. While anyone can have a problem and want—and legitimately need—to talk about it, you have to learn to recognize the pattern of people who drain you or who always take but don't return the support. There comes a day when you have to say to these people, I've listened, I've been understanding, I've given you my suggestions. Please either take my suggestions, show me where they aren't usable, or don't complain anymore.

Often their reaction to this is hostile. They're likely to call you insensitive and cold. Suddenly, it's all your fault. You become a target for their anger because you've caught them in their act. It's like catching a liar in a lie; watch how quickly they blow their cool. People who are caught in something dishonest will overreact; the whole idea of overreacting is to make you feel guilty for having caught them. But you don't have to feel guilty. Say, "Yell at the wind. I'm out of here." You'll save yourself a lot of time.

It comes down to this: For every person you help who doesn't want or respect that help, you're keeping your attention from a person who would accept your help and become a stronger person for it. It's like feeding a fat person who is moaning because they haven't had a meal in the past two hours instead of giving the food to a person who is starving to death. There's a limit to what we're capable of giving. So don't be afraid to qualify what you're giving. You have the right to do that. Sometimes guilt keeps us from doing that, but you have to get beyond guilt.

Give your time to people who respect you for it. You'll know intuitively that something good is coming from it. There's a bond that develops between people. You'll feel it.

One more thing on the subject of helping others: There's a big difference between helping people for the right reasons and using the act of helping as an excuse to hide your own inefficiency at living by acting as if you're some sort of saint or martyr. People can get caught up in what I call the wounded ego syndrome. They've been hurt and made to feel worthless. They have taken this seriously and now all they do is immerse themselves in other people's problems, hoping that everyone will think they're a nice person. They're always helping and never have a moment for themselves. This is not healthy.

Do the Things You Do Feel Natural and Honest?

I know a man who, two years ago, was in crisis. He had a successful practice in corporate law but found that his clients were not ethical people. He felt trapped by compromises he had to make in order to protect their interests. Although he was well-paid and only doing what every other lawyer did, he could not respect his own decisions. He realized that he'd been considering his income first, rather than his ethics. As a result, he woke up one day and concluded that he couldn't live this lie anymore. His work was dishonest.

Now the things he does are honest and natural. He's left law altogether. He works in a northern California spa showing people how to take care of themselves. He gave up the $300,000 a year and the high-class lifestyle to live in an adobe hut. It doesn't make sense to others, but it does to him. That's because he's being honest and doing what's natural. He feels great working with people without having to compete against them. He doesn't have to be mercenary and hurt people. He's happy.

Unfortunately his family is not happy with his version of success. Can you imagine a family saying you're wrong for being happy because the way you're doing it doesn't make us happy? His father, who is also an attorney, has been angry ever since he made the change. He won't talk to his son; he just yells at him. But then his father never talked with him anyway. He *always* yelled at him. The mother would not interfere with the father, who was a very dominant man.

It was easy to see how my buddy got caught up in believing that he had to prove himself by being a tough corporate lawyer, making money, and being successful. He was saying, "Hey dad, have I done enough to get a hug?" But he could never do enough. When you're insecure, there is never enough.

Now he's a different human being. He looks ten years younger. His body is different. He used to run to win. Now he runs because he likes to run.

What Drives You?

Our passions are what drives us—that is, assuming we allow ourselves to express or experience passion. If, for example, you want to learn a particular craft, and you spend the required time studying and apprenticing to master your craft, and then one day someone asks you, what motivates or drives you to give this type of commitment to this craft, what is your answer? If it is because you simply enjoy it or you feel good doing it, that's fine. If, however, you are doing it to prove to someone that you deserve respect or attention, or that you love them, your drive is motivated by a need for self-validation. So ask yourself what drives you. What do you expect to get from your efforts?

How Do You Spend Time Alone?

How do you feel about spending time alone? Your attitude determines whether that time is constructive, positive, and invigorating, or depressing, anxiety-provoking, and lonely. If you adopt the first attitude, your life is in greater balance than if you hold the second view.

When you feel good about spending time alone you can use that time to read, create, study, focus, clear out, unclutter, and set new priorities. But if you feel anxious about being alone, you end up squandering your time. You keep the television or radio on or spend too much time on the telephone to keep feelings of loneliness at bay. Your precious time becomes wasted.

How Do You Sublimate?

Determining the ways that you sublimate will identify the parts of your life you're not honest with and not finding fulfillment in. What are the most common ways men sublimate? Sports are important for a man. Football, baseball, and basketball are the most popular sports for men, and what do all of these have in common? They're team sports. Men love the fellowship of other men.

But as things work out in our culture, once you become a family man you lose the comfort of other men. That's one of the tragedies of our society. One of the biggest mistakes the institution of marriage has ever created is the demand for full time and attention. I can't tell you how many men get married and then can no longer retain their best friends. They never seem to have the time to get together with them. Or they do have the time but there's the thought that the friendship is competitive with the marriage, especially if the friend is a single man.

There should be no reason for that. If a person is a friend, he should always be a friend, and you should make time in your life for friends. A very important part of being balanced and healthy is to have quality relationships with men and women. I do not believe in monogamy as we now know it. I'm not referring to sexual monogamy, but rather to an exclusivity of time and attention. It's unnatural. Many crises in marriages and relationships are the result of one person trying to be all things to another person. The woman tries to become the mother, the mistress, the soothsayer, and all other things, when it's not possible. Similarly, a man cannot be all things to a woman. Why can't people be smart enough to realize this?

For a man, the loss of meaningful friendships is terrible for his sense of self-esteem. There's a betrayal of the masculine bonds that historically have kept men together. That's why sports, even though they may seem barbaric, are ways men identify what is uniquely masculine in the effort to pursue a state of excellence. Men identify and feel like they're one of the team; that's why men adopt a team. That adoption becomes a part of the extended male family. When men take time on a Sunday afternoon to watch a ball game, they're not just watching a sport to distract themselves and waste three or four hours. They're continuing a bond that identifies what is uniquely masculine and lonely in them. They are showing that they're still connected.

Everyone needs more than one person in his or her life to communicate with. You need a variety of people with which you can share multiple ideas and multiple energies because you have multiple energies to share. So regardless of whether you're married or not, you should establish what kinds of friends you need. Ask yourself, what do you want to share with your friends? If you don't do that, then the part of you that seeks friendship has to sublimate. It has to go somewhere. Unresolved energy must find an outlet, and it always will. Whether it's a disease process, or a manic process, or something constructive, an outlet will emerge. Your outlet might be, for example, compulsive work, so that you end up having no time for yourself.

If you are married, ask yourself whether you are honoring the institution of marriage, or perhaps an unquestioned and old conception of it, instead of being spontaneous and honest and honoring what is natural. Institutional beliefs tend not to be natural; after all, the whole idea of an institutional belief is that the institution is controlling us. Ironically, the institution can become like a service industry. The institution services our dysfunction. And what is the cause of our dysfunction? Not being happy with how we feel in the institution!

Sometimes our whole behavior gets bound up in negative

patterns instead of positive ones. This is what happens in sublimation. Overeating, taking drugs, smoking, and working compulsively are all ways of sublimating.

A healthier idea is to ask yourself, what are you really missing in life, and how could that need be met if it weren't being sublimated?

Describe How You Honor What You Value

How do you honor those things that matter to you? For example, I honor health every day by getting up and doing something good for my body. My diet and my mind and my exercise honor my body because I value it. Likewise, if I value my friendships, I honor those by engaging in them in the best ways I know how. I don't engage in anything that would destroy the friendships or dishonor the personhood of my friends—that is, that would infringe upon the sanctity of their inner beings. This may sound simple, but it pays to remember that your friend is first and foremost a person, not just a friend. In other words, I can't assume that because a person is my friend I have the right to say anything. I can't just show up at my friend's house and assume that because he's my friend he has no boundaries. On the contrary, by honoring his boundaries, I am honoring his personhood and thus the friendship.

If I value creativity, then every day I'll set aside time to create, even if only an hour. I'll make that time. And for whatever else I value, I'll make more time. Of course that means I will not put time and attention into things I do not value. If you ask me to do something I do not value, I won't do it. Those are the choices that make a difference in how I define my life.

Ask yourself what you value. Then ask what you do to show it.

When You Work Hard, What Do You Really Want?

What are you really looking for from all that hard work? You may be looking for satisfaction, pleasure, and finally recognition. But if you're *only* looking for recognition, something's wrong.

Do something you really like and you won't need recognition from it. Do you ever notice how many times an artist will work on a piece of work, no matter what it is. It isn't for the public. It's for herself. It doesn't matter if it's never shown, never sold. She does it for herself, to honor her inner spirit.

This idea can be applied to any area of endeavor. If you're living a life in which you're paying attention to what honors your inner needs, then you don't really require recognition. The public is of no consequence, because the doing itself is the recognition. You feel good about every moment so you don't have to say, can I have some recognition now? Did I do what I was supposed to do?

Stop and think about how many times you did something for other people because you needed the recognition in return. You had a hidden agenda, and thus the time and energy you spent on what you were doing was not honestly spent. The problem is, without honesty there is no effortlessness, nothing natural; everything is manipulation. What you are doing is putting a lot of intense energy into something that ultimately imbalances you.

Natural processes keep you balanced and focused. They keep you going in one direction, and something positive will come from that.

One more thing: In the normal course of life, you *will* get a response from the decent people around you. It is natural to respond. I respond to things people do that I consider special; I'll always acknowledge them. Most people are going to do the same thing. The point is, if you find that you absolutely need that reinforcement in order to keep doing what you're doing, then you have to ask yourself whether you're working hard on the wrong things.

Where Do You Need To Organize?

Do you need to organize in discipline, focus, or attention? Take a total inventory of yourself. As part of that, each week ask yourself, "what have I done?" If you haven't done anything worth noting, you're obviously not willing to take control of your life. You're still waiting for someone to fill in the blanks. There was a time, by the way, when I would do that. I would fill in all your blanks for you. I'd tell you how to get discipline and I'd tell you about your fears. Well, I didn't help anyone. I was trying to take on something that people had to do for themselves.

It's your life. You've got to not only fill in the blanks but also create the blanks to fill in! That's because you don't learn primarily from the quality of your answers, you also learn from the quality of your questions. There's far more profundity in the question than there is in the answer. So you have to figure out the best way to ask the questions. Once you do, you're on the right track.

A simple organizational chart might assist you in better managing your time and projects:

Date
Time—over the next 12 months
Project—sell everything I don't need
Goal—get out of debt
Short term
    (a) get estimates of current market values
    (b) get rental rates for comparable space
    (c) hire a specialty broker

Research

1. estimate current income, saving, expenses
2. what are my buying habits?
3. what do I own that I don't use, like, or need?
4. how much more would I save if I stopped buying stuff and sold what I don't need?
5. where would I like to live?
6. how would I like to live?
7. how much time do I spend working to pay down my debt?
8. what would I do with the extra free time?
9. how well do I manage the stresses caused by my standard of living?
10. do I need help doing any part of this?
11. list the support groups that I could go to

After reviewing your chart, you may change your priorities, but at least you know where you are headed and how you are going to get there. Or if you need focus and attention, there are Buddhist classes that are phenomenal for getting focus. Just look in the phone book under Buddhist.

There's always a resource to help you if you are at least honest in knowing what you need help with. It's not necessary that you do it all yourself if you have others who can help guide you into change. Combine your energy with other people to mutually enhance all of your lives.

What Is Divine Within You?

Define that which is divine or the eternal spirit within you. Then you can honor it. We can get very caustic and very down on ourselves, and as a result we forget that we are divine beings filled with a divine energy. You are that energy. What are you going to do with it? How are you going to nourish it and manifest it? One thing that almost everyone has experienced is being around people who manifest their divine energy; there's a comfort and joy in just occupying the same space.

You can become the person that gives comfort and joy to other people because you will be able to provide this energy simply by manifesting it in yourself.

I feel that everyone has enormous reservoirs of passion for life that just remain locked inside them. It's as if people have a lush oasis within them, but instead of tapping into it, most wander through the desert of trying to live their lives based on the wrong premise. Use all the wonderful energy inside you instead of reverting to blaming, anger, disappointments, sublimations, and dysfunction. Just let go of the negative so you can find what works, and realize what is divine.

What Was Missing When You've Felt Bad?

Frequently I find it helpful to ask questions that are the opposites, or the negatives, if you will, of what one would normally ask. Thus, if someone comes to me and says, "I feel bad," I don't say, "What made you feel bad?", but rather, "What wasn't there?" Their response is often the quickest answer that will give them the truest insight. What wasn't there is what they weren't working on, what they didn't pay attention to but perhaps should have.

So when you feel bad, something is missing. What is it? Otherwise, when you feel bad, what do you feel? You feel sadness and despair. You feel those because something isn't there.

An example: you knew someone was stealing at work. Everyone else knew also, but kept quiet. First, you confronted the person who was stealing and told them to stop or go elsewhere. They told you to mind your own business, so you told the owner. The other workers were angry at you. So for honoring your ethics, you did the right thing, even if others didn't like you for doing it.

If you've ever felt good about a particular situation but were conditioned to feel bad about it, you have to make the choice about which attitude to trust. Can you trust yourself to create answers and solutions even if you were taught that when something bad happens you just have to accept it? People get into this self-deprivation and self-destructive pattern instead of saying, I feel bad because I'm lacking something. I'm going to look for what I need to feel good and I'm going to find it or create it.

Do You Judge Yourself by What's in Your Heart and Mind?

In most cases you judge yourself by your accomplishments. It's easier and usually what you were taught to do. But in doing so, you lose focus on the inner self.

Few people learn what it means to feel something from the heart, or from their inner being. We're taught to focus on external factors, and these become the all-important features of life. But if you get caught up in judging your life by your experiences, you'll start to constantly anticipate the next experience. That, in turn, is going to make you think about the consequences of the experience, as opposed to just experiencing it. So the sense of dread, loss of control, or fear of something negative happening can take over.

Do you find that long periods of your life are simply wasted waiting for an experience to happen? You wait for the good experience that you feel will redeem the time you have been in the limbo of waiting. You get overly focused on what is mundane when you keep on this experience-seeking path that has no purpose and no end.

What Areas of Free Will and Freedom
Do You Use?

How do you use freedom? Make a list.

1. to be your own person
2. to take responsibility for your own actions
3. to actively seek the right goals for your true inner needs
4. to let negative people know that you won't accept negative energy
5. to commit yourself to causes that make you feel good
   a. environmental action groups
   b. men's or women's study groups
   c. adult education classes to broaden your knowledge
   d. political and religious action groups
6. to unclutter your life—give it away, throw it away, or use it wisely
7. to organize your time so you count
8. to let go of unnecessary responsibilities

This very important exercise will tell you an awful lot about yourself. For instance, when is the last time you did something completely out of character, spontaneous, and different from what anyone would expect from you? It was probably a really long time ago. Why? When did you use freedom last and how did you use it? If you don't use the freedom you have, it's like muscle tissue that turns to fat.

The whole idea of being free is to express what's in our hearts and minds. Of course, with freedom comes a responsibility not to abuse others. With that in mind, if you're not afraid of what's in your heart, then you will find other people who will acknowledge that and honor it as well. I've never found a situation where I couldn't find someone who was interested in freedom, and who wouldn't be interested in what I am. When two people share an understanding of their own freedom, they have endless ways of demonstrating that freedom. The people who are afraid of freedom within themselves are the people who are invulnerable. You can know them for a hundred years and never know them because they're never going to reveal what's really inside.

What are you doing with freedom? How have you expressed it? How have you used it? How are you making it work for you?

I talk a lot with cabdrivers who tell me that in their native countries people don't have any right to freedom. They can't express their feelings, emotions, political views, sexual views, religious views, creative views. They don't have any of this. And here so many of us just abuse freedom. We think freedom is just an opportunity for gluttony or for being a loudmouth or for being selfish. How sad that more Americans don't use freedom in a constructive way to help society and experience growth in the process.

Write down the ways you use your freedom.

Can You Live With Uncertainty?

Uncertainty creates fear, which limits free will. As long as you're uncertain about who you are, what you want, and what you need to get what you want, the uncertainty becomes that big bugaboo that stands right in front of you. Perhaps every day you get up to do something and you're uncertain. I don't know if I should go back to school. . . . I don't know if I should move to San Diego. . . . I don't know if I should change my diet. . . . People are very confused in our society; they're uncertain of everything. And they don't like it.

But is cast-in-stone certainty really an asset in life? The need for constant certainty means that you will never change. Why do you think conservatives are so conservative? They have something to conserve! People who are in positions of power need certainty in all things because they don't want to change. They can't have a society where people express themselves openly and freely. They can't have people manifesting change because then they would lose control and power.

Here are some examples of a counterproductive need for certainty: when you have to find a friend that's good before you'll drop the "friend" you don't really like; when you have to develop a relationship that's better before you'll get out of a bad relationship; when you have to have a body you really like before you'll start exercising. You end up defeating yourself in each case.

People don't change any area of their life unless they have confidence that the change is going to be beneficial. This makes sense. The problem comes when they're not willing to let go of anything—even the bad things—and replace them with something unless they're certain of success. So they start looking for input that allows them to feel some certainty that the change is going to work, some certainty that the business is going to work or that the relationship will, or the job, or the career, or the move, or whatever the change is. The trouble is, nothing in life is certain.

The need for certainty breeds a contempt for uncertainty, yet it's only with uncertainty that we can change. Learn to be confident with uncertainty. Learn to feel the discomfort that accompanies change without focusing on it, and that discomfort will disappear. This will allow you the flexibility and freedom to be yourself and take the consequences of whatever happens. When a person is healthy and balanced, she or he will take whatever doesn't work and simply say, it's okay. Nothing in life is meant to work all the time. I took a chance and tried; it didn't work; I'll try something else. Healthy people, and people who are kind to themselves, are not afraid of uncertainty. They make it work for them, and—here is the key—they learn from it.

Feeling Passion and Desire

At some point in your life you finally decide to get out of your own way and go after what you want. You begin knowing what is important to you. Yesterday no longer exists, you've let it go. You've realized that what it takes to survive is an adaptive mind; the nonadaptive mind stagnates, trying to honor allegiances to things it was taught to accept in the past, and you don't choose stagnation.

Now you've got a whole new mindset that you're learning to take control of and you want to move with it. You want to do something with all this insight, energy, and power.

Even now, though, when you start to do something, you may get in your own way by saying to yourself, "Hold on, I don't know if I can handle this. I'm not sure I really want to redirect my life. I've been this way for so long that I'm used to things as they are. I'm used to this kind of mess in my life. I'm used to the excuses I give. I'm used to the patterns of emotional malfeasance that I indulge in." When this happens, don't wait for the old self to react. It will just stand there and say, "I don't know." What kind of option is that?

The new you says, "I don't want to argue with anyone, least of all myself. What's the point? I'm going to examine the consequences of my actions. If I get up and exercise, then my metabolism is going to improve. If I go out and look for new ways to share my energy, then I'll stop repeating old patterns. I know what it feels like to be stuck in the same old place, and I'm tired of it." When you hit a barrier, the new side of you will say, "Take a break. Go to the beach, hang out, and then come back and start over." The new self seeks positive change. It won't let other people influence or stop those changes.

When it's time to start organizing your life, start with mini-goals that take a week or two to achieve. Tie several together to form larger goals. Take your ideals, ambitions, and dreams, and pull them together to consolidate them into the strength you need.

When you set larger goals, you don't necessarily have to see the end product; goals can just be formulated as the things you want to change without a final solution. Maybe your goal is to live someplace else in a year's time. You don't have to know where that someplace is, but you can use your time to explore until you find a place that feels right. It's a world of adventure; life should be fun. Instead of concerning yourself with what you're trying to secure, focus on creating balance. You should find nice people and opportunity everywhere. If not, you can make that another goal.

So often, people fight change merely to protect their egos or to cover up insecurity. But as the saying goes, "The wise water moves around the rock." It doesn't go up against it and become stagnant. Set a year or six months' goal for yourself, asking, "In that period of time, can I be the person who will have the competence and inner resources to take control of my life?" When you hit a barrier, you're immediately going to think of several options to get around it. In my opinion, you need to have five options for fluidity in any situation. If you start thinking of options, you will create alternatives.

How Do You Share Your Special Qualities?

Do you share different parts of yourself with different people? Perhaps as a child you learned to clown around at home and make people laugh. Although you're still able to amuse your friends, you close yourself off to having fun at work. You think a serious image is needed at all times to gain the trust and respect of others. As a result, you cut off an important side of yourself.

Notice where you feel safe and where you don't. Maybe life taught you that being yourself in the professional world makes you vulnerable, and easy prey for others who are looking for an opportunity to knock you down so that they can get ahead. Unfortunately, this is an overly competitive world, and you may tend to fear that others will take advantage of your openness and use that against you. So the things you would like to say are kept inside. You say only what you believe others are going to accept. Although you may be protecting yourself in this way, you're also denying an important part of your nature.

What if you had just one personality all the time? Think of how simple your life could be. Other people could accept or reject you for what you are and you wouldn't need to constantly adjust what you say and do just to please them. Some people would hate you for it, but you'd learn from that to weed them out of your life.

I would rather have no friends than false friends. I would rather have intelligent, sensitive conversations with myself than with a bunch of bubbleheads that I'm trying to somehow placate. I would rather have the connection with my own heart than with other cold, embittered hearts. What is the purpose of cluttering up your life with people you can't communicate with honestly and compassionately?

Ask yourself, how much of your real self do you actually share? Do you share your essential nature or a manufactured, contrived personality? Do you share some of both, depending upon whom you feel safe with?

When you love yourself first, you share your life only with others who treat you lovingly. Whatever you are is enough. You don't have to be two, three, or five different people. You don't have to be placate others' insecurities and prejudices. Nor do you have to honor their belief systems when they don't represent how you feel. You are able to communicate your real needs to friends by clearly defining what their friendship means to you.

If a person is intimidated by your honesty, he or she might think, "Are you telling me that if I ask you something you're just going to say what you feel? That's scary. I don't want to hear what you really have to say. I want to be around people who give me a false sense of being okay because I'm insecure about myself. I want you there as a false sounding board. You're my psychoanalyst for free. I want us to spend twenty years together sharing the same nonsense. You're telling me that you're going to be honest with me and going to share love, but I wouldn't know love if I saw it because I was never given love, only conditional responses. If I did well I was given a reward. If I didn't I was punished. I'm a product of all that and I use it as an excuse not to change my life. Therefore, I surround myself with people who dislike me. You're telling me you're going to be different—the one person in my life who's going to be radiant, joyful, and always happy. I can't handle that." And that's how it often works.

Conversation, which ought to express your true beliefs, is easy when you're not worried about what the other person thinks of you. If that person isn't looking for the kind of friendship you have to offer, so be it. There are enough healthy, balanced, joyful people out there wanting a friendship based on truth.

Notice your special qualities by looking at different areas of your life. What have you done to make different parts of your life work? What parts of your life don't work because you have neglected them? Ask yourself, "How can I apply my special qualities to these areas of my life?" Determine where you are able to share wit, charm, compassion, insight, wisdom, self-lessness, courage, and trustworthiness.

Can You Accept Another Person as He or She Is?

People usually have certain qualities that you can relate to and others that you cannot. Does this mean you have to accept someone totally or avoid the person altogether? Not necessarily.

Few people will agree with you on every issue. If the differences between you and someone else are not interfering with your peace of mind, you can still enjoy being with that person. As long as the person does not in any way undermine who you are, you have the basis for a relationship. I might have friends with different political philosophies. One might be a communist, another a capitalist, and the third a socialist. It is our ability to respect each other as people—and not for our politics—that is going to determine the quality of our friendship.

Look at your relationships to see whether your differences are frustrating the affiliation or not. Are you comfortable around the other person or do his or her beliefs make you uneasy? If they make you uncomfortable, you need to draw the line and reconsider the relationship.

Are You Giving Mixed Messages?

You may be in a relationship where you want to share something with the other person but don't know how. You're afraid that your passion and desire are more than the person can bear. You're terrified of being rejected. As a result, you end up never really feeling completely fulfilled with the person.

The other person may have the same thoughts and may also be afraid to impose them on you. Both of you are frustrated. Your relationship becomes superficial.

Relationships become meaningful when both people's desires are met. You should be able to tell a person what you're thinking right up front.

We're a society that fears being honest about our passions and desires. Partly it's because people tend to gossip, which makes it hard to confide our innermost thoughts. In the back of our minds we wonder, who else is going to know about this?

You've got to let the person know that what you're sharing with him or her is only meant for that person. You're not sharing this, with their girlfriends, boyfriends, mother, father, or work associates. You don't want what you share to be the topic of discussion. Let the person agree to honor that privacy before you share anything at all.

A person who betrays your confidence is not a person you should have in your life. Yet the reality is that a lot of people out there will betray you at the drop of a hat. Somehow we've forgotten about trust and honor. We seem to have become motivated by fear and by the desire to satisfy immediate needs, which has led us to a largely mercenary attitude, with our own interests superseding those of others, or the community. We should often give pause to reflect: What are my actions, thoughts, and deeds going to mean to those around me? But we don't do this, which makes us a dysfunctional nation, at least ethically.

Are you able to share confidences with anyone? If not, is it because you don't trust the people in your life? Are you a trustworthy person yourself?

Make a List of the Things You Wanted to Do But. . . .

Make a list of things you wanted to do but never did. Choose one item from your list and create a program to make it happen. Maybe you wanted to be a ballerina but. . . . It doesn't matter that you're not going to be performing at the Met. You can become a ballerina in your dance class. Give yourself time to make it happen, even if it takes a year or more.

Whatever you want to do, there is a way to make it work. There are support groups, adult education courses, books, everything you need to bring your dream to fruition. Right now, in New York City, there are hundreds of study groups, classes, and social groups of all types. Every one of these groups started with one person saying, "I'm not going to say, 'I wanted to but . . . ,' I'm going to make it happen."

I know a man named Rupert Ravens. At one point in his life he was a drug addict and an alcoholic who was wasting a great young life. He had been a top athlete in high school and then he postponed his life for about 15 years while he engaged in addictive behaviors. He was working as a house painter to make a living, although he was a very gifted artist, and the fumes were racking his body and affecting his immune system. The first step he chose to change his life was to detoxify his body.

One day he said to me, "Gary, I don't have any money. I can't buy vitamins or even organic produce. And I hate the idea of eating pesticide-contaminated produce." I suggested that he call some suppliers and start a food co-op. That way he would be able to get food at cost.

He got a group of people together and started a food co-op.

They were able to buy produce at a fifty-percent saving (cheaper than buying food in a supermarket). Instead of being helpless and not having the money to buy food, Rupert buys more healthy food at a lower price.

His confidence has reached new heights. The co-op has 100 members and is on the way to becoming one of the largest in New Jersey. It has more organic produce than any health food store in New York City. What's more, in a period of four weeks, Rupert formed art classes and health support groups to encourage other people, including a running and walking club in southern New Jersey. These things benefit and honor Rupert's community but he is helping himself in the process by honoring his spiritual self.

I'd say that's pretty good for four weeks. If he can do it, why couldn't you? Why couldn't anyone? He could just as easily have hung around bars for the rest of his life, but he chose instead to self-actualize. He chose to enhance the best that he is instead of condemning himself for what he is not.

All this is the result of one man deciding to do exactly what I'm asking you do to. Make a list of all the things you wanted to do but. . . . Then create the reality. Fill in the blanks in your life. Work alone or find other people who share your goal. When two, three, four, or more people have common goals, think of how much good they can do. Perhaps you have a talent and someone else has the money. Why not get together and make things happen even faster than they would if you worked separately? As long as there's a basic sense of trust between you, you can make it work.

Where Do You Turn for Solutions to Your Problems?

You've started on your journey by analyzing who you are and noting your positive and negative qualities. You've begun the process of preparation and have created the hero within. You're inner-directed, self-empowered, and all set to change.

To whom do you turn for help in this effort? Who will help you with your creative, emotional, spiritual, mental, and physical challenges? And are the people you turn to in fact providing you with the right catalysts? Consider whom you turn to when faced with each of these challenges.

Creative Challenges

If I want to do something creative, whom do I seek out for support? Creative people. Look for people who have succeeded at what you're attempting to do. An uncreative person has no framework. If you're interested in learning about medicinal herbs, you're not going to ask an orthodox doctor who doesn't even know what an herb is. He won't understand herbs because he has no background in them. You go to a holistic doctor who has been using herbs for years, because she or he will be able to help you.

When you find a person whose life is working, don't be afraid to ask that person for help. The most selfless people, the ones always giving of their energy, are the ones doing the most. It's easy to do more when your life works. The person whose life doesn't work is the one who is bitter and not willing to spend time with you.

Spiritual Challenges

Who are the people best able to help you with spiritual issues? Look within yourself, not out there. All the answers you need are within you. You can touch the spirit when you let go of fear and you let go of the material.

People spend their whole lives looking for spiritual help by running to evangelists or gurus. We try strange ways to connect with our inner self. We go everywhere but inside.

Why not look inside? Why not trust what's in there? One explanation might be that in your life you've never been allowed to be the authority. Authority, you learned, comes from somewhere else. You, like most people, don't have either power or control. But if you understand that all you need to know is within, you will spend time sitting in quiet contemplation to find the answers.

You've been taught, however, to seek out experts, such as psychiatrists and other doctors, or priests, rabbis, or lawyers. But why is everyone an expert about your life except you?

Beware: Experts can take control of your life and negate your intuition. A doctor might say, for example, that you must have a radical mastectomy. You respond by saying that you were under the impression that a simple lumpectomy is a safer, more effective option. The doctor, in turn, will negate your knowledge by replying, "When did you get your medical degree? Where do you come off challenging me? Nobody does that. I have to dismiss you for being a bad patient." But you're not a bad patient, just an empowered one. The difficulty is in trying to talk with someone in power about anything that challenges that power. It causes a reaction that is not necessarily based on reason.

When you look at spiritual, as well as emotional, mental, and physical areas of your life, often you're your own best teacher.

List New Possibilities

Look at the possibilities in different avenues of life. Look at all the possibilities that exist for each of these factions of your life.

For Yourself

What possibilities can you see for yourself? What would you like to make happen? Make a chart and map it out. If you want to move to a new location, place that at the center of your chart. Then write your reasons for moving around it. Perhaps you want less clutter and responsibility. That will tell you that you're now in a place where there is too much clutter and responsibility. You might feel the need to start unloading your possessions.

Then you can start taking action. After deciding what things you no longer need, you can start the process of disengagement by bagging or boxing things and giving them away. In a short time you will have the freedom you desire and moving will be easy.

You can decide where it is best for you to live by listening to your heart. Visiting possible new locales will give you a feeling for what different places are like. For instance, in Boulder, Colorado, you might find intellectual energy and beautiful surroundings. New York might attract you if you plan to advance your career. If you're an artist you might enjoy living around Taos or Santa Fe. If you want to live quietly you might enjoy Tucson. If you want a combination of culture and ambience, you can go to Dallas. If you want to be where people are laid back and having fun with life, you can go to San Diego. If you want to be a part of a close community with intense intellectual activity, you might decide to live in San Francisco. If you want to be where people are more adventurous and poetic you can live in Portland. Find the place that feels comfortable, where you can meet people like yourself. Once you make the move, you will find it easier to make your life work.

For Your Family

Define possibilities for your family. That might include new ways of relating, connecting, healing old wounds, and communicating. It might mean having more time for your children.

In your marriage or your primary relationship, it might mean recapturing the romance you once felt. Go back and remember the passion and excitement of your romance when you were captivated by each other, and joyful just being together. Having fun, as opposed to materialistic concerns, was all-important. If you could do it all over again, would you choose to have all the things you've accumulated, or quality time to share your passion?

One time through is all you get. Think of that when you create new possibilities for yourself, your children, and your relationships; it may impel you to change your priorities. You may want to replace false responsibilities in your life with possibilities built around love.

For Your Friends

What are some new possibilities with friends? Making new friends might be one. What qualities would you look for in new friends? They might have similar interests, enabling you to do things together. They might be people who love you for being you. They might have positive attitudes and compassionate hearts.

They will not be people who undermine, criticize, and talk about you behind your back.

For Your Work

What new possibilities can you envision at work? How about creating your own ideal job? Self-employment is an exciting, exhilarating experience. But what about sharing your business dreams with other people who have similar desires? Working together can create a synergy; a lot more happens when two or three people are working together. You can do it on your own—many people have—but it's a lot of more fun and a lot more efficient to work with other people that you trust. When each person helps out and there's no selfishness, everyone's needs can be met.

For Society

What are some new possibilities for society? As a part of society, you need to involve yourself with it. There are a lot of members of the baby boom generation who don't do a thing for society; they're too busy focusing on themselves. I can't imagine being in a society and not contributing to it.

You could choose to make one day a week available to helping some segment of society. As an example, you can give one day a week pro bono, based upon your profession. If you're an attorney or an architect, you can donate time to any number of church centers that fund charities for the homeless. Or you could become a Big Brother or Big Sister to one of the six million orphaned children in America. You can also donate time to the local school system or to other public causes. Commit to making it work, just as you do on a personal level.

For Nature

What possibilities allow you to reconnect with nature? Everybody loves nature if given the opportunity to experience it; I always notice how, when people come down to my ranch, they spend half the time with the animals. They're fascinated by them. Think of all the things in nature that you haven't experienced yet that are there to explore.

One of the most powerful experiences people have at my ranch is participating in a Native American sweat lodge ceremony. People love it. People with all types of religious beliefs benefit from the experience. There is no philosophy taught, merely experiences shared. People have a chance to see another belief system and are just blown away by it. It changes their perception of life. That will happen when you allow yourself the chance to get close to nature.

Where Do You Belong?

You need to look within for spiritual guidance to get an answer to this question. The conscious mind alone won't be able to help you. Ask yourself where, of all places, do you belong? Don't try to think through the answer—feel it instead.

Once you know where you belong, focus on being there. Affirm your answer by saying, here's where I feel I belong. Then it becomes a real possibility. Remember, with possibility there is action. With passion you create the action. With desire you create the passion and are able to get there.

The movie *Field of Dreams*, a metaphorical film about a midwestern corn farmer about to lose his farm, is a good example of this. The farmer keeps hearing a voice that says, "Build it and they will come." He follows his intuition and builds a little baseball field, and long-since-deceased players come back and play the game. His passion leads him to take action, and he makes an impossible dream happen. It's like reliving the fantasies of youth, where anything is possible.

You'll find that people who listen to their intuition and follow their dreams attract other people who support them in their efforts. Throughout the country you'll find people who did what no one thought was reasonable and succeeded because they had the support of someone else. It's that other person's way of reaching for the dream too.

How many times in your life have you heard a little voice inside you say, "Do the impossible, think the impossible, follow your dreams"? How often have you listened? When have you not?

What Things Do You Fear?

I believe that you can live in a fulfilled and happy way and make anything real, if you have the courage and confidence to try. That is what life is about. Once you define your new possibilities, you have set the stage and are ready to start your journey.

You may not get there right away, but with planning you will get there. Don't give yourself an unrealistic timetable; it takes time to let go of things, unclutter your life, and heal from the elimination of the negative things you were attached to.

In the process, you are going to face changes that you fear. So ask yourself, what fears may keep me from getting started on my journey? Take on one thing that you fear each day. Write it down where you can see it. Look at what you've written and resolve it by affirming, this is how I'm going to deal with this fear today. Take action and you will be able to put fears away once and for all.

What Would You Do Differently if There Were No Punishments and No Rewards?

How much of what you do in a day is based upon punishment and reward? Looking at life that way helps you to see what you do to please others instead of what you do for yourself. It may get you to start saying what you need to say instead of what someone else wants to hear. You have every right to let people know if what they've giving you is enough or not enough, or whether it's right or needs to be changed.

Identify what is essential to your well-being. Don't be afraid to express feelings of excitement. People often think that as they grow older they should dull their passions, when that's not true at all. You should explore your passions with the innocence and honesty of a child, and make everything a wonderful journey.

Part of you might say, I'd like to have this, but I'm not sure it's acceptable. You might think what you want is too immature, so you hide your feeling of desire. But how do you know? Based upon what? Are you allowing someone else to tell you what you should want and believe in? Only you know what you need.

Do You Live by Opinions or Knowledge?

A recent issue of the *Medical Tribune* reports a range of opinions that doctors have regarding vitamin E. Some of these doctors say that vitamin E is worthless. Others say you should have just the Recommended Daily Allowance. Still others think you need more. But no one has presented the fact that the scientific literature is filled with hundreds of examples of how vitamin E, at levels higher than the RDA, has benefited people with all kinds of conditions, from intermittent claudication to coronary heart disease. Knowledge ought to supersede opinion, yet many people speak their opinions without investigating whether or not they are based on truth.

Here's another example. People commonly accept as true the opinion that as you age you lose your libido. This is not necessarily so; there is no age at which your sex life necessarily diminishes. Society doesn't like to think of older people having a sex life, though, so it perpetuates this opinion. You see images of older people in movies as little old men and ladies in rocking chairs, or in advertisements as people troubled with hemorrhoids, or in a bathroom holding up their adult diapers.

These images lead to your forming a one-sided opinion about older people that is not based on truth.

Think of all the beliefs you have that are based on opinion and not knowledge. For instance, you may believe that blacks are not as smart as whites, that women are not as emotionally stable as men, that going to an Ivy League school makes you smarter than others, that rich people are more successful than others at living. You may start equating money with happiness based on your opinion.

On the other hand, what have you done recently to gain real knowledge? When you gain knowledge, you gain power. And power gives you the confidence and courage to move on.

What Excuses, Emotions, or Feelings Do You Use as Distractions?

Do you distract yourself by getting angry, blaming, or becoming confused about what you want or need? These distracting feelings come from not trusting your inner guidance.

You need to trust your inner feelings about what you really want in all areas of life. Ask yourself, what kind of life do I want? Your age and other so-called limitations are immaterial. The only thing that matters is knowing what you want from your life. Once you know that, you can get anything.

The false starts come from not trusting your inner voice. You continue doing things you believe you should be doing but they don't feel right inside. This comes from following someone else's suggestions instead of your own.

Life is not a child's game of choice played with a blindfold on. You can look around at what you may want. You can make your choice and then create a life around it. Otherwise, you're living a life limited by your circumstances, a life of adapting—to your environment, to your job, to your social responsibilities, to your family—in short, to everyone else's needs. Constantly adapting distracts you from your own vision of life. Then your life doesn't work, and it doesn't get any better tomorrow, next year, or ever.

So you've got to decide what you really want. You alone know what that is and you alone can choose to build a life around it. If you envision a certain type of house, for example, you will find a location and proceed to build your house. Otherwise, you might accept somebody else's dream and end up living in a well-manicured little suburban prison instead of the house in the country you envision for yourself.

You need to create a life based upon your own vision. Forget the excuses, such as, nobody ever told me I could; I'm not smart enough; I don't have the resources. If other people can follow their dreams, so can you.

If Rupert Ravens, the man whose story I described earlier in this chapter, can create a food co-op, a health support group, a holistic health center, and begin a new book project—all in four weeks, with no education in that area and no money—think of what you can do. All you need is the desire and the willingness to follow your dreams. And of course you've got to get rid of what doesn't work and focus on what does.

Many people live busy lives but the busyness is nothing more than a series of distractions. They're not in touch with what they need to be doing for themselves. Rather, they're engaged in things that don't matter much and won't amount to anything.

Can You Imagine Your Ideal Job?

Imagine creating the type of job in which everything you put into your work matters, where what you do meets your real needs and fits your images and ideals. If it doesn't exist, create it, like in *Field of Dreams*. Build it and it will come true. Once you create the ideal job, people will pay attention to what you are doing. We're a service-oriented society. If you create the right service, people will want to support you.

Think of the people who have become successful just by doing the unusual. I talked with the owner of Celestial Seasonings, the tea company. He started his company in Boulder, Colorado, by going out with his knapsack and picking herbs from the sides of hills with a bunch of friends. He never let go of his ideal and now has a large, successful company.

Look at Ben & Jerry's ethical ice cream company. They've created a good quality product that comes from a company that is socially conscious. They cared enough to create an organization based upon high standards.

People tried to discourage them from starting a company by telling them they were going to fail. But they listened to their inner voices instead, and succeeded despite the naysayers, because they believed in their dream and had the passion to follow it through.

There are many people who will support you in your dreams if you have the courage to honor and embrace them.

Eliminating Self-Defeating Habits

There are several ways to go about overcoming self-defeating habits. One is to take an honest look at the part of your nature you generally try to hide, even from yourself, so that sometimes you are unaware of what you say and do and the consequences of your actions. Recently, for example, there was a rally in New York City against the Food and Drug Administration. It had a pretty good turnout—I'm guessing there were between 500 and 700 people present. Some people told me they had never protested at a demonstration before, and I complimented them for being there in order to encourage their efforts.

Then I started thinking about all the people who weren't there. At least 600,000 people listen to my radio show and knew about the rally's significance, and yet they weren't there. They never protest anything in their lives because they choose not to create discomfort.

I know the owner of a health food emporium who chose not to protest. I said to him, "Surely you know that your freedoms are being impinged upon. Since you sell vitamins, why couldn't you take the time to show your support?" He answered, "I was with you. . . ." I immediately jumped in, "No, don't tell me you were with me in spirit. Either you participate in something or you don't." Although this man's livelihood is threatened if a law passes that bans vitamins, he chose to risk losing that rather than risk causing discomfort.

This seems analogous to the way many people live. They deceive themselves and try to fool others. They like to believe they are doing something when in actuality they're not. They like to believe they are really committed to changing what is wrong, when in actuality they never get around to doing anything about it. They keep practicing their bad habits even as they complain and whine about their problems.

Men and women usually perpetuate bad habits differently. Women will generally talk openly and passionately about what is not working with their lives. They'll vent their feelings and discuss their problems, but not do anything to resolve them. In our society, women are encouraged to empathize with other women, which, up to a certain point, is a good thing. After that point, though, the conversation becomes pointless and frustrating.

Men, on the other hand, rarely complain about what is not working in their lives. They tend to intellectualize their problems away to keep from showing they are vulnerable. Men generally express few emotions. They show some joy and anger or rage, but are otherwise silent about their feelings, even among other men.

Let's begin with the idea that if you're going to make real changes happen you need to face your problems and do something about them, not simply vent them or pretend they're nonexistent. Start by looking at what you care about.

What Do You Care About?

Look at some issues that are important to you that you do nothing about. Our society professes concern for the environment, for example. Corporations now say they are environmentally conscious, although few really are. Most corporations' actions speak otherwise. For example, many of them dump more pesticides into the ocean than ever before.

The environmental movement in this country is very small. Maybe a thousand people in the entire nation work full-time to support an environmental cause such as Greenpeace, Friends of the Earth, or the Audubon Society. Only a thousand people remain between total abuse of the environment and our health.

Since the environment affects us all, why aren't we more committed as a nation to healing it? Why isn't it more of a priority? Why does an entire infrastructure have to disintegrate to the point at which it no longer functions before someone pays attention to it?

Again, there's an analogy on the personal level. The environmental situation can be compared to waking up one morning, looking in the mirror, and exclaiming, "My God, how did I get this way?" Nothing happens overnight. You don't get fat overnight. A marriage doesn't disintegrate in a day. You don't become alcoholic instantaneously. Things fall apart gradually as a result of neglect or abuse. If you wait too long, you no longer have a problem—you have a major, grade-A crisis.

Why not change what doesn't work? Why not be open and honest with yourself and decide what you really want from your work, your relationships, and your family? Why not simply change your priorities, since there is only so much time, energy, and emotion you can put into anything in one given day?

That may sound reasonable, but most people focus on the obstacles, such as how their changing will affect others. People also tend to complacently accept their situations. I grew up in a town where the men never complained about anything, except maybe the outcome of the local high school football game. Everything else they accepted as a given. They were supposed to work in polluted factories, even if that meant inevitably contracting emphysema or lung cancer. To complain was unacceptable; it would be perceived as weak, unmasculine behavior.

These anti-change messages start early in life, when you're commanded to do as you've been told. You're a helpless, vulnerable little child. All you can do is feel; you can't yet intellectualize. You quickly learn that if you disobey, you will be punished, and if you obey you will be rewarded, even if the reward only means not being punished. As a result you learn to contain the real essence of your being. What should be expressed isn't.

As an adult you continue to play by the rules in order to feel included. If you're the only person at work really working, you may be confronted with chidings such as, "What are you doing? Slow down. Do you want to make us look bad?" Since you don't want to rock the boat and make enemies, you start to slow down. Fear of exclusion can be a powerful force.

What do you care *about* that you have neglected to care *for*? What would you like to see change? What action can you take to effect change?

Do You Have Outside Support?

Your fantasies can make you different. They give you the impetus to explore your dreams. They make you feel you can be anybody. You believe you contain the power to change anything.

Then one day you wake up and are told that you can't do anything. You have to stay in your place. Families are frequently the first people to give you that message. Instead of giving support, they tell you you're wrong for feeling different. If you start living up to your potential you become a reflection of what they might have been had they tried. You remind them that they didn't have courage. You're threatening them by saying, in effect, that they've lived an un-actualized life. They never became who they really could have been, but instead chose to be who their father, mother, and others told them they should be. They were obedient, and now they no longer feel the pain because they've anesthetized themselves to it. They've lost touch with anything vital and essential to their own natures and they've forgotten their real needs.

You, on the other hand, want to be who you really are, so you don't feel conflicted and contradictory. You don't want to walk around in a thousand bits and pieces; you want to feel whole.

Search out people with goals similar to yours. Associate with people whose standards are better than yours or more specific and stronger so that you have to raise yours. They'll make you stretch and reach new heights. When I train, I want to train with people who are better and faster than I am. That pushes me. When I have a conversation, I want to talk to someone who is smarter than I am and who has something to add.

The whole issue is one of self-actualization. Shouldn't you count? Shouldn't your time and energy be prioritized around what is important to you? When it isn't, two years, five years, twenty years fly by and you still haven't spent time on you. Everything else has gotten your attention and emotions but you. As a result, you feel angry and resentful. Then you start to burn up and implode. To call that scenario unhealthy is an understatement.

Write about a dream that you want to actualize. Have you shared that dream with anyone? If so, have those people given you negative feedback, or support? What is the result of that interaction? Dreams are fragile; be careful about whom you enlist for support.

Why Are You Attracted to Someone?

One reason you're drawn to another person is that you're seeing a reflection of what you ideally see in yourself. The other person becomes the surrogate you. You fantasize about what the other person will fulfill for you, and the idea of that fulfillment keeps the attraction alive.

You can be attracted to someone for any number of reasons. Sometimes they're the wrong reasons; sometimes the right ones. It's okay to be attracted to someone because he or she is good-looking. There's nothing wrong with that. But of course you also have to care about what lies beyond the looks. You have to evaluate the nature of the person to see whether she or he has a warm heart, if he or she is caring and accepting. It's okay to need things from people if those things help you to be a more healthy, happy person, but it's destructive to need things that result in a disempowering relationship. Be clear about what you need.

One of the biggest problems that can come up in a relationship is dishonesty.

Honesty and trust are basic to a healthy relationship. It doesn't matter if your partner is sexy and fun to be with if you know the person is going to betray you. I know men who will stay with women who betray them because all they're concerned about is having good sex. That's all some men think about. I know women who choose to be with attractive, sexy men, without asking themselves what other qualities an ideal mate would have.

You may stay in a relationship to have someone take care of you. The price you pay is becoming dependent rather than self-reliant. You become limited because you've never attempted to expand your horizons to see what you are capable of becoming. Instead, you only continue to perpetuate basic skills. Your position in your family becomes all-important.

What happens, though, when the children grow up? Many stay-at-home mothers go through a crisis when their children leave home. It's because they have no one to be dependent *for*. If the purpose of your relationship was to have a family and you haven't made any life for yourself, one day the family is gone and you're forty or older, feeling empty, alone, and abandoned. Some mothers continue to attach themselves to their adult children, trying to play a role in their lives that goes beyond that of a parent. They meddle and try to make decisions for their children because they haven't developed a life of their own.

Do You Fear Intimacy?

Most men in our society have a terrible time expressing intimacy because of the intensity of relating that accompanies it. They want autonomy and intimacy at the same time. They want the benefits of attachment and relating and having their needs met, but they also want to be able to step aside and say, "I don't feel like being intimate now."

Women, generally speaking, are conditioned to enjoy intimacy and openness within a relationship. They have no problem sharing their feelings. These differences between women and men in our culture may cause difficulties within a relationship. One person sees intimacy as a positive thing; the other uses intimacy as a way of establishing that he's needed, but then takes a step back from the relationship. You can see the possibility for problems when you have two styles of relating that don't mesh.

Being sexual is not the same as being intimate. Intimacy leaves you open and vulnerable. It is more difficult than being sexual because it allows others to see your imperfections. Men generally are afraid their vulnerability will be used against them. Women don't want to be too open as a rule because they fear rejection. If you're telling people what you really think and feel about things that are essential to you, and others reject your thoughts as unacceptable, it's as if they're rejecting you.

Your beliefs about yourself dictate how freely you confide in someone. Once, I was out running with a bunch of guys. One of them, an artist, said some things out of the blue that two of the other guys were shocked at hearing. Later, one of the guys said, "I can't believe he told us those things." I said, "Why not? He's a very open person. Also, his belief system is autonomous. You and I will not affect the way he thinks. He's not afraid of us, nor is he in competition with us. Therefore he's willing to be open and to share his innermost feelings."

I added, "Wouldn't it be nice if you could tell your innermost secrets without fear, knowing that there was no way that you would be rejected because of them?" He replied, "Man, I have too many things I can't tell people. If I did, they would think I was some kind of kook." Yes, the likelihood is that you will be rejected and scorned for many of your innermost beliefs. As a result, most people show one side of themselves and hide another.

Some time ago, I did a special about who goes to prostitutes. I interviewed about fifteen street prostitutes, some call girls, and some escorts. The most interesting interview was with an escort who told me that her primary clients don't have sex with her, at least after the first time. The first time they think it's a prerequisite. Once they feel confident and comfortable with her, they just talk.

I asked her what they talk about and she said, "Simple things. They talk to me about things they're afraid to talk to their wives or buddies about." I asked her who these men are and she told me they come from all walks of life. A lot of them, however, are in management and government positions. They're afraid to talk openly with people around them because they have an image to maintain. What they tell her shows that these men live with fear and uncertainty. They're afraid to project their vulnerabilities. Even their families have this idea that these men are good providers who are strong, forceful, and dynamic, when that's not who they are at all. She said, "I know some men who the world perceives as dynamic and outgoing, but to me they're terrified little boys. They come to me because I'm the only person who is not going to use that against them." She added, "It's interesting how much better they feel after talking to me. It's as though I'm their therapist. I feel bad for them." What a society we have when people are terrified of telling anyone about their real feelings for fear that they will be used against them!

Are you able to express intimacy? Is it easy or difficult for you? In whom do you confide?

Where Do You Yearn to Belong?

If you are like most people, you want to belong to something. Belonging verifies who you are and makes you feel connected. You may be a loner, but if you join a club and go to meetings, you are, in a sense, no longer alone. Suddenly you count because you're a part of something, even if you're one member in a million.

I do not mean to imply for a second that you shouldn't belong to a club or organization. Joining one is a completely legitimate thing to do. I do, though, want to bring up the question of your maintaining the autonomy to make decisions for yourself while being a member. Some organizations allow you that and some don't.

The danger is that, in order to stay in an organization, you may have to give up your critical feelings about what doesn't work. Usually, you can't stay in an organization and at the same time oppose it. There's an understanding that if you're going to join anything you'd better accept that which you are joining almost unconditionally. So, for instance, if you are supporting a presidential candidate, you have to accept that person completely, even his or her obvious limitations. You must overlook these because you have committed yourself to a cause.

If you look at what a person belongs to, frequently you can get a good handle on who the person is. Some people, for instance, belong to non-mainstream movements like vegetarian societies, or the yoga movement. They will adapt much of their lifestyles to embracing the principles of their particular cause.

All of these movements have something important to contribute.

This doesn't mean, however, that the people running them are always balanced or necessarily doing the right thing. Often they're concerned only with maintaining power and control. This frustrates people and results in their leaving organizations that, ideally, they'd like to be committed to. I've met people who have gotten out of the animal rights movement because of some of the acts committed by people within the organization, such as throwing dye on people wearing animal furs. Such assaults go beyond expressing one's philosophy to transgressing a boundary, and, as a result, a lot of people won't join the animal rights movement who otherwise might have.

Groups may benefit you to a point, but be careful not to lose your identity. Joining an organization for a period of time may give you valuable information and link you to others with similar beliefs, but don't automatically take on the group's values. Question what you are told, and accept only what feels right to you. The important thing to remember is that you must not feel compelled to accept what doesn't work for you. Take what works, use it, and let go of what doesn't.

Look at where you yearn to belong. When you feel very alone and you're unable to express your ideas, you will generally join an organization that helps you feel more powerful through mutual support. The more helpless you feel, the greater the energy you need from the organization.

The same is true in a relationship. If you feel weak and unactualized, you're going to look for qualities in another person that compensate for your deficiencies. You want someone to say, for example, "Don't worry. I'm successful. I have the intellect to figure things out." That person will try to be responsible for you and many people find comfort in that. But that doesn't guarantee that that person is going to take away your problems or pain.

Again, we should always be asking questions. What do we care about? What are we bringing to that area of life? Are we rejecting what we should care about? In joining something, or in a relationship, are we allowed to be autonomous or not? To what degree do we want to be autonomous? To what degree do we want to be empowered?

Once we answer these questions we can begin to make changes, and be attached to the right things openly and completely, without fear of intimacy. When we have an open and intimate relationship we can thrive. That's where happiness and balance occur.

Stop Blaming, Start Growing

❖

Frequently we try to achieve goals that other people set for us. We take courses in college we don't want to take but think we should. We work in jobs we really don't like but think we should keep because other people tell us we're lucky to have a job. I interviewed coal miners in England and found that not one out of 200 was happy with life. In fact, they thought that my question about happiness was a stupid question. They had no concept of creating a happy, fulfilling life, and thought that the way past generations had lived was the way they should live. It was all they knew, and they saw no other options. They would even justify their way of life. "I work myself to the bone for what I have." "I don't have very much as it is." "If I tried anything else I wouldn't have anything." "How would I support my family?" Not one person I interviewed expressed a passion for living. Their mood was somber. Life was terrible.

To a large degree, it's the same way in America. People learn not to have desires because the moment they express them someone makes discouraging remarks. When you envision changes, you are told, "What are you thinking about that for? How are you going to pay the rent?" You start thinking they're right, that it is indeed foolish of you to have a desire. It's easy to see how desire gets lost.

People start to give up and live in an escapist fantasy world, which is why so many people mail in sweepstakes entries and invest in the lottery. People have stopped believing in their own creative initiative. They want something more but don't know how to go about getting it.

Why not choose to make your life different if that's what it takes to make it work? Who says it has to be difficult? I believe the opposite is true. It's really easy to make your life work. I find it's easy to be healthy. Just eat what is natural and real and leave the rest alone. It's also easy to be with people by confronting situations as they arise instead of holding them in. On the other hand, I find it difficult to hold on to something that doesn't work and then try to justify it. It's also difficult to think negative thoughts, project negative deeds, do destructive things and then try to rationalize them. These activities don't make any sense to me, so they're difficult for me to engage in.

Dealing with life honestly and openly becomes progressively easier. You get into a pattern of making the right decisions each day. You need to tune into the little voice inside of you that is connected with the subconscious mind. People are used to hearing the conscious mind all the time. That's the mind that makes almost all their decisions. The conscious mind is rational. It tries to project a public image. But the subconscious mind is always honest. It has not been changed by conditioning. It is eternal.

In order to master life you've got to be honest about what you do that keeps your life from working. Then you can focus on what will make it work. Again, it starts with desire. At the top of your list, note what you've always desired, but not paid any attention to, because you felt guilt from the conscious mind telling you all the reasons you couldn't follow through with your desire. Desire is not the pathology you've been led to believe it is.

First of all, stop having the idea that you have to justify your life. If you're like many people, about half your time is spent justifying yourself to other people, for the work you do, the emotions you have, or the relationships you have. This continual justification is a big distraction that causes you to lose focus on what you're doing. And focus is important. The most productive people are the ones who can maintain their focus on whatever work they're doing at the moment, the way a professional ball player keeps focused on the ball.

Start by honoring yourself: It's your life. You're the only one who is going to live it. No one else has the right to tell you who you are, what you are, and how you're going to live. So give yourself room to breathe by letting others know how they're affecting you. Be upfront with people. Say, for instance, "Mom, don't call me every day to see if I'm getting married or not. It's my life, not yours. I'm the one who's going to get married if and when I want to." All it takes is the courage to say to someone, "Sorry, but if you didn't call to support me and share something positive, please don't call. I'm not angry; I have started to take control of my life and I need positive reinforcement so that I can grow."

Sure the status quo of your relationship is going to be threatened when you do this. But threatening the status quo is sometimes part of the challenge of mastering life.

No matter what happens each day, I never lose my focus on what the day is, what it can mean, what I want the day to mean. I have a desire to make that day work. Do you think I'd be doing my radio shows or this book, or all the other things I do, if it weren't for the fact that part of what I have to do in life is offer service to society? I don't feel bad if people are mad at me for trying to help them, because I never lose my focus. I don't get angry either because anger would only be a distraction from that focus.

Be confident in your ability to make the right decisions. You have to go inside to do that. Learn not to be afraid of what other people will say when you make the decisions that are right for you.

How many times have you refrained from doing something because you were afraid the other people in your life would not approve? You were more concerned about their approval than you were about making the right decision. How many times in your life have you made the wrong decision because it was more important to have someone accept you than it was for you to accept the right thing for yourself? It happens all the time, because being accepted is very important to people.

Honoring your true self seems to be a secondary consideration until something is lost—until you end up overweight, for instance, or until you end up stressed and in a crisis. Then you realize that you've been making the wrong decisions, and that it's time to start making the right ones for a change. For this, you need support.

Where Does Your Support Come From?

As you grow and change, you're going to need support in many areas. Consider where you can get support for each of these aspects of your life.

Emotional

Make a list of the people and groups who give you emotional support. Are you getting enough, or is it lacking? If you need emotional support for the changes you want to make, there is no shortage of places that offer it. There are twelve-step programs, for example, and all kinds of other groups, that support change. For every homemaker who wants to get out of the home, there are women's advocacy groups that are out there to help her. There are men's advocacy groups helping them to understand what it is to be a real man and not just a superficial stereotypical model of one. It's easy enough to locate these groups: simply look in the Yellow Pages under self-help or support groups. A recent scanning found more than forty different ones.

Remember, change is a long-term process, and you've got to have emotional support you can count on. If you don't have it, look for it. It's not going to come to you. You're going to have to be assertive and find the people who will support you without criticizing, condemning, or trying to manipulate you.

Financial

Getting financial support from people means more than getting money from them. Frequently, it takes the form of advice that will help you improve the quality of your life. Someone might listen to me lecture and respond by saying, "It all sounds nice, Gary, but I'm living on $32,000 a year. Sure, I'd really like to change; I do feel stagnant. I've lived in the same place for so long, and I'd like to be someplace else. I've got some things I'd like to do. But I can't afford any of them."

My response would be, "You're right and you're wrong. You're right in that you can't afford change if you're not looking for options. You're wrong because people without much money also try to change their lifestyles, and many succeed. I can show you people who have wonderful lifestyles. They're deprived of nothing they feel they need, and they're living lives radically different from those they used to live. They've learned to change and do without many of the unnecessary trappings of life."

Let me tell you about a technique I use each year. You may or may not find this useful. I never start a new project before stopping an old one. I even give up things that are profitable. I stop them and just let them go. People think this is the dumbest thing in the world. "My God," they say, "you took so much time and energy and commitment to create something and now that it's succeeding you're giving it up? Why?"

I feel that if I start doing more things than I can reasonably take on, then I don't have a balanced life. And I believe that having a balanced life is so important that I'm willing to give things up to support that balance. In doing so, I have more time for myself, and I have the opportunity to do something different.

As I start a new project I ask myself, do I want this to be a one-year, two-year, three-year, four-year, or five-year project? I don't do anything longer than five years. I can't see doing anything longer than that.

Think about what would be different in your life if you were told you had five years to live. Would you start doing things differently? Frequently what you would start doing is what you really want to do. Find ways of doing it now.

Part of the art of living and mastering life is the art of letting go. The more you let go, the more you have room and freedom for better things. Every year I try to give away as much as I can. This is a big challenge when you come from a background where you never had anything. I come from a very poor background. I've been working since the age of eight, and nothing has been given to me at any point in life, so to be able to give things away is a challenge. Being strict about getting rid of things makes you realize what you can live without. If you don't learn to let go of things then you just have clutter.

A friend of mine recently went through a major crisis over his uncertainty about his career of twenty-two years. Finally, in one absolutely nerve-wracking weekend, he let go of his career and went through withdrawal, crisis, and a lot of depression. Two days later, he was offered an opportunity to do something that was wonderful for him, even though it was only a six-month project. I advised him not to look for projects that were going to take him through the rest of his life, but for projects that act as transition points, that will take him to a new level.

Right now he's living in Arizona on a dude ranch. Here's what's amazing. We were watching the film *City Slickers*, and all through the film he kept saying, "I'd love to do that." And then the day came when someone gave him the opportunity to do it. The first words out of his mouth were all negative: "I don't have the money and I've never ridden a horse. . . ." I said to him, "Hold on. Give me ten reasons why you would like to do it, and how you could. If you had stopped with the negatives you wouldn't have done it, but you went ahead and showed that you can do it." That's what I'm talking about—look for the reasons why.

Intellectual

What education do you need in order to do what you want to do? One nice thing about the United States is that we have more classes, workshops, and adult education than any other country in the world. We are a nation filled with rejuvenation and growth. Look at the Learning Annex here in New York City. Look at all their classes and workshops. Look at the 92nd Street Y and all their lectures and workshops. You can get any skills you need. And you can barter for services if you don't have the money, through a practice called creative scholarship exchanges. There's always something you have that will help someone else, and they in turn will help you. Virtually every organization, individual, or group has a need for part-time assistance—helping with mailings, answering the mail, filing, and the like. Generally, if you approach the office manager and explain that because of a temporary shortage of funds you're not able to pay but would be able to work part-time in exchange for the classes, they can probably accommodate you. After all, the lecture is their "product," and having one more person in a class does not take away any of their income. Speaking for myself, I have never given a lecture or workshop or retreat where several people didn't approach me to say that they wanted to attend but couldn't afford it. I never refused a soul and am sure others are of like mind.

List Your Special Attributes and Skills

Often you're not even aware of how special you are. You're not cognizant of your skills and attributes. Write them down. Many of your attributes may be the result of having gotten through crises, or the crises may have shown you that you had them all along. Think of all the crises in your life that you've weathered. In all likelihood you've already weathered the very things you've feared the most. You've probably already gone through separations, deaths, firings—a lot of things that are traumatizing and high up on the stress scale. You've survived and are stronger for your experiences. If you think along these lines, nothing should create fear now.

We've all experienced humiliation; we've all gone through these processes and survived. That's what's nice about an AA or an OA meeting. You get people to stand up and say what they've done and how they have survived. They're acknowledging that they have a life beyond their crippling experiences.

What have you survived? How are you stronger from the experience? What special attributes did you learn you have as a result of what you've been through?

Do You Sabotage Your Own Efforts?

Watch to see whether you sabotage your own efforts. The moment you start feeling a little depressed or unfocused, do you undermine your efforts so that you need to start all over? An example of this would be going on an eating binge when you've been trying to reform your diet.

Watch out for the process of self-sabotage. List ways you engage in it. If you have a really close friend, or if you're part of a support group, let someone know what you do to sabotage yourself. Ask the person for help when you start hurting yourself. A little support goes a long way. Hopefully, in time, you'll be your own best support system.

Do Your Inner Beliefs and Outer Realities Complement Each Other?

Believing in one thing and doing another generates conflict. It creates a psychic spasm. Check to see whether you live according to your own beliefs or according to other people's. How many times have you adopted behaviors inconsistent with your inner feelings because you felt you should be loyal to people? You need not honor them out of some bizarre loyalty. Think of how many people on the inside knew that our country shouldn't have been involved in Operation Desert Storm. They went along with it because everyone else was wrapping themselves up in loyalty to the flag and being patriotic. They were living a double standard and causing conflict within themselves.

Don't be afraid to commit yourself to whatever you feel in your heart, even if you feel that you're in the minority. When you acknowledge what's in your heart, you are getting in touch with spiritual truth. If spiritual truth is on your side, you're a majority of one.

Are You Able to Forgive?

What unresolved conflicts are you still holding onto? Unresolved conflicts keep you from getting on with your life because you give them all your attention.

There's a time when you've got to give them up. You have to stop feeling sorry for yourself and angry because someone betrayed and used you, or because you didn't do more with your life. Start perceiving unfortunate things that have happened to you as nothing more than learning experiences, and let them go. Now you're right on track.

There are a million ways to forgive. Every religion and every belief system has a way of forgiving. But in order for forgiveness to happen, you first have to realize that you no longer need to invest in the pain that came from the original indiscretion or abuse. You have to make your life more important than your pain. The original pain is gone. All you're living with now is the memory of that pain. That's not very smart, is it? And it's not being kind to yourself either. It was bad enough that you were abused, disregarded, or hurt as a human being. Now you're compounding the damage by living with something long after the experience. You're revolving your life around painful memories. That keeps you from expressing your true self and functioning as a whole, dynamic, integrated human being.

Give it up. You don't need a lifetime to do it. You don't need thirty-five workshops with all the currently popular leaders out there telling you all about your mother and father and what they did to you. You know that already. Just say to yourself, "My life is more important than the memory of that pain."

You're more than just your experiences. You're a living entity with a capacity to create, feel, and grow. Yes, you have experiences that you can draw feelings and emotions from, but you shouldn't become merely the feelings and emotions of your experience. I know a woman who was raped by a black man on the subway when she was sixteen. Today, she hates all blacks. He didn't rape her because he was black; he could have been any color, but in her heart she formed a hatred against all black people. Her whole reality has become distorted based on her perception of what caused her pain.

Experiences can give you an understanding of life, and you can learn just as much from negative experiences as from positive ones. That doesn't mean that if you have a bad experience you yourself have to become negative. You don't have to start feeling bad about yourself just because someone says something to you that's uncomplimentary. That would be allowing the person to manipulate you, which doesn't make a whole lot of sense. Your self-esteem goes down when you allow an experience to be more essential to you than your own inner dynamics. All that an experience should do is give you a greater understanding of life.

Once I was invited to participate at a feminist meeting, but I never got the chance to talk. If I had gotten a chance to, the audience would have heard about the spiritual feminist perspective as viewed through a male perspective. But the people at that meeting were not into hearing anything of a spiritual feminist nature. In fact, the woman who headed the meeting had a very hateful attitude toward men. I did not overreact to the situation. I felt the woman supported a particularly radical political and sexist position, not a spiritually and humanistically feminist one. But she had a right to that. I know that another workshop that I'm invited to will have a completely different perspective. What I'm saying is that you shouldn't jump to angry or defensive stances based on individual experiences. Allow them to be what they are—individual experiences.

Living defensively keeps you from mastering life. You need to be vulnerable. Otherwise you have all sorts of problems. You become fat, stressed out, angry, locked in the past, and full of excuses. You blame the world because your life isn't working.

Where in your life do you live defensively? You've got to deal with this, so look at your biases, notice your conditioned beliefs, and acknowledge them for what they are. Clean them out or you'll be carrying them around forever.

When you defend wrong beliefs you become defensive about it. When people want to defend the merits of their beliefs they pass a law. The state of Illinois passed a law, for example, that made pregnancy a condition that doctors exclusively must treat. The law passed despite a New Mexico health study done over an eleven-year period that shows midwives to be more effective at helping women give birth, at far less cost. Their death rates are lower and they have a five-percent cesarean section rate as opposed to the twenty-seven-percent rate that obstetricians have. The state of Illinois ignored the evidence and excluded midwives from participating in the birthing process with their new law. That is simply a wrong belief. And the fact that it is law institutionalizes it.

Once something becomes law, people start to think it's beyond question. Of course, the law can be challenged and amended, but that's quite difficult because, unfortunately, people tend to be more focused on obeying the law than on examining its merits, or asking whether it is just. The average person won't challenge the law. In fact, most people won't challenge anything that's wrong. They won't challenge the quality of their food, air, soil, or anything else. Instead, they've come to accept things as they are because they haven't challenged their own lives. If you're not challenging your own life and what doesn't work within it, you'll certainly never challenge what is outside of your own life.

How do you react to negative experiences? What can you learn from them? List the feelings you have that are not completely reasonable and rational. What experiences are you reacting to?

Whom Do You Blame for Your Problems and Feelings?

If you're going to master life and live happily, you've got to stop blaming. People who want to master life don't blame; they take control of their lives. Did you ever notice that the people out there who are trying and learning make more mistakes than anybody else, yet they never blame anybody for them? They just get back up and try again. I counseled a woman last year who blamed everything on everybody and everything. She projected her anger onto others instead of taking responsibility for making her life work. She spent all her time blaming and had no time left for action. That person was no better when she stopped counseling than when she started.

Blamers are people who, when they try and fail, seem to fall in cement. They get stuck in their failure. All they look at is the pain and anger of their failure, and who they can blame for it. If you get caught up in blaming, you stop growing. Show me someone who blames and I'll show you someone who hasn't grown since the day they began to blame. Their life stops; it's like they're dead. People blame because they're looking for an escape. Blaming is just a way of keeping their minds from looking for constructive solutions.

When you make a commitment to do something new, accept that you're going to make mistakes. It's alright to fail. That's a part of life. It's how you'll grow and learn. Once you stop blaming, you'll have room to grow. You'll become more interested in what you're doing than in the consequences of not doing it right. Something good happens when you take on that attitude.

When you develop the right attitude you're not going to be afraid to take some major risks. The people I know whose lives have succeeded have taken lots of risks. They've had many failures, but a lot of rewards too. In fact, I've never met anyone who succeeds at life who doesn't take risks. At some point you have to realize that without risks there is no reward. What risks are you willing to take? No risks? No reward. Small risks? Small reward. Take a big risk, get a big reward.

What risks are you willing to take to get where you want to go? Does fear of failure stop you? Do you blame others when things don't work out, or do you see it as part of the learning process?

Are Your Limitations Real?

Is your whole life bounded by limitations? How real are they? Who put them there? How long have these limitations been there? What have you done to adapt to them?

People tell me what they can't do. They never tell me what they can do. The moment they say, "I don't think . . ." I stop them and say, "Then why are you here? If you talk that way you'll never get anywhere."

I work with people who say can do, will do, here I am, let's do it. It's no big deal. It's simple. The people who want to do, do it. The people who don't, make excuses.

Start to listen to how people talk. Listen to the excuses.

Limitations should not be set before you try something. Otherwise your conditioned responses, which come largely from the experiences and the input of other people, will dictate what you're willing to try. This places artificial limitations in front of you. Think of how many senior citizens in our society never set foot inside a health club because of a social image they adhere to. They don't believe they ought to mix with the younger culture. Working out isn't something they should be doing. They think that instead of keeping fit they should be staying at home rocking on their porches and taking medicines. Because of an artificial limitation they've placed on themselves, they're missing out on something that could be of enormous benefit.

What would you like to do but feel you can't? What limitations do you perceive? Look for role models to follow if that's what it takes to get started. Look at where you've been successful in your own life despite your conditioning to the contrary. What have you done that you were not expected to do?

What Price Do You Pay for Success?

We've been talking largely about failure. Now let's consider success. You are probably successful in some area of your life, perhaps several. What price do you pay for your success? Are you stressed out, for example? How does that stress affect you? Does the stress equal the benefits? Is it balanced by the success?

It's rare to find a person we call successful in our society's conventional sense that doesn't end up paying a big price for that success. I've counseled many successful people. This past summer I worked with an internationally known artist who was enormously stressed. He was afraid to turn jobs down even though he was overworked. He couldn't say no to all the commissions. I asked him why he didn't just take a year off. After all, he had plenty of money. He said he was terrified of taking a step backward. Someone else might come in and take his place. This man is a prisoner of his own success. His drive to go on and on creates a pressure that will ultimately destroy the quality of what he has succeeded at.

Our society tends to praise successful people, often giving them more praise than they deserve. Two people will go into a boxing ring to beat each other up and get more praise and recognition than all of the Nobel Prize winners in history. In America, success gives you access. People suddenly pay attention to you, whether you deserve it or not.

Once successful, people become fearful of losing this attention and try to hold on to that success more tightly than ever, like the artist I counseled. They're afraid they might lose it all. If you don't fight, you get stripped of your crown. In broadcasting and television, with rare exceptions, the moment you go off the air, no matter how popular you are, it's almost impossible to get back on. The same is true for writers. Once you stop publishing, you're forgotten. As a result, most successful people don't know how to say no.

Seeking success to gain public approval will make you insecure and apprehensive. The public is fickle, and if you start to fail in any way it will withdraw its support of you. Just as we're enamored with people climbing up the ladder of success, we don't like to associate with someone on his way down. Once you're down nobody will help you get back up; we're very hard on people who are trying to make a comeback. So people end up constantly striving, terrified of losing status.

We make success almost impossible to sustain while staying happy and healthy. I think it's because our society doesn't encourage people to make mistakes and learn from their failures. We don't allow people to show their flaws once they've attained a hero's status. For instance, we want to keep Pete Rose out of the Hall of Fame for betting on his own team, even though that has nothing to do with his status as a great athlete.

We need to keep balanced and realize that success is more than financial, more than public adulation. Success is how you grow on nonmaterial levels as well. Success can be internal. It can be learning to relate to people well, growing spiritually and emotionally. You can be successful in any area of life. Go forward because you want to learn and enjoy life. If you're only motivated by your fear then you're still a prisoner, you're not balanced, and you're not mastering anything.

What Have You Had It With?

An effective way to focus on changing your life is to write on a piece of paper the things you've had it with. In a prominent place, such as on your mirror or refrigerator, or on your desk at work, place a little sign that reads, "I've had it with _____."

That will focus your attention on what needs to be changed. In that moment when you say, "I've had it!" you are facing your life truthfully. You're being honest. You're saying, "I'm out of here. I'm changing this." You've reached your limit. It's the last straw. You've tolerated too much abuse, indifference, or imbalance, and you've had enough.

Do this each day. Ask, what have I had it with? What am I going to change? This exercise eliminates a big buffer zone for excuses and adaptations. Remember, you're extremely adaptable. You keep adapting to what doesn't work. If something doesn't work, you twist, you turn, you contort yourself emotionally because you've adapted to so many different things that aren't you. Straighten up and say, "I've had it. I'm not wearing anything that I don't like. I'm not saying anything I don't believe. I'm not doing anything that doesn't honor me. I'm not relating to people who don't respect who I am."

Making an "I've had it" list each day will not only help you see what works and what doesn't work in your life, it will give you the courage and the impetus to actually make change happen. A friend of mine had been overweight and a hypochondriac for over twenty years. One day I asked him, "Have you had it?" and he said that he had. He made a list of the things he had had it with and one of the things on his list was compulsive overeating. He ate a lot of junk foods. I said, "Now that you've made a list, do you want to change?" and he said yes.

We took the food from the cupboards and threw away everything that wasn't good. We threw away *everything*. His heart was palpitating as I chanted, "Junk, junk, junk." Not only did we throw food away, we stomped on it. I even put food on top of the toilet as a symbolic gesture. I said, "This is crap. It belongs down the toilet, not in your body." When we finished I said, "Now that you've got it all out, keep it out."

This was a painful process for my friend, who was actually sweating as he let all this go. It was traumatic for him, but at the end of the day he had a whole new kitchen full of healthful foods and cookbooks that we bought. He later hired a person to come in once a week to cook lots of good food and freeze it for him. He joined an overeater's support group and each day called someone to make sure he stayed on his plan. He took it day by day.

Today he is of normal weight, in perfect health, and wouldn't go back to his old ways for anything. It took him over two decades, but it started on the day he said, "I've had it."

Make a list of the things you've had it with. During the week, select one item you need to change. When you feel balanced in that area, deal with the next item on your list.

Creating a Healthy Goal

Do you stop yourself short of your goal? Perhaps you allow whatever feelings you wake up with to dictate your actions for the rest of the day. If you wake up feeling good, then everything seems possible. If you start the day feeling bad, you hold yourself back. You don't believe you can do what you set out to do, and you make excuses to keep yourself from getting things done. In effect, you make something or someone out there responsible for how you feel inside. You wake up waiting for bits and pieces of light to hit you and make you feel good about who you are, instead of affirming that you are always in the light. The trouble is, once you take a step past the light you're back in the dark again. Now it's just another day, there's another person to deal with, another occurrence; that nice little ray of sunlight is no longer hitting you.

The danger in thoughts like these is that you start to believe that you can't motivate yourself. In the absence of self-sustained positive energy, you become helpless and hapless. You start looking for excuses to justify your lack of initiative and, as a result, you never fulfill your personal goals.

Life becomes different when you realize that every step you take in life is illuminated with eternal love and joy. This is something that preceded you and that will be here long after you are gone. Knowing there is light and love within you wherever you go promotes a true sense of happiness.

This knowledge kindles the desire to take appropriate risks for the joy of it. Every action you take naturally sets off a chain of events. If something good happens and you receive a reward, that's fine. But if it doesn't, that's alright too. What you do is not going to be predicated upon whether or not it makes you feel good. Instead, you will already feel good when you wake up, and you will sustain that good feeling no matter what happens.

Don't wait for someone or something out there to acknowledge that you're okay. Get out of your own way and make a life for yourself. Learn to use your mind positively and don't worry; worrying never accomplishes anything. Use the mind in a relaxed, natural way. That allows you to explore life for the curiosity, wonderment, joy, grace, innocence, and honesty of it. Dare to be different. Life is about taking appropriate risks. They're what make it worth living.

Let's explore some reasons why you may get in your own way and keep yourself from creating and achieving healthy goals.

What Are You Uncertain Of?

Uncertainties can keep your life in a state of perpetual postponement. So it's important to look at what you're uncertain of and then deal with it. Look at the following areas of your life to determine how uncertainty holds you back.

Fantasies

Fantasies will impede you if you retreat into them instead of using them as a catalyst for constructive change. If you're working at a boring job, for example, you could fantasize about working someplace else but not follow up and make plans that can lead to change. You could stay there, spending most of the day engaged in escapist thoughts. But imagine what could happen if you were to put effort into making your fantasy into reality. Who's to say it couldn't happen?

The mind is powerful. It can take you to new heights, but it can also constrain you. The other day, for example, I worked with three people who have just committed themselves to racing nationally. They want to be as healthy and as fast as they can possibly be. These are not elite athletes; they're just normal people who dream of becoming athletes. I pushed them very hard. One person said, "I can't go a seven-minute mile. I've never gone faster than a nine-minute mile." Ten minutes later when I had the treadmill on, I didn't tell him what he was doing. I just encouraged him to go a little faster. He was working at a seven-minute mile pace and was keeping up with it.

After the first mile, I said, "Now I'm going to take you into the seven-minute range." He gasped, "I can't do it; it's too hard." He had already done it at that time but when I put it into his mind that he was going to have to do it, he pulled back.

He was completely surprised when I told him he already did it. That's the power the mind can have over the body—it's not always a positive power. The demon inside says, "Can't do it. Can't do it. Can't do it."

If you ever think you can't do something because you're not as talented or capable as someone else, perhaps you don't know what you are capable of doing. The only thing standing between you and your higher self is you. Don't worry about what other people are doing. All you can do is the best *you* can do. Honor that, whatever it is. You may even learn that you are more capable and talented than you ever realized. But nothing will ever happen until you allow yourself to actualize your creative fantasies.

Intuition

Intuitively, you know what feels right. The problem occurs when the conscious mind tries to rationalize your feelings away. Inside you know the honesty and integrity of the people you're dealing with. The internal self never lies. It gives you a signal to either stop or go.

Are you able to differentiate the signals your heart sends from the signals of the mind? Notice how the mind steps in and creates chaos, pain, and confusion that blocks you. Let your intuition be your guide; don't be a prisoner of the rational mind.

Commitment

You may feel uncertain about what you want to commit yourself to. You may not know what to do with your life. Remember that commitment is not just a matter of enjoyment but integral to your growth as a human being. It allows you to connect with something greater than your own life, something spiritual. It gives your life meaning.

If you don't commit yourself to something higher than yourself, then you are committing yourself to your lower nature, concentrating on such things as indulgences and distractions. Distractions are acceptable as long as they're kept in perspective. But when money and other signs of outward success become your focus, then you don't really have a life. One day you wake up, look in the mirror, and think, "My God, look how old I've gotten, and what have I got to show for it? What have I committed myself to?" You've devoted yourself to wrong values and wrong decisions based upon insecurity, invulnerability, and being a prisoner of the rational mind. You have all the things you thought would make you happy and you don't have happiness.

The key is, can you be happy with none of the things that you've worked so hard to get? If you can, then you're a truly happy person.

Think for a moment. What is the most important thing you've committed yourself to in the past year? Is it something as important as, or more important than, your own life?

Are Your Expectations Realistic?

I was helping a racewalker train when he commented that he wanted to start running instead of racewalking. I asked him why and he responded that he didn't think he was a fast racewalker. I reassured him that I thought he was fast. We discussed the fact that if he ran he would probably run a 6.5-minute mile. Since people in his age group are doing between 4.55 and 5.05, he'd be running long after everyone else was finished. Without self-confidence, he would give up before long. However, if he continued racewalking, he would remain in the top group and improve his self-esteem.

My suggestion is to first do something you can do well and that you like doing. That gives you a chance to develop confidence. Establish some short-term goals for yourself. Once you accomplish those you will gain an inner fortitude that will enable you to take on new goals. I suggested that the racewalker continue in order to feel what it's like to excel before starting to run.

Once you succeed at one thing, you have greater strength, which makes it easier to work toward something else. You've got to be realistic about your expectations. It may take years to get to your destination. If you plan your strategy properly, with short-term, intermediate, and long-term goals, you'll be able to note different points in your development. You'll be able to say, "I've really accomplished something." Your progress will be more satisfying if you note improvements along the way.

What Expectations Do You Have Of Others?

Once you start experiencing success you expect other people to have equal success. You want other people to join you in your success. You're motivated and you want other people to be motivated as well. Your life is happy and you want other people to have a happy life too.

It's fine to want that but, again, your expectations must be realistic. Is the other person capable of doing what you would like her (or him) to do? Is that what she wants in her life? If not, don't blame her and don't interfere with her life. Accept people for who they are.

One of the worst things you can do is to force your expectations onto another person. A friend of mine contacted me, asking for work. I hired him, first, because he was a friend in need, and second, because he could make a legitimate contribution to my office. He was honest, and told me that because of his addictions he had not worked more than two hours a day for twenty years. He was highly anxious, and explained that because of substance abuse he was hyper, and could only stay focused for short periods of time before looking for distractions. As a result, I suggested he begin by working two hours per day. I felt that to expect more of him than he expected of himself would place immediate stress upon him. Instead, I proposed that he add one hour per day each week, so that by the end of six weeks he would theoretically be working eight-hour days. He agreed to give it a try. At the end of six weeks, he was able to work four hours per day. By some standards, this was a failure. By my standards, this was a partial success. Within nine months he was able to remain sober, drug-free, and not gamble. He had also gone on an exercise and health program, and was attending support group meetings—as well as staying focused on his work.

Look at the people in your life and ask yourself, what are they honestly capable of giving me? That's all you should expect. If they choose to give you more, fine, that's a plus. The point is that having reasonable expectations of people will help you avoid a lot of pain in your life.

Or simply don't ask anything of others. Give without the need to receive. Then you will never be disappointed.

What Are the Consequences of Your Thoughts and Actions?

There is a consequence to everything you do in life. Do something positive and you'll create a positive result; do something negative and you'll create negativity. If you're bitter and cynical, expect bitter and cynical returns. There's no mystery to this; what you do is self-fulfilling.

Everything you do or say affects someone else at some level. Either you're helping someone or you're causing him harm. If you're not helping someone through your thoughts, actions, and words, *stop* before you affect him in a negative way. Pause and look at the effects you're having on the other person. You have no right to denigrate the human spirit.

If You Had Only Five Years Left to Live, What Would You Change?

I live my life in five-year cycles. I change entirely every five years, giving up much of what I've accumulated during that time so that I can accomplish other things. Only by letting go of things do we have the freedom to move forward and do something else. The problem is, we're terrified of what's going to happen if we let go. We're afraid, for example, of the high rate of unemployment. In reality, many of the people ultimately beset by unemployment are people who have had ample opportunities to develop alternate careers, skills, and attitudes, but chose not to. While they were working, they never considered the possibility that they could ever lose their jobs. When they lose their jobs, rather than look for opportunities for self-improvement, many of them choose to blame. They sit at home and overeat and are angry. They watch television and wait for someone to come and take them back. They want someone else to be responsible for their working again. That's a welfare mentality. That's saying, I don't want to do it for myself. I want you to do it for me.

What about people who do want to do something for themselves? For every ten people who victimize themselves, I'll show you someone in the same situation who goes out and has a life because he or she has a focus. As long as you have some desire, that desire will motivate you to get a focus, to get an image of what you want.

A sixty-year-old salesperson I knew had burnt himself out. When I asked him, "Where do you want to be?" he said, "I'm sick of the cold climate. I'm sick of all the hustling. I'd like to be in a nice, warm climate where there are positive people who can accept me for just being me."

I suggested that he look into Hawaii. Hawaii is full of adventurous, positive people. It's full of beautiful places to live. It's nice all year round.

He's been there for a couple of years now, and he's as happy as can be. He's managing a surfing show on television. He's not making a lot of money, but he doesn't need it. He's not counting the dollars; he's looking at the happiness. He's in the environment he needs to be in.

For other people, New York might be the perfect environment. It depends upon where you see yourself and what your needs are.

How Do Others Respond to Your Actions?

There will always be both positive and negative responses to your actions. I spoke with Tony Brown, who had featured me on his TV special about AIDS, about the response to my appearance on the show. He had gotten a lot of positive feedback and some negative reactions as well. One doctor was very angry when he called. "How dare you have Gary Null on the show!" he said. "Where did Gary get those documents? I want those documents. I have a right to those documents." Tony answered, "You don't have a right to anything. Gary got those because he did his homework. Why don't you do yours?"

You see, the doctor was angry because I had held up documents onscreen showing that a person with AIDS had improved using vitamin C drips, ozone therapy, a natural foods diet, juicing, meditation, and guided visualization and prayer, all of which the doctor claimed had no relevance to health. If I hadn't shown the documents, anyone could say the documents didn't exist and keep the AIDS myth going. They could say no cure exists because there's not a shred of evidence that it does. But I had the evidence. Now all they could do was denigrate me for not giving the evidence to them.

Another man called, angry about the fact that I wouldn't see him personally about his AIDS. I had spoken with 1800 people. I thought that was enough. If all I do is speak with people all day long, I don't have time to do any of the other things that allow me to help more people. I gave him the names and phone numbers of doctors in his area who could help him, but that's not what he wanted. He wanted hours of my time. But that wasn't reasonable. If he were to call a lawyer and ask for free time, I don't think he would really expect to get it. Since I don't charge people for my time, some people assume it's not worth anything.

What I'm getting at is that you need to act based on your own convictions, not in response to other people who would have you act to fulfill their personal agendas, which may be in opposition to yours. Do you act in ways that are in accordance with your own inner convictions, or do you act to try to please others?

List Your Assets

You may feel you can't grow because you don't have the necessary resources. You think you can't get out of your rut because you're not capable enough. I say that's not true. You're just unaware of your assets.

To become more aware of what they are, list the assets that allow you to grow, enjoy life, engage yourself on all levels, and make your life happen. Write down your assets in each of the following areas of your life.

Spiritual

What are your spiritual assets? Whenever you have any problem, your spirit helps you to overcome it, change, face the crisis. It gives you inner strength more enduring than that supplied by any outside influence. It lets you know that no matter what, you're still okay.

If you acknowledge your spirit, you honor the hero that's inside you. A true hero holds the spirit in high esteem. There's a true sense of sacrifice, not fear. In battle, people often become heroes, and in sports, athletes with the warrior spirit become heroes. In Somalia, volunteer doctors trying to help people are heroes. There's no publicity. They're not doing it for any gain. They're doing it because they're honoring the spirit. And it touches us.

When your spiritual self is guiding you, then everything you do stems from unconditional love. You don't manipulate, lie, or deceive. You don't do anything that dishonors the human spirit and hence you don't dishonor other people. There is no hidden agenda.

Getting in touch with the hero inside you allows the best part of your nature to emerge. You instantly know what is real and true. One of the ways to grow is to honor the inner spirit—the warrior, the hero, the healer. Every human being has it. So acknowledge it, let it out, and discover that suddenly you're a different human being because you don't face adversity in the old way. Panic, desperation, overreaction, anger, and anxiety leave. Instead you can deal with life and every problem that arises. You keep your balance. You're confident that you're going to be okay no matter what. That spiritual component is an important asset. Use it.

Intellectual

What are your intellectual assets? Your intellect is what allows you to reason, to look at all aspects of an issue, and thus to find solutions to problems. Intellect gives you the ability to discern choices and the judgment to value certain choices over others. It provides you with perspective so that you don't have to feel overwhelmed. You can choose to do something in a way that is reasonable, considering your needs.

Emotional

List your emotional assets. Can you express your emotions to other people? Do you understand your own emotions? Healthy emotions are accompanied by an understanding of what you're feeling. You might, for instance, feel upset every time someone questions you. Instead of reacting to your emotion, stop yourself and ask, "Where does this emotion come from? Why is it every time this happens I feel this way?" If you don't get in touch with what you're feeling, you might find yourself re-peating an undesirable pattern of behavior.

Educational

Most people assume that their education is what they've learned in school. But formal schooling is relatively insignificant to your education. Most of what you learn in school has nothing to do with whether you succeed in life. Most schools don't teach the important lessons, such as interpersonal communication, problem solving, conflict resolution, and critical thinking. You learn these lessons in life, and they are critical to your well-being. Quite simply, everyone has gained some unique skills, knowledge, or insights from their education. These can be used to your advantage. Don't downplay them.

Location

Look at the assets your location has to offer. Many people, for instance, downplay New York. A woman sitting next to me on a flight from Texas hated New York and told me everything wrong with it—the crime and violence, for instance. I told her she was both right and wrong. Yes, there is crime, but every city in America has crime. And there's violence everywhere too. What she neglected to notice was that New York has better career opportunities than any other place in America. There are also some beautiful environments in New York and many wonderful people. There are more museums than in any other place on earth. All of these assets, plus New York's uniqueness, color, and vitality are the reasons I choose to live there.

Think about where you live. What are its assets? And do you take advantage of them?

How Have You Used Your Assets to Enhance Your Life?

Have you ever asked yourself, what is the best that I can be? Have you ever pictured yourself without any constraints, moving beyond what you now think is possible? You can't undo your limitations to a certain degree. You either shed your limitations or you don't.

Make a note to yourself that starting tomorrow, you're going to create the ideal self, the ideal job, and the ideal relationship. Maybe you have it all now. If you do, fine. Then honor it. If you don't, then gather up all your assets, focus on your ideal self, and work toward what you want.

Honoring Your Assets

With every asset comes a responsibility that you must honor. You honor your assets by using them. Each day that you don't use an asset, you weaken yourself. This morning, for example, I did a speed workout along the Central Park Reservoir even though there was a 37 degree below-zero wind chill factor. Why? My physical fitness is an asset, I honor it, and I want to keep using it—daily. (By the way, when you start moving, your body warms up, so that five minutes into a speed workout you can be sweating. In many cases what you might anticipate to be problematic—in this instance the cold—turns out not to be a problem at all.)

Create a Plan to Increase Your Assets and Decrease Your Liabilities

Notice the liabilities that keep showing up in your life—fear, lack of time, anger. How might you limit these? The first step is to know what you don't want in your life. If people keep wasting your time, for example, you can simply let them know how they make you feel by saying, "Sorry, I don't have time to give you."

You can overcome your own fears by facing them head on. You'll find that most of your fears stem from your imagination more than from reality.

For example, many people fear financial failure. But if you envision the worst that could possibly happen, you can dissipate that fear. Does losing what you have change you as a person? I know people who live on ashrams or other retreats for periods of their lives, with no material possessions whatsoever, to better understand their spirituality. They own nothing. They eat a frugal diet and sleep on mats in a communal room. These people give up everything to practice techniques that enhance their spiritual awareness. When they feel a renewed inner strength that connects them to a larger vision of life, they go back into the world. What these people find is that what they have in the world is not as important as knowing who they are.

People in the most economically distressed circumstances can live a completely fulfilling life. I would rather have a fulfilling life that allows me to feel good about myself as a person than have financial or material security. Of course, this attitude requires taking risks.

I met a man on the street who came from a Wall Street background. He said that one day he found himself homeless because he had waited too long to change. After he lost his job, he waited and waited to get rehired. He used up all his money and wasn't able to pay his mortgage. His friends and family stopped lending him money. One day he came home and his door was locked. They had taken all of his belongings. Everything he had feared, everything he had worked so hard to keep from happening, happened in that instant.

He spent three days on the street in a state of shock. He wouldn't go to a shelter even for food.

On the fourth day he thought, "What the heck am I doing? I've got a mind." He started going through garbage and recycling things. He got giant garbage bags and did ten times the recycling of anybody else. From this he made $60 a day. He was able to do that seven days a week and earn $420, which is more than most people in America take home.

He was able to get back on his feet. In two months he had a small apartment. He started a home-based business, and began attending night school. Now he has a whole new career. Ironically, it's the career he had always wanted but was afraid he couldn't do.

Now he's not afraid of losing what he has, because when the bottom fell out he survived. He's a stronger person for what he went through. He realizes that when things fall apart, they fall apart for a reason. On Wall Street he hadn't been content with his life and had needed to change. But he'd been afraid to let go, to take risks. He was living by his fear, not his strength. Now he has a life he enjoys.

Ask yourself if you hold on to old ways that no longer serve you because of fear. Are you able to let go and trust that something new and better will replace the old? Once again, look at your assets. Notice what you are capable of doing and focus on that instead of on your fears. Life is as self-fulfilling as you imagine it.

Create Both Short- and Long-term Goals

Goals help you to become more balanced and whole because they give you a sense of purpose and direction. You become engaged in the process of your life.

You should have both long-term and short-term goals. The long-term goals should be slightly beyond your reach; the short-term goals should be those you can attain if you keep your sense of focus.

Give yourself one week to create a short-term goal. Each day, take time to create your plan. Use the input you receive here, as well as from the many other resources you have. What you learn only becomes meaningful when actualized.

Then create a long-term goal. When I write a book I don't just wake up one morning and jot down the entire thing off the top of my head. I start with a plan of action. One project can take me two to three years to complete. Research and planning take time and patience, but I know that as long as I keep focused, I can do it.

You must be willing to acknowledge that you will make errors. You'll fall off track at times. We all do that. As long as you get back on track, you'll be alright.

Do You Become Excited by the Possibility of Change But Fail to Actualize It?

You may think you are ready to change but never actually take action. You make excuses instead. You are going to start a diet tomorrow. You're prepared to throw out all the sugar, meat, caffeine, and everything else that's bad for you. Then you think maybe you shouldn't get rid of it. After all, it cost you seventeen dollars.

Forget the seventeen dollars! You have to do something each

day to affirm your commitment to change, and one of the easiest things for you to do is to toss away all the bad food. Select a goal for the day in the area that you specifically want to change. When you wake up in the morning, the very first thing you need to do is work out a strategy to achieve that goal, whatever it is. Write it down. Work toward that goal every single day, seven days a week. That helps you to focus on what you need to do for yourself.

Make that one small goal the focal point of your day. Make everything else secondary. Your goal becomes your reason for waking up in the morning. That motivation will help you achieve what you want.

At the end of the week you will have achieved seven minor goals, and at the end of the month, 28 to 31. In one month, three months, six months, and one year you can achieve goals of increasing magnitude. In a year's time you will have accomplished a life goal, as well as 365 minor goals, 12 important goals, four major goals, and two long-range goals. Think of it: all of this in just a year, by concentrating on one thing per day.

Once you achieve your goal, don't take a step backward. If your goal for the day is not to have sugar, don't have sugar. This is not unrealistic if you are concerned only with honoring your body and mind. You're establishing new priorities. In effect, you're starting life over with the issues that you want to focus on and the ideals you want to create. Since you're the architect of this new scheme, you're going to honor it.

If you should fall back, don't beat yourself up over it. Analyze what went wrong. Do something nice for yourself, such as going to a movie, taking a walk, meeting friends, or cooking yourself a special dinner. Reward yourself for being human, but in a positive way.

To What Do You Feel Naturally Connected?

When you feel naturally connected to what you are doing, the activity comes easily to you. Honor that feeling. In other words, realize that where passion and excitement are is where your life should be. If your passion is helping people and your career doesn't offer that, then take the time to learn the necessary skills to make a career change.

If you follow your natural passion and excitement, you will automatically know what you want to do with your life. I'm willing to bet that, inside of you, a voice has told you a million times what you really want. It's tried to draw you to the real self through feelings and fantasies, but getting in the way of your accepting those were a lot of other images, e.g., you had to be the family man or wife, the responsible member of society, or the successful professional person, when perhaps these weren't you at all.

I'm not suggesting for a second some radical detachment from life as you know it. I'm not asking that you push a significant part of yourself into a guillotine. Rather, I'm suggesting that you think about preparing yourself over a period of time for what is real, new, and essential. This will allow you to extend one energy forward and at the same time retract the other energy. At some point—in one, two, or three years—you'll be fully into your new life and the old life will be gone. The process should be gradual as you do what is natural and healthy, at a pace that is natural and healthy.

List the things you feel naturally attracted to. For example, what makes you feel excited, interested, and passionate? If these feelings persist and your interest grows even more, then this is your inner self sending you messages to follow your bliss. It's not important whether you are educated or even skilled in the area. That can always come later. Alongside, list the things you feel pressured to accept, and the things that feel unnatural and intuitively wrong, so that you can start to disengage from those things. I call this constructive disengagement; it's constructively letting go of the things that are not a part of your natural self. Look at what you have made yourself responsible for that feels artificial, and constructively disengage.

Be Prepared to be Judged and Rejected

Be firm about what you are doing even in the face of objections and rejections from others. Before I go into a meeting, I try to anticipate most of the objections that are going to hit me and I prepare answers for them in advance.

For example, recently I gave my publisher a book I wanted published that wasn't a part of my contractual obligation, knowing in advance that he would say, "Well, you know, Gary, this isn't. . . ." I had already anticipated his negative responses and had answers prepared that would justify publishing the book. After I answered all his objections, there was a turn-around. They will be publishing my book. Had I not prepared for his objections in advance, my book would not be on its way to publication.

When you believe in something, be affirmative about it. Hear a "yes" in your mind even before you start the conversation. Think of possible reasons that people will have for rejecting your ideas, and build into your plan an answer to every possible rejection. Otherwise, people's disapproval may kill your ideas before they get off the ground. If you do your homework, there will be little room for rejection.

There is No Final Destination

Do you believe that at some point you arrive at your final destination? Or do you understand that you never arrive but continue your journey after each brief interlude when you reach a new goal?

Most people think their goals will get them to a certain fixed point in life. At that point, they assume, they will no longer need to grow. A doctorate or a master's degree will prove they are smart and can stop studying. A job, a bonus, or a pension will mean that they have made it.

When people reach a goal they often try to build a protective barrier around themselves to keep the world out and prevent any further changes. Their attainments become a fortress. This is akin, though, to taking free-flowing water into a pool: The pool remains clear for a day or two but soon becomes a cesspool and dies. Our life putrefies in the same way when we remove ourselves from the flow of life.

You have to set new sights and move on. It's fine to pat yourself on the back to acknowledge yourself for attaining some long-sought-after goal, but life does go on. It's a continual journey.

My life is always changing. I'll be altering a major segment of my life over the next few months. I'm going to have a lot of new and exciting things happen that will enable me to reach a lot more people. But to do that I have to live by my philosophy of never taking on a new project until I give up an old one. Think of what would happen if you did the same thing.

I worked very hard to establish the first holistic gourmet natural foods restaurant in New York City. It was called The Fertile Earth. I had it for five years. Then I opened another restaurant, called Gary's Place. It had great food that was beautifully presented. I hired a French decorative chef whose only job was to decorate each dish before it came out of the kitchen. Every single dish looked like a work of art. In fact, people couldn't believe basic dishes could be so beautiful, and yet remain inexpensive as well.

Then one day I was asked to do a television show. It wouldn't pay anything. In fact, it would cost me $100,000. But I would be able to reach a lot more people with my message. I agreed to do it.

The next day, I sold my restaurant. It was that simple. I needed to move forward, and in order to start a new project I had to let go of an old one. If someone else wanted to carry on what I had started, that would be fine. If the public is aware of what you're doing and feels a need for what you've created, they'll carry it on. Otherwise, it has had its time. Life is a matter of things coming and going. Some things stay and get carried on; others don't.

I did 165 television programs that aired in Connecticut, New Jersey, and Massachusetts for six years. That served a purpose. Then I started another project and gave up the television show. The idea is to start something, do it, enjoy it, and then let go and do something else. This directly contradicts the popular idea of finding your niche and holding on to something for the rest of your life. Where is it written that you have to spend your life doing just one thing? You can do many things in your life—as long as you don't do too many things at once.

Don't take what you do too seriously. Just know that everything you do is the best that you can do. Even if what you do isn't as good as you would like it to be, know that if you strive a little more you will do better. You're not striving out of anxiety or fear. You're not working for ego gratification. You're not trying to gain approval from the world to prove to other people that you're alright. You're doing it as part of a natural process of growth. Watch a horse run in a pasture. The horse is not running in order to win a trophy. It's running for the joy of running. It's natural to run. We forget to do what is natural, to honor our natural energies.

You May Not Know Your Goal Until You've Reached It

Sometimes you don't know what your goal is. You may think you've reached it when in fact you're only at an interim stopping-off point on a longer journey to a very different kind of goal.

For example, my good friend George, whom I grew up with, seemed to have it all at one point. He was the very successful manager of an advertising agency. He had an upscale house in the suburbs, and a beautiful wife and children. However, it had all come too easily. He seemed to have succeeded on the basis of his personal charm and ability to inspire trust. Because he was likeable and somewhat glib, he'd managed to do well financially, but there was something hollow about his life.

George became a gambler, dropping vast sums of money and jeopardizing his family's savings. He also became an alcoholic and a drug addict. He was diabetic as well; in short, not in good shape. Despite all his problems, and despite the fact that these were keeping him away from work for days at a time, he was able to hang on to his job for almost three years, mainly by force of his compelling personality.

Yet he was spinning downhill all this time, and when the company changed hands, George finally lost his job. He soon found himself in a halfway house, working in a chair factory.

I hadn't seen George during this downhill period, and when I met up with him when I was in town for our thirtieth high school reunion, I was alarmed by how awful he looked. He was puffy-faced, overweight, haggard, smoking. At the reunion I noticed how our cohorts' smiles of greeting to George turned to disapproving frowns as soon as he walked away. He'd been in town for a month before the reunion and many people knew his story. People have difficulty looking compassionately at golden-boy types who self-destruct.

Shortly after the reunion, I went over to George's and asked him, "Do you want to get out of this stagnant recovering-alcoholic, recovering-drug-addict thing?" "Sure," he said. So I arranged for George to visit my ranch to learn about health and nutrition, and to revamp his habits. He did this, and for the first time in years, George began to wake up each morning with joy in his heart.

Then he came to visit me in New York. He had a positive attitude and was appreciative of everything new and exciting the city had to offer. There was just one problem. George didn't know how to be politically correct! He's the type that tends to say what's on his mind, and he's not sensitive to boundaries. In a city where keeping your distance is practically an art form, George offended people fairly regularly.

He knew that he and New York City were a mismatch. The upshot of all this is that George has gone back to the ranch, this time to work helping others who are going through personal crises involving drug addiction, relationships, or other problems. His personality attributes—the ones that kept him going in his advertising job—are being used in a modified, more humane way, in a counseling capacity.

George has reinvented his life. He's a wonderful, totally honest human being who is motivated by the joy of living. He's a sensitive and compassionate listener. He knows how to make each day work because he's learned many lessons by living them.

The Chinese have a proverb—"to travel far you must travel light"—and George, who has shed a lot of the material trappings of his earlier "successful" life, is an inspiring example of this.

Being Autonomous

Most people don't decide whether or not to pursue their dreams. They consult other people and wait for their approval. If their ideas are rejected, chances are they'll give up their dreams rather than oppose the people who advised against it. Even if they do go ahead and do what they want, they allow the influence of other people to make them feel fearful and guilty. They don't approach their dream with an open heart and mind, and this breaks the flow of energy.

You generally consult the same people for support, advice, and acceptance. So in time, you begin to know in advance what these people will accept or reject and, as a result, you begin to edit your thoughts. You don't share real feelings, desires, and ambitions. Instead, you say only what you think the people want to hear. That way, you will be accepted.

But what happens to the part of you that no one knows about? It becomes secret. In time, it can manifest as a pathology.

When you betray yourself by neglecting to honor your dreams, you lose control of your life. You let someone else get into the driver's seat and control your life. You can change that, however, by identifying which people you seek permission from and asking, why do I need their blessing?

Do what's important to you. You might explain your intent to others, out of courtesy, but keep in mind that only you know what is best for you. You are going to go through with your decision whether anyone else supports you or not. Hopefully, some of these people will comprehend what you need to do for yourself. If they don't understand, they are entitled to their feelings, but you don't have to accept them.

Paradigms Can Blind Us to Possibilities

A thirty-year-old professional woman admitted to me that she had had many relationships but that none of them had been fulfilling. She decided that she would like to be freer but still be part of a relationship. The question was, how do you combine the two? Either you belong to a relationship and are devoted to your partner, or you are free. At least that is the model set forth by our society; a relationship in which you *are* free is not generally viewed as an option. This woman is not the only person with this quandary. Many people are dissatisfied with the standard sort of relationship they are taught they need in order to be happy. Yet they stick with what they are taught, and stop short from looking at other possibilities.

The same holds true in other areas of life. Your mind is conditioned to react in specific ways, thus eliminating your internal reasoning. You learn to shape your reality around being Catholic, Jewish, Islamic, Republican, Democratic, and so on, and to take on all the trappings of that identity. You accept or reject information because you are expected to respond to it in a certain fashion, not because you feel it is inherently right or wrong.

You become attached to the facade you create—a personality, a persona, an ideology, a religion—in order to feel more comfortable and safe in the world. While belonging helps you adapt to the circumstances of your existence, it doesn't help you to transform your life. You may, for instance, choose to live in an area that's flooded or burned down year after year instead of moving to safer ground. What keeps you there? What keeps you in the same predictable patterns leading to the same results every single time?

To understand your behavior, you have to appreciate the power of the paradigm. Paradigm comes from the Greek, paradigma, meaning pattern. Picture a circle inside of which all your needs are supposed to be met, and every question you ask is supposed to be answered. That's what societal paradigms attempt to do. Let me be more specific. Belief systems are the central catalysts of every part of society. Most groups try to centralize their power, and reward those who honor their belief system, while punishing and excluding those who disagree, and in general exhibiting a very low tolerance for change in any of the fundamental beliefs.

A major example of this would be in medicine. Doctors are taught what is considered the scientific basis of medical practice, the assumption being that they are the sole experts on the cause and treatment of any condition, from heart disease to AIDS. As a result, medical organizations have, for more than fifty years, fought a protracted war against cancer—and with few exceptions, have failed miserably. In such instances, protocol often becomes more important than the patient. If, however, you're on the other side of the medical paradigm, it's easy to see how doctors have gone in the wrong direction by looking for a viral cause of cancer, rather than expanding research into multiple causes—environment, diet, and behavior—all of which can be changed. But because the paradigm of the medical belief system has excluded these factors as "unscientific," there's no chance that serious research will be funded. As a result, vast amounts of money continue to be spent in search of an elusive virus, while the bodies mount up—over 500,000 per year. Paradigms that include alternatives, such as diet, herbs, vitamin C drips, and that recognize the culpability of ozone levels, have shown enormous benefit in both prevention and treatment—while being derided by the medical establishment as not being "real science." Truth in science, then, is determined by who controls the power base; and until their minds are opened to new ideas and asking new questions, nothing will change. So, to the degree by which you are directed by an institutional belief system, your reality, perceptions, and truth will be merely an extension of theirs. They serve as models for behavior and thought—thus, the relationship model, or paradigm, of the woman I spoke with was one of codependence and lack of freedom.

You may know the paradigms you've internalized are inherently wrong, but lack the confidence to challenge them. You may listen to my radio show and read my books, for example, yet run to a standard doctor at the first sign of sickness. You are afraid to trust your feelings. Instead you adhere to the paradigm that you were conditioned to accept, that traditional medicine has the only true solutions.

I've been curious for a long time about many of life's contradictions. In the area of medicine we say that we want to do anything possible to alleviate suffering. Yet when someone comes up with a new and innovative idea that helps people, and that certainly would help more people if given wider exposure, it is immediately attacked because it is outside the accepted paradigm. So benefits people claim to be receiving are completely ignored.

On the other hand, the scientific community condones ideas that have not produced successful responses from patients. Dr. Robert Gallo of the National Institutes of Health decided in 1984 that the cause of AIDS was a single retrovirus called HIV. That theory became dogma overnight. If you want to get a grant for AIDS research, you have to accept that HIV is the cause. So an enormous industry has emerged around the virus.

Nowhere in medical history have anomalies been more apparent. Look at the following contradictions:

- People are told that AIDS is a highly infectious disease that will reach epidemic proportions throughout the world. But when you step away from the hysteria and look at the actual statistics of people with proven AIDS, as opposed to people with AIDS-like symptoms who actually have malaria or TB, you can see that the disease remains mainly in its original risk groups of fast-track homosexuals, hemophiliacs, and IV-drug-using heterosexuals.

- People are told to wear condoms to keep AIDS from spreading. But condoms only prevent bacterial sexually transmitted microbes from being transferred. They do nothing to prevent viruses, such as HIV, from passing through latex. Viruses are smaller than the pores of the latex.

- People are told that they will die within fourteen to eighteen months of being infected. Yet people have been living with AIDS for fourteen or fifteen years.

- People are told that AIDS has a long latency period. That defies all scientific logic. There is no known virus that can destroy the entire immune system, create 29 separate diseases, and be latent for indefinite periods of time.

- People are told that the mere presence of HIV antibodies will cause AIDS to manifest. Yet antibodies are known to protect and immunize people against disease. This is true with polio, measles, mumps, smallpox, and chickenpox. This is the first time the presence of antibodies means that you are going to get the disease and die. There is no basis for this in science.

People who best survive AIDS use alternative therapies. They change their diets and lifestyles, use vitamin C drips, ozone treatments, vitamins, juices, and homeopathic and herbal therapies to cleanse and strengthen their immune systems. People often become HIV-negative after adhering to these protocols for a period of time. And even if they test positive for HIV, their blood is normal in all other aspects.

Society tends to ignore these success stories. When I held a press conference in New York City, the room was full of people who had been diagnosed with advanced AIDS. They chose holistic treatments and were able to reverse their condition. At the time of the conference, these people were healthy, with normal blood chemistries.

Every major news organization in the country was invited to attend, but not a single one showed up. If I had been presenting a drug that kills viruses in a test tube, it would have been a different scenario. Everyone would have been there and the story would have made front-page news. But the media wasn't interested in stories about people triumphing over the disease process without the aid of conventional medicine. The information fell outside the accepted paradigm.

I had the identical experience years ago when I held a press conference to introduce survivors of inoperable cancers. Five, ten, and twenty years after diagnosis these people were completely cured. I had medical records showing the original diagnoses and reports verifying how well they were doing. But all this didn't seem to matter. No one in the media paid any attention to the event.

I've seen other successful modalities ignored as well. Dr. Marshall Mandell was censured for curing upwards of eighty-five percent of his arthritic patients with rotational diets and detoxification programs. Doctors using chelation therapy, vitamins, and changes in diet have high success rates curing heart patients. But their work and patients are ignored and the doctors are attacked.

I've also seen contradictions occur outside of medicine. Look at the following examples:

- People are told to be innovative and work for themselves. Bureaucratic rules and regulations, however, make it almost impossible for most people to open their own businesses.

- Candidates for government office often proclaim a need for campaign reform. They say it's unfair that only the very rich are able to buy enough air time to get elected. Candidates should not be allowed to use private funds, they claim; they should all be given an equal amount of money and media time. That way, just normal, average people will have a chance to be elected to office. But the moment these people are elected to office, they stop being interested in campaign reform.

- People in the media claim to be working in the public interest, yet they're constantly selling the public everything from alcohol to cigarettes, and providing them with violent programming.

Everywhere I look I see discrepancies between what people say and what they do.

One of the problems is that no matter what we think, we are part of a belief system that determines our reality. Let's return to the field of medicine. If you're a physician, you have been trained to believe that medicine should be practiced in a certain way. You're given a standard set of rules about what causes disease, and you're given a standard set of tools with which to treat it. Society rewards you with social acceptance, financial security, and public trust when you follow the canon.

Here is the irony. If you use the therapies you're instructed to use and every patient you have dies, you are still rewarded. No one questions your choice of treatment. You are not held accountable. The protocol, then, is more important than the patient. The patient is there to serve medicine's larger ideology.

Patients tend to look up to their physicians and to believe what they are told. They are expected to be submissive. Obedience on the part of the patient is crucial for the system to continue, and people are taught to respect those in charge.

Even when they know the authority is wrong they tend not to want to offend them.

When a patient voices uncertainty by questioning a therapy—"Can you show me five cases of people who have been cured with this technique?"—the doctor will try to put the patient back in his place. "This is your only hope," he might say. If a patient continues to inquire about holistic options, the doctor will try to intimidate the patient into accepting standard methods. He will say, at best, that alternatives are unproven and regarded as ineffective. This is intended to discourage the patient from pursuing other possibilities and to keep the patient from losing confidence in the system.

This does not mean that the doctor doesn't care about his or her patients. It means that he is being guided by a certain set of beliefs. The doctor's psyche is indoctrinated with the idea that anything that is not part of the system must be rejected. His immediate reaction to anything foreign is to call it quackery. If it were legitimate, he thinks, he would know about it. It would be written up in medical journals. Researchers would test it and doctors would talk about it. After all, he reasons, doctors want to see a cure for cancer. Their daughters, sons, wives, and parents get cancer too. If the doctor doesn't know about it, it must not be valid.

Think again. People with vested interests in maintaining paradigms hate to be challenged. Look at the following scenario:

A doctor sees patients getting well after going on a detoxification and stress management program. These patients make changes in diet, drink fresh vegetable juices, eat raw foods, and take large amounts of selenium, vitamin C, and other nutrients.

The doctor realizes, "My God! I've been doing it all wrong. This patient is not sick because of a gene or virus. He has an immunosuppressive disorder. He's been living under chronic stress in a toxic environment and eating a poor diet. Clearly all these poisons are accumulating and causing cancer."

Now the doctor understands how a person can progress toward wellness. He no longer sees disease as a noun, a cancer, but as a verb, or a process. The doctor is excited and talks to his colleagues about his findings.

If alternative treatments help patients, then standard therapies and medications become suspect. They may be causing symptoms that get confused with the symptoms of an illness. It's difficult to differentiate characteristics caused by a disease from those caused by medication. In the case of AIDS or cancer, symptoms caused by chemotherapy become confused with those caused by the AIDS or cancer. In a depressed patient on medication, suicidal behavior might be related to the patient's depression or it might be medically induced.

In short, it's not in the best interest of the status quo to allow doctors to dissent from the norm, especially when the dissenters are getting good results. These doctors must follow the rules or be punished.

Thus doctors who praise, use, and research unorthodox approaches are first warned to stop. If they choose not to listen, they are admonished more strongly. Further persistence results in the doctor being isolated from the medical community altogether. The doctor will lose his or her privileges at the hospital, and will no longer be allowed to publish in peer review journals, or obtain research grants.

What happened to Dr. Peter Duesberg is a good example of this. Dr. Duesberg was considered a golden boy of American science, one of the best retrovirologists, and a scientific genius until he had the boldness to suggest that the HIV does not cause AIDS. Although he gave very plausible explanations and backed up his statements with good scientific reasoning, he was excluded from the scientific community for his outspokenness. His funding dried up and his teaching was restricted even though he taught at a supposed bastion of intellectual enlightenment, the University of California at Berkeley.

There are many doctors right now who are losing their licenses. A lot of these physicians had stellar reputations in the medical community until they began incorporating approaches to treatment into their practices that were not part of the accepted medical model—approaches that, ironically, earned these doctors the reputation of quacks even as they were helping patients and eliminating iatrogenic (medical-treatment-induced) problems. So these doctors now wake up every day knowing that the other 600,000 practicing doctors in this country will not come to their support no matter how many cures they can show and how many successful cases they have. Instead, they will be thrown out of the establishment, proving the old saying that no good deed goes unpunished.

Why, when they're successful helping their patients, are these doctors being selected for chastisement? If they used standard treatments they'd be hurting their patients. On the one hand, this scenario doesn't make any sense. On the other hand, it's easy to understand if you remember the power inherent in belief systems and when you realize that there's nothing more threatening in any belief system than an idea that cannot be controlled.

Once on the outside, doctors are able to see, more objectively, the limitations and false notions of the belief systems they participated in at one time. If they are able to move forward, they become the pioneers in a new system of medicine and are able to look at old problems with an open mind and a new point of view. So the doctors getting the best results treating AIDS patients are not part of the orthodoxy. The scientists doing the most to understand its cause are not looking at HIV. They are looking at multiple causes, such as drug use, repeated unhealthy sexual acts, and chronic abuse of the immune system. These doctors who have stepped back from the medical "party line," if you will, are able to be more objective and are therefore better able to help patients.

Society accepts only one ruling system. Even though various people uphold that power, they represent the same set of principles. It's like being the president of the United States—it doesn't matter whether you're Democratic or Republican. There is really only one party—the business party—and both groups honor the business mandate. That's not necessarily good or bad, but it's the reality.

Another contradiction: We say that we want equality, yet we don't encourage it. We say that people have the same opportunities, yet people in positions of power never let others get a taste of it. We almost never see wealthy people associating with the poor, educated people befriending illiterate people, people fraternizing with people of other races or even other age groups.

Our statements are politically correct but practically void. We don't acknowledge the contradictions and inconsistencies in all areas of our lives. We don't take things in the larger context. We don't see the consequences of our actions. We don't visualize a larger way of living. Then we wonder why nothing gets better.

How Do Paradigms Function?

Paradigms prescribe values. You learn to care about things you are constantly told to believe are important. For instance, our culture endorses a paradigm that encourages spending, along with the creation of artificial needs. People are taught to continually buy, in order to support the "supply side" of our economic system. If you don't have the means, you can still buy on credit. You can buy fashionable clothes and dispose of the ones your paradigm tells you are too old and no longer stylish. You need new clothes in order to feel good, the fashion industry says.

There's nothing wrong with feeling good or having nice things to wear. The problem lies in your being made to feel you always need something new to feel good. You then begin to devalue what you liked at one time. So you have fifteen pairs of shoes but wear only two. You have twenty dresses but wear three. If you lived in France you would have four dresses and wear all four. The French save until they can afford something they really like, while the United States is a society of disposables. It's all part of our economic paradigm.

People defend their paradigms even when they're harmful. A good example of this phenomenon is the issue of smoking. It was profitable to start people smoking, and the cigarette industry worked hard at it. They even paid doctors to promote smoking's supposed safety on television. Doctors would say that cigarettes were safe according to scientific studies. People felt comforted by that, because if their doctor said smoking was alright, it had to be so. As a result, smoking became an acceptable part of their paradigm. If they later got emphysema, people were caught in a paradox. Did they trust their own experience or the doctor's message? Often they might trust their doctor and not their own experience, since a physician signifies authority.

Paradigm followers also tend to blame people outside of their own belief system for problems that arise instead of questioning their own beliefs. So conservatives attack liberals, liberals attack conservatives, and so on. The problem is always the outsiders—never the insiders' assumptions.

Belief systems tend to establish a wall of accepted thought beyond which you must not venture. Orthodoxy tells you to stop all your questioning at this wall. That's because those who have an interest in maintaining certain points of view must discourage you from questioning, since if you investigated the beliefs you've been fed, the likelihood is that you would go beyond them as you found their weaknesses. You would start to see the paradigm's limitations and say to yourself, "Hold on a second. I can't accept this."

How Do You Work Outside of a Paradigm?

Realistically, you'll probably need to find a way to work within the existing paradigm while taking care that your beliefs are not compromised. You can't just change everything about your society, but you can change your part in it. For example, if you feel uncomfortable with your work routine, you could start a

business from your home, as an alternative to fitting into somebody else's nine-to-five framework.

I recently spoke with someone about a magnificent business
he started. He said to me, "Gary, I've got a great business and
I want you to tell people in New York because maybe they can
do the same thing. Everyone is interested in health and looking
for an easy way of maintaining it. To help them, I've made up
a menu of juices. I make fresh juice each day and go around
to corporations, businesses, and restaurants, where I sell it in
containers. It's easier and quicker for people than if they made
it themselves, and it gives me a nice income. I enjoy this work
because it allows me to offer something healthful to society.
I'm doing something good that I like and making some money
in the process. Plus I'm maintaining my autonomy by setting
my own hours and working for myself. Sometimes I work
longer than I would in a nine-to-five job, but I don't mind
because I'm working for me."

What a great idea. And this is just one of a million ideas
that are coming to light in America right now. People are actualizing their ideas. If you're creative you can come to grips
with any problem. Instead of adapting to a bad circumstance,
transform it to work for you. How much better this is than
escaping and running away from things you don't like.

Does Authority Limit You?

Authority exists everywhere. It influences every aspect of your
life. You consult a counselor before making a career change.
You see a doctor to determine whether you're healthy.

Established experts act as if they're the only credible source
of information and advice. In our health care system, for example, people who suggest you can be healthy with the aid of
yoga, meditation, tai chi, wheat grass, or guided visualization
are disempowered by the mainstream, and you're discouraged
from seeking advice from them. Their charges are not covered

by health insurance. The media ignores them or makes them look laughable. The scientific community overlooks them, and they're not given academic acceptance.

Most authorities are concerned with self-preservation. Therefore, they are limited in what they can tell you. You may speak to a hundred experts, but if they've all bought into the same paradigm, you're hearing the same words from a hundred different mouths. This doesn't mean that authorities from the prevailing paradigm are bad people or that they don't want to help. It just means they may be limited in the aid they can offer and in the information they can accept.

A highly regarded physician called me. He told me he is suffering from AIDS and cancer and from the side effects of chemotherapy. I asked him if anyone could assure him that the chemotherapy was going to work. He explained that he had no assurance. I suggested that he try a protocol that would build the immune system rather than destroy it. He said he couldn't because he is an orthodox doctor.

This doctor is a victim of his own limited beliefs. He refuses to try something new even in the face of life-threatening illnesses. That's how powerful belief systems are. That's how authority limits you. A reasonable question could be asked to the effect of: Why would the doctor call me and ask for my advice if he had no intention of using it? This happens all the time. My assumption is that by at least calling he was assuaging some guilt for not having looked into everything. But looking and learning about a therapy is not the same as engaging in it. He was keeping it on a linear, left-brain, very safe analytical level, and I suppose that if someone asked him, "Have you even looked into alternative therapy?" he could say, "I called Gary Null, I even spent time listening to him. I just wasn't convinced that what he had to offer would work."

You need to be the authority in your life. Go after what you really need.

What if You Broke Out of an Accepted Pattern?

Let's say you've decided to be single at a stage in life when this is not quite the thing to do. Being un-paired often threatens people who are paired. If you enjoy being alone you may become a threat to people who derive security and meaning from being in relationships. When you are no longer married, notice how quickly most other married people exclude you from their lives. You may have been friends before but now, no matter what you've shared, suddenly you're out of the loop.

I've counseled numerous people confused about why no one wants them around once they're single again. Sometimes the reason is jealousy. A single person's lifestyle is different and often more engaging. They have freedom that their married friends can't relate to. Most married people don't want to hear about a fun party or an exciting rafting expedition if their life has no place for those. They don't like to acknowledge something that they can't share.

Is fear of losing acceptance holding you back from being more independent? Or do you have faith that you will meet new like-minded people? Are you able to let go of the old, if necessary, so that you can live a more self-empowered life?

How Do You Hide Your Loneliness or Sense of Not Belonging?

As a society we believe that we must belong to something, so we tend to join different groups. We identify with these groups. There's nothing wrong with that, provided we don't lose our own identity. We shouldn't use groups to hide our loneliness.

Since you were taught that you must be connected to something to feel whole, when you're not connected you tend to feel isolated and abandoned. Sometimes it's hard for people to cope with this sense of abandonment. But remember that aloneness is not synonymous with loneliness. Think of the things you can do alone. You can meditate, relax, do things for yourself, and have time to put your life in order. Quality time alone can give you a much-needed new perspective. In this chaotic world, where everything seems to require our time, isn't it nice to have time alone?

When you choose to be with people, make sure your time is spent with people you enjoy. Don't seek company just so you won't feel lonely. That isn't enjoying the company. That's hiding from the loneliness. If I'm with someone it's because I choose to be with the person, not because I'm lonely. If I'm with someone just because I'm lonely, then I'm not really accepting or appreciating that person. She or he is merely the means I use to help me overcome my loneliness, and that's devaluing to us both.

What Are the Advantages of Being Single or Married?

Whether you're single or married, list the best parts of the experience and the worst. Then ask yourself an honest question. Do you feel good about your status? Does your life work? Are you happy?

Maybe you are unhappy being single only because your conditioning tells you that you should be married at your age. Your friends and parents pressure you to meet someone or to get more serious in your current relationship. You really like being alone, but this is unacceptable to others.

Perhaps you are unhappily married and feel pressured to make it work. In your heart you know you would prefer being on your own.

You may, on the other hand, be happily married. If being married makes your life work more successfully, that's fine.

Being single or married is not, in itself, good or bad. Acknowledging your true feelings and honest needs is what's important. Make a list of these. This list will help you create balance.

How Do You Respond to Uncertainty?

Making changes in your life will undoubtedly lead to feelings of uncertainty. If uncertainty makes you uncomfortable, your first reaction will be to avoid unpleasant feelings. You might back away, scurry into a relationship, or keep chronically busy. Then you're never going to get around to projecting your new self. You're always going to find something else that's a priority.

When you feel uncertain, you may revert to childlike behavior. You might feel you need to be taken care of or to be told what to do and how to do it. A sense of abandonment and rejection can keep you in an unhealthy situation, even an abusive one. You may resort to childish behavior out of a misguided desire to be needed and accepted.

Notice how you respond to uncertainties. If you respond in unhealthy ways, you can work to change that.

Where Do You Go to Have Your Needs Met?

You'll almost always go to the people inside of your paradigm for answers. A problem arises when your needs require an alternative perspective. You may not even realize that you do. For instance, if you have breast cancer and you talk to traditionally-minded women friends and doctors, they're all going to tell you pretty much the same thing. You won't consider talking to someone with a different viewpoint who can present different, maybe life-saving, options. Your paradigm limits you.

How Might You Treat Others Differently?

I know a selfish person who only considers his own needs. His world begins and ends with him.

Long-time friends finally rejected him for being that way. If these people had responded to him differently from the start, they might have helped him see the way he was. They might not have had to wait for a crisis to occur where they rejected him for being selfish. At the very beginning they could have said, "I will not accept you, nor will I share anything with you, because I find your actions and attitudes selfish." But instead they ignored his selfishness until it became too much to bear. They blamed him later. That's the way a lot of people are.

How might you change the way you respond to others?

What Messages Do You Tell Yourself?

Listen to the messages you tell yourself. These are messages you should pay attention to. Talk them out in your mind and actualize them. If you say, for example, "I know I should be healthier," think about ways to make that happen. Affirm, "I'm going to be healthy," and create a program to change. Change your attitude, your beliefs, and your support system to encourage health. Then you will change the silent voice to an empowering one that helps you to actualize what you want to become.

Change Only Those Attitudes, Actions, and Beliefs That You Don't Like

You probably accept a lot of beliefs that you don't like. Identify them and write them down. You may believe, for example, that politics can never change anything. As a result, you have become cynical, and never put your energy into making change happen.

If you want to live a more positive existence, you must acknowledge that change is possible and that your input does make a difference. If, for instance, you decide that you want to become a vegetarian, you can start associating with other like-minded people. You can encourage friends who want to become vegetarians to do so by showing them that they can refrain from meat-eating and be optimally healthy. By doing so, you'll be developing a small paradigm which in time can become a very powerful one. In the 1960s there were only several hundred thousand vegetarians in this country. Today there are twenty million. People influenced each other and caused a positive change to occur. They responded to a vegetarian Mr. America and to great athletes who didn't eat meat. These new models gave them the confidence to change.

It becomes more difficult to change certain attitudes and actions without the support of friends and family. If your family disagrees with your wanting to become vegetarian, changing is going to be much more difficult. You have to be very self-motivated and confident; only the autonomous person can succeed. With autonomy, you can find the inner strength and support you need to make positive change happen.

Anger can sometimes be a strong motivator for change when channeled constructively. A woman I know just ran the marathon. But three weeks ago, this woman had been about to give up because her family had been opposed to her spending time and energy in training. They'd made her feel guilty about doing it.

She came to me one day and said she wasn't going to race.

I asked her why and she replied that she just couldn't do it. I told her she was right, that she was obviously not emotionally, spiritually, intellectually, or physically able to succeed. Then I told her good-bye. She just stood there and looked at me. I asked her what she wanted from me. I wasn't going to encourage her to do something she didn't feel capable of doing. She said she was physically able to do it and I disagreed. I told her she wasn't or else she would run. I said, "You obviously just can't do it. You tried and failed and it's alright. Now you can go back to being all the things you were. You can gain back your weight and your negative attitude. You can become cynical and bitter and let all your friends and family affect you. That's obviously what you want because that's the choice you've made, and it's okay. Make that choice. Live with it."

She got really angry. And I said, "People sometimes work extremely hard to climb a mountain. They almost reach the top. Just a little further and they would suddenly see every vista that's in front of them—all the unlimited possibilities. But they allow other people and their fears to just drag them right back down again. You came that close."

The next day she called me and said, "I told my family and friends that if they opened their mouth to me today I would smack them." She said, "I'm going out and I'm going to stay by myself until I get through this race." And she did. And they were there cheering her on.

Today, she's a hero in their minds and in her own. Voices of uncertainty no longer hold her back. Once you break free and become autonomous you gain inner power. A transformation occurs when you see positive change occur. Your perspectives and attitudes change. Then you notice that people who were against you are now on your side. The same people who denied you support are now looking up to you and even bragging about you. I can assure you that on the day of the race the family of the woman who ran the marathon, who did nothing but badger her for months, told everyone they knew about her accomplishment. Now she's a paradigm leader. Remember, a paradigm can be as small as your own life, or your relationship, or your family.

How Did Your Parents Treat Each Other?

Look at the way your parents treated themselves and each other. You learned from them as a child and are now, perhaps, a reflection of who they were. Have you incorporated their qualities—the best and the worst? Identify these qualities so you can change the ones you don't like, keep the ones you do, and, in the process, become more truly yourself.

Do You Take Responsibility for Your Attitudes and Actions Regardless of Who Is on the Receiving End?

How do your attitudes affect other people? Does it feel good being at the other end of what you're sharing? If it doesn't feel good, then change it.

People in positions of power don't usually think this way. If they are "above" someone else, they assume a superior attitude. People with less status aren't given equal respect. All around you see the ritual of inequality. Our society accepts that. You'll be standing in line and a rich and powerful person will walk right in front of you and get immediate attention.

All this is a façade. An attitude of superiority has no power if you don't acknowledge it, since power is an illusion. It doesn't exist unless you acknowledge it's real. When I counsel a member of a royal family of Europe, which I have, they come to me without their title, just a person. I don't use titles. I don't call myself doctor and I don't use titles with anyone else. A person is just a person.

Can you imagine how you could communicate with people if you felt you were equal to everyone you met? You would be removing the distance between yourself and others and relating person-to-person. Respecting people's differences is fine. Respecting their uniqueness is fine. But respecting their so-called superiority is not. In our society, differences are equated with superiority or inferiority. And that has to change.

Define the different systems that you accept or belong to in which you feel inferior. Find those systems or relationships in which your attitudes, beliefs, and actions are always considered of secondary importance to someone else's. Acknowledge that you are equal to every other person. Becoming aware is the first step in changing the process.

Forgiving: Letting Go of Pain

❖

I ask people attending my workshops about the challenges they face in their lives. One person said he feels conflicted about what he really wants. Being conflicted is like saying, for instance, I want intimacy and solitude, or I want to eat healthy food and junk food.

How do you reconcile these? It's simple. You recognize that, at any given moment, every single thought has its opposite in your consciousness and you determine the advantage of each side.

Acknowledge that you have opposing thoughts and desires. Otherwise, you'll bury unwelcome ideas. They'll remain inside of you and are likely to come out later. That's where you harm yourself and others. You may do things and then think, how could I have done that? A part of your nature may emerge that you didn't consciously realize was there.

You will know exactly who you are by understanding what you are capable of doing. Then you can decide how to act in your own best interest. If you're trying to be a happy, whole-some, healthy person you won't entertain the dark thoughts and feelings that are there. Once you get into the habit of making the right choices for yourself it becomes easy. You start to know when you're making the correct decisions.

Of course, being human, you sometimes choose wrong options. That's okay as long as you can recognize what you've done and learn from your mistakes. You'll scream at someone, you'll do something that in retrospect is stupid. And then you'll say, alright, I acknowledge that I made a mistake. What can I do? Forgiving yourself is key to rebalancing.

So is forgiving others.

The whole idea of forgiveness is to allow yourself to go forward. If you don't forgive, you are stuck with the anger and pain of the event. You honor that pain more than your right to go forward without it. All of the love and kindness in you and directed toward you will mean nothing if you're not willing to acknowledge why you're in pain. Forgive the pain and get on with your life.

Who Creates Your Pain?

Although you may blame others for the distress you feel, your pain is your own doing. You create it. If you were to write me an insulting letter, for example, calling me arrogant, conceited, and self-righteous, I could choose to become very angry. I could strike back in an attempt to retaliate or I could go to the other extreme in an attempt to prove how nice I really am. I could internalize what you say and become depressed. With any of these responses, I am causing myself pain by reacting to what you've said.

Another possibility exists. Before reacting, I can take a step back and think about the situation. That way I'm distancing myself from the immediate conflict and putting it into perspective. I can look at the letter you sent and think about your possible intentions. I might decide that I took what you said out of context. Maybe I'm misinterpreting and assuming something that wasn't meant.

If you react to a situation without thinking it through, it's difficult to later change your mind about what happened. Once you become emotional and retaliate, you start justifying your actions. Your ego tells you that what you did was right. Unnecessary conflict arises.

Realize that people have the right to their feelings. Some will like you and some won't. That has nothing to do with you. As long as people don't spread lies to hurt your reputation or physically harm you, they are entitled to their opinions.

When you start to feel distressed, take a step back and ask yourself, what is really happening here? Do I have to accept this situation as painful? Must someone's negative feelings toward me affect how I feel about myself?

List the Old Hurts You Still Feel

What old hurts do you still keep alive? Which ones come up over and over? Perhaps some of these sound familiar: Your mother wasn't there when you needed her. You were abused, rejected, ridiculed, or abandoned. Someone stole from you. Something that was supposed to have been given to you was given to someone else.

You must give up old hurts to be free to live more fully. Otherwise, the pain from the past influences the present. You keep yourself from relating to others because you were abused or abandoned earlier in life. You want to be open and trusting, but you have painful memories of being manipulated and taken advantage of. So you hesitate to be yourself. You keep your relationships from working because of the way you were treated previously. That happens when you don't let go of the past.

Living life fully involves taking risks. Unless you take chances, your past fears prevent you from growing.

Examine the hurts that keep reappearing in your life. See what makes you emotionally imbalanced. Notice the patterns. Resolve the hurts and they will stop reappearing. It may seem easier said than done, but you are put into painful situations for a reason. There are lessons you need to learn. Work through your issues and in time you will resolve them. You will regain balance if you work at it.

How Do You Deal with Hurt or Pain?

Do you hide it? Scream it out to the world? Distract yourself? Go into therapy? Chronically complain and whine? Share pain with someone else?

If you deal with pain in any way except by making constructive changes, then you are keeping your hurt alive. Therapy tells you that your hurt is real. While the right kind of therapy has the potential to do you good, sometimes therapy can serve to reinforce your pain, making it more genuine. When this happens, your whole immune system becomes depressed. You start manifesting physical symptoms. The pain grows and becomes as tangible as a tumor and takes on a life of its own.

Therapy can also make you dependent on someone else. You start to feel you can't resolve your own problems. It's disempowering to suggest that unless you're being helped by someone you're incapable of positive change.

I see this often in the recovery movement, where people must acknowledge their dysfunction and then go through a program involving several steps. Everybody has to go through the same stages. People are discouraged from dealing with problems on their own, even if they feel capable of doing so.

You may distract yourself from pain by looking for things to take its place, such as food, drugs, or being overly responsible. But a better approach than distraction is to take quiet time every day during which you can be introspective. This allows you to face what's bothering you, and to put your problems into perspective.

Sometimes you want to share your hurt with others, but after a certain point, this doesn't do any good. I have friends who always want to share their problems with me. This is fine, except when it's the same problem over and over and they never change anything. Then, I simply ask them what they're trying to achieve. Are they talking just because I'm willing to listen? They share the same thing over and over, until I don't want to hear it anymore. Finally I tell them, "If you're not willing to change, don't share your problems with me anymore."

Perhaps most of the pain you now experience is not real but you make it appear real. Is that possible? Be honest. Perhaps much of what you're calling your physical crisis does not exist but is self-created. Is that possible? If it is, remember this: Until you let go of self-created or self-perpetuated pain and no longer treat it as a real problem, it will continue to live.

Intellectually you might understand this, but nothing will change until you actually let go of your pain and fill your mind with affirmations to reprogram your body and mind. Tell yourself that you're pure, whole, complete, healthy, positive, lovable, and an ideal human being who deserves all the good things life has to offer. Until you do, the old messages will supersede the new ones.

Once you start believing in yourself completely, you'll be amazed at how far you can go. Where you didn't think you had the resources, your self-confidence will enable you to accomplish what seems impossible.

People ask me how I do all the things I do. I've written fifty books and done 165 television programs. I've produced sixteen documentaries and thirty-five specials. I've built resorts and detox centers and have owned and operated health food stores and natural food restaurants. I have done more than 7,000 radio broadcasts and helped over 20,000 people race thons. How do I do it? I've never gotten around to believing that there's something I can't do. I believe that I can do anything. As a result, anything I want to do I just do.

The only person that can stop me is me. The moment I listen to anyone else's doubts I stop myself. People might say, "Gary, you can't do that because you don't have the education, support, or money. You don't have the institutional systems behind you." Maybe I don't, but I don't need those. I don't accept what people say I can't do. In my belief system, I make up the rules.

Some people try to stop me. I've been called a quack, a charlatan, and a fraud. Some people even try to make me appear crazy. But there's no way they can convince me that I'm anything other than a perfect human being. As I result, I continue to go forward. I don't waste my life in frivolities and fear. I'm not motivated by what I can't do but rather by what I can. So everything people say can't be done I end up doing.

I believe the human spirit is perfect. As long as I'm in touch with that spirit in my body, mind, and soul, I realize my perfection. I just have to trust enough to connect with it.

At some point you might say, "Gee whiz, if Gary's done all these things then maybe I can too." Of course you can. I'm no more special than anyone else. I wasn't born or raised differently. I have as much dysfunction in my background as most people. But I choose not to identify with that dysfunction. I don't let myself be a victim sitting around feeling sorry for myself. I could be like most people who are in therapy three days a week, reinforcing their dysfunctions. But why hold on to that?

This is your journey. There's no other support system you need. You need only you. Look for resources out there to help strengthen you, but don't depend on them.

Now is the time to look at the pain you've held onto, and let it go. Reaffirm every single day that you do not need that pain in your life, and give yourself something in its place. Create small goals, intermediate goals, and major goals. Focus on achieving those. Don't let anyone tell you that you can't do anything that you want to do. If anyone else has accomplished something then you can do it too. Recently, there was a news story about an eighty-six-year-old woman who just raced the marathon. She started training at the age of seventy. Who would have believed it? The fact that she did it means others can too.

Become the hero in your own life. Have the courage to go out there and make changes. You will meet obstacles, of course. You just have to differentiate real from imagined obstacles and reject the imagined ones.

What Do You Enjoy?

Notice what you enjoy doing and engage in those activities often. Enjoyable experiences will give you the confidence to continue doing things that are good for you. That's why I've been running marathons for twenty years. It feels good, and it reaffirms my right to be strong, disciplined, and integrated in body, mind, and spirit.

Are you happy in your work situation? I never work at a job I don't like. Yet many people feel stuck in their work. They argue that they must stay there; they have no choice. These people justify their actions with questions such as, "Who is going to pay the mortgage?" "Who will feed the kids?" "Who is going to pay the health insurance?" Their concerns go on and on. Thus they rationalize being stuck in an unhappy situation.

Ask yourself, do I enjoy my surroundings? Recently, I visited the southwest to see some old friends. I did a workshop in Santa Fe where I got to talk to some ex-New Yorkers.

I spoke to one woman who is a jewelry designer. She makes costume jewelry and jewelry from platinum, gold, and silver. This woman loves her work and enjoys the pace of life of Santa

Fe, the cleanliness, being close to nature, and the people. Most Santa Fe residents will let you be whatever you want to be; the whole community acknowledges freedom of expression.

I also met a third-generation police officer. He told me how difficult it was for him to convince his Irish Catholic family that he wanted to do something else with his life. He does landscape architecture, which he loves. His life is fulfilled. He feels balanced. As a result, he no longer suffers from migraine headaches. He has lost weight. He's happy in his marriage.

These people weren't afraid to make changes. Think of how your life would change if you did things that made you feel good and were around people who supported you. That doesn't mean that what you are doing is not what you should be doing. I'm just suggesting that if you feel trapped you may need to go forward.

If you find yourself unhappy in your living or working environment, take a step back and look at both sides of the issue. Fold a piece of paper in half and on one side write about why you stay put in the same location, the same job, the same lifestyle. Why haven't you let go of your pain, anger, disappointments, and hurt? Why do you continue to blame yourself?

On the other side, list what you would ideally like to do. That way you can focus your attention on it. Write about the resources you will need to achieve what you want to do. Maybe a year or two of schooling is necessary to get the skills, credentials, and support system you need. Your written ideas will give you a plan of action. You'll have goals to focus on.

Selecting a job or a place to live based on what gives you the greatest pleasure may be a difficult concept. Society doesn't teach you to associate happiness with lifestyle. You've been taught that you can only attain so much. You are told that you are limited because of your education, class, gender, culture. Your belief system says that what you have is the best that you deserve and the best you should expect.

You have to stretch your beliefs to go beyond that notion. Why should you accept a barren little island as your reality when you've got a whole continent to explore? You probably do so because you've been told that's what you can expect. You're middle class. You come from a certain background. Everyone else does it this way so you've got to do it this way. Your whole life becomes circumscribed by your supposed limitations.

It's easy to lose sight of possibilities that can enhance your life and bring you greater enjoyment. If your family has never gone to the ballet, for instance, you don't go to the ballet. If they have never gone to an art exhibit in SoHo, you don't go either. If they've never been hiking, you don't do that either. You don't do anything outside of what is expected.

If you accept the expectations that everyone lays down for you they become as formidable as an impenetrable, un-scalable prison wall. These limitations don't really exist, but you make them seem real. Instead of taking a step back to differentiate between what's real and not real, you are prone to staying limited. You'll say things like, "We're in a recession." "I can't change." "The only jobs I can get are jobs I don't like." "I'm stuck in my ways." "I'm too old." "I have to live with it."

Such words justify your lack of motion. Instead of changing you become frustrated and start to sublimate. You indulge in alcohol, food, television, or sex. You find endless ways to distract yourself.

Experiment with new experiences and behaviors you might enjoy. Once you identify what you do enjoy, create a support system with people that enjoy the same things. One of my friends likes to cook and watch movies. So do I. We've watched movies for six hours at a time. His energy is compatible with mine, and we have enough in common to build a friendship. You want to be with people you feel comfortable with, who reinforce a lifestyle that makes you comfortable.

Doing what is natural requires little effort. It feels as though you are doing what you should be doing. Ask yourself, what do you feel good about doing? What do you look forward to? What gives you great joy? Build your life around these things.

What Do You Gain by Letting Go and Forgiving?

Write down the following: I'm going to forgive _____ because I will gain _____. This exercise allows you to see how you will benefit from giving up the pain and anger connected to your feeling hurt. It shows you there is a reward in giving it up.

Once you can let go and forgive, you can get on with your life and move forward. The more you release, the freer you become. Life is an educational process. With each lesson you learn to live it more constructively. You keep rebalancing yourself.

Decide what you want to change. Then find the strength and resources to make the conversion, step-by-step, day by day. Remove something that you don't feel you want and put something that will work in its place.

What Have You Learned From Your Pain?

There's a lesson in pain. Pay attention to what it teaches you. Once you learn the lesson you're not going to repeat it. You can share what you've learned with others and help them in the process. The lesson of pain can be learned by examining who first creates the situation which results in a reaction of pain. For example, you say something without thinking or knowing that it will provoke a reaction in someone; then, when they do react, you feel pain. Another example: you're frustrated, but instead of dealing with the frustration in a constructive way, you overeat something that's bad for you; then, the next day, you feel an inner pain for what you perceive as your weakness in relying on your old, self-destructive behavior patterns.

Remember a difficult time in your life. What did you learn

from that experience? How have you grown and become better for it?

If You Could Be an Unbiased Mediator in Your Own Conflict, What Would You Suggest Both Sides Do?

List your major conflicts. Now take the role of arbitrator and assess the pros and cons of both sides of your conflict. Let's say you have a conflict about being married. First note the benefits of being on your own. You are free to make up your own mind. You can live for yourself. You won't be part of a codependent relationship. You have time for yourself. You can make mistakes without being criticized. You can create your own schedule instead of working around someone else's. You don't have to wait for someone else's approval before doing things.

The negative part of being on your own might be that you feel incomplete. In our society you're nobody unless you're a part of a relationship. You may feel insecure being alone. You may think you're unlovable and that something is wrong with you. People do not expect you to be happy being single.

Then look at the other side of the issue. What are the benefits of being married? You have the security and companionship of another person, someone to wake up with and grow old with, a person that will share love and affection with you.

The down side might be going into debt buying things you need to have as a couple. Things may become more important than the relationship. You may go into debt buying a house you don't really like or need. Soon the relationship may exist to pay for the mortgage, the furniture, and the children. The stress will put a damper on the relationship, and it will no longer be joyful.

When you look at everything from the positive and the negative aspects you will clearly pin down what the ideal situation would be for you. Then you can make your move.

What Gives You An Adrenalin High?

Most people live their whole lives remembering the one or two rushes they experienced early in life when they were willing to take some risks. If you start taking some chances now, you can feel charged all the time. You can become the adventurer in your own life.

Think of times you felt excited to be alive. Perhaps you were going down rapids, starting a romance, beginning a new career, seeing the Grand Canyon, or going down a roller coaster. Find ways of creating new highs for yourself and you will have something to look forward to every day.

Letting Go of Fear

Fear is a primary reason that people don't progress. I talk to many people who read good self-help books, seek counseling, attend workshops and seminars, and yet remain stuck in their problems. Nothing changes until they break through their fear.

Sometimes fear is justified, but most of the time it is the result of illusion. I'm going to try to differentiate between the two types of fear—real and illusory—and show you several ways of dealing with each. You can approach real fears pragmatically. Illusory fears need to be eliminated from your mind.

(Note: My answers are not the only solutions nor are they necessarily right for you. Rather, I hope they will inspire you to think of answers that are personally meaningful. In addition, my questions should help you generate questions of your own. Some thoughts will appear immediately, whereas others will come to you later.)

This section will help you to explore what you're afraid of and analyze how you manifest your fears. It will encourage you to think about ways of letting fear go so that you can live a more full and vital life.

What Are You Afraid Of?

Many factors can cause fear. See which of the following makes you fearful.

Fear of Losing Self-Esteem

You lose self-esteem when you fail to live up to your image. Athletes who lose a game posture themselves in a humiliating fashion before the public. They don't say to themselves, it's just a game. I'm not going to lose any sleep over it. It's not all that important. They take themselves seriously and take losing to heart.

Where in your life do you strive to maintain an image for fear of losing self-esteem? You may feel bad about not getting a promotion, for example, or about not being able to appear responsible.

Fear of Being Out of Control

If you're like most people, you're terrified by the possibility of your life getting out of control. When was the last time you really played? If you're part of the baby boom generation, there's a good chance that the answer is, a very long time ago. Does this sound like you? Every minute of the day is purposeful. You work too hard and never have time just to enjoy yourself. You become successful at doing things but not at just being. I meet a lot of people like this. They always feel the need to be responsible and productive. They can't spend the weekend just hanging out and having fun. They always feel the need to be doing something. They're afraid of losing control. Even their vacations are planned out and timed from beginning to end. They'll go to Cancún and spend a half hour playing tennis and a half hour scuba diving. An hour after arriving, they're wondering if they could make a deal on a condominium. All their meals are during meetings.

When I go to a resort, I'm nowhere to be found. I'll be on a hammock somewhere, resting. I go away to rest. I don't want to do any business. I don't want to think. I just want to relax and play.

Being out of control asserts that you are different and independent and not just like everyone else. Allow yourself to be out of control. Be creative in a way where you do something spontaneous and completely out of character. Let yourself go, and use being out of control as a way of growing.

On a societal level, being out of control can have positive implications. I constantly work to break through barriers in order to make people aware of their alternatives. Five years ago I said on television that AZT was hurting AIDS patients and that alternative therapies were helping people stay alive. I was out of control in the sense that I was saying things that other people wouldn't dare speak about. They were in a controlled situation, but I wasn't. Of course, in the long run, there is no controlling the emergence of the truth.

Most journalists will not risk being out of control. They have too much to lose going against the system. People such as Mike Wallace and Tom Brokaw are bound by fear. They're afraid of losing their jobs and their power, and—as a result of these losses—their self-esteem. Think of what would happen if more people didn't play by the rules. We could progressively move forward as a society. Until enough people break those barriers, fear will keep us trapped.

Fear of Loss of Place

You may fear losing your place in different areas of life. In a relationship, for example, you become jealous and hurt if your partner tells you that he or she has met someone else. Jealousy has always puzzled me. I've never understood the concept. If I were in a relationship where someone didn't want to be with me anymore, I would feel fine about that. It wouldn't be a problem. I would get on with my life rather than feel hurt and betrayed. I wouldn't compete against anyone or fight for someone. I don't see the point in that. I would just move on.

As a student, you may have feared losing your place in school. People are put under a lot of pressure to perform well in school. Remember the people who were always competing for A's? Their lives were often imbalanced. They had to give up developing other areas of their lives in order to become school-smart. There's a type of person who always strives for goals but neglects the process leading up to their attainment, and this is sad. The person achieves something but learns nothing in doing so; everything gained boils down to a trophy to be displayed, and it's only through the trophies that the self-esteem is manifested. I see this all the time.

Fear of Authority

Authorities want to dominate you. They make you feel that you must comply with their demands—or else. In any confrontation with authority, you may feel afraid, and you react by humbling yourself. The IRS sends you a letter and panic sets in, followed by anger and helplessness. How can you fight an institution that has everything on its side? You're just one person. You allow this insensitive, uncaring bureaucracy to affect your life.

Or you get pulled over for a traffic violation. Whether you are guilty or not, you feel helpless and act childlike. You answer the officer's questions obediently and try to act humble instead of standing up for your rights.

Fear that Your Real Needs Will Not Be Fulfilled

Most people live unfulfilled lives. They learn early in life that their own needs are unimportant and carry that belief with them into adulthood.

Parents often live through their children instead of helping them discover their own interests and attain things important to them. As a result, children may become ego extensions of their parents' dreams. A high school student becomes a football player because his dad wants him to be an athlete. Perhaps the child wants to be an artist. He is actively discouraged from doing so. His father tells him that art is something girls do. The boy's need to explore life through art is supplanted by his father's need for him to become an extension of his ego. Conversely, a child might want to become a football player but not explore that possibility because his parents fear the sport is too brutal and unnecessarily competitive. Once again, the child is acting out of a need to be accepted by his parents.

Most schools distance children from their own interests as well. They program pupils to learn things that have no relevance to their lives. A curriculum board that is out of touch with students dictates what the children are supposed to be learning. Teachers force them to regurgitate facts instead of exploring what is interesting and important to them. As a result, the student's natural curiosity is killed early in the game. Children either learn to become school-smart to get good grades, or drop out if they see nothing in it for them. Either way, they are never encouraged to explore and fulfill their own real needs.

So you can grow up with your real needs never being met. You may learn to be a certain kind of person who acts and reacts in certain predetermined ways. But maybe those ways aren't you. Maybe the real you has a different voice. If you are still in touch with your real needs, you end up living a surreptitious existence where you keep a real part of yourself hidden from others lest they judge you harshly for it.

Fear of Manipulation

You may be fearful of manipulation, and with good reason. Often, people don't accept you into their lives without wanting you to be a part of their agenda. For example, they're lonely and want you to fill the void.

The best way to avoid being manipulated is to be very aware of how someone makes you feel. Don't just listen to what a person says; look at her or his actions. If a person tells you that he accepts you for who you are but tries to get you to do things that are against your nature, then you're dealing with a manipulator. That person is using you to get something for himself.

Sometimes two people manipulate each other. They overlook the way they are treating one another because they want the relationship to supply them with something else they need, such as good sex or financial security. Two egos are working together, but each is working toward its own end. Sooner or later, people suffer as a result. Honesty, compassion, decency, and ethics are ultimately more important than the other things you think you need.

A lot of people are in recovery programs where they are acknowledging having been used or having used other people. They are learning to be upfront with others and not to be afraid to tell others what kind of person they are. They're learning to say to someone, "This is what I need and expect in a relationship."

Fear of Failure

You may be afraid to do something for fear of not doing it correctly. Therefore, you don't even make an attempt. If this describes you, ask yourself, what is the worst that can happen? Consider that most people don't do things perfectly the first, second, or even the tenth time. That doesn't mean you shouldn't try. It is only through doing that you learn. Keeping something in your head until you can execute it flawlessly will never work. That's not how humans function. Learning is a process that involves practice through doing.

If you were encouraged early on to do things regardless of the outcome, then you probably felt accepted for yourself. You tried things and did the best you could. You probably attempt new things with little anxiety.

Most of us, however, were not so fortunate. As a result, we've become a nation of spectators. We sit on the sidelines and pay good money to watch people who've conquered fear perform. More people would be actively engaged in things if they didn't have to combat the fear of doing them wrong.

Fear of Not Being in a Relationship

So many men and women have suffered in relationships that made them feel trapped. They were living in a war zone, stepping gingerly around emotional minefields. They were scared to say or do anything that might trigger some unwanted reaction. As a result, they would edit their thoughts, feelings, and actions just to keep arguments from erupting. They would do things just to please their partners, regardless of their own desires. They would go to a movie they didn't want to see or entertain people they didn't like. Everything they did was to accommodate the other person.

This happens frequently if you feel a need to be in a relationship, any relationship. You may feel unacceptable being alone. The average man or woman feels that he or she must be married by thirty or thirty-five. Otherwise they worry they'll be considered strange, or gay. People may discourage your legitimate right to be by yourself. If you are susceptible to a fear of being un-paired, you may get into a relationship for the wrong reasons and end up feeling trapped.

Fear of Speaking Up

I know people who keep silent about other people at work who are goofing off, doing bad work, stealing, or lying. They won't say anything because they're afraid of confrontation. Or they're afraid of what people will think, say, or do to them.

Keeping quiet about your point of view hurts you. The situation stays with you when you keep it inside. Part of you knows that you have to have enough courage to stand up and speak out when something is wrong.

A man once walked into my office when I was out. He acted obnoxious and rude to the people there but nobody said anything. When I heard about what had happened I asked why they had kept quiet. They said they didn't want to offend him. He might have been an important businessperson.

The next time this person came to the office I was there. I confronted him and he was shocked. I asked him if he would treat his daughter or his wife this way. Then I said that the people in my office were wives and daughters too. If the only person he was going to treat with respect was me then I couldn't do business with him. I couldn't trust him.

If you're like most people, you keep quiet because of your conditioning. You're taught to keep your mouth shut, to stay in your place, not to rock the boat, not to stand out. You become constrained by fear.

I'm suggesting that you correct or challenge situations as they arise. You can't change everything, of course. You can't make other people change. But you can let them know where you stand. And you can be an example for others. When you stand up, suddenly someone else will follow. You will help another person find the courage.

Fear of Incompleteness

Do you ever feel as if your life is incomplete? Perhaps you're filled with regret because time has passed you by and you realize that there are certain things you wish you had done differently.

Maybe you thought a relationship would make your life complete. So you devoted most of your time searching for the ideal relationship instead of looking inside and strengthening yourself.

There is no perfect relationship. You have to start a relationship with yourself. You need to be a friend to yourself before you can be a friend to anyone else. Love, honesty, patience, and understanding begin with you.

Fear of Aging and Dying

When you're young, you think you have an unlimited time in which to live. As you get older you accept that you do not have that kind of time. We do have a lot of information now about how to live longer. With what we know we can easily live to ninety healthfully. If you're very disciplined, one hundred or one hundred and ten is possible. That's realistic because the average life span has increased from sixty-eight to seventy-four in just twenty years. We can add another sixteen years to our age span in the next twenty years. Over the next forty years we should add at least another twenty or thirty years to that.

If you're forty, you're not even halfway there. At that point you've gotten your pace and direction. You have greater knowledge, patience, and willpower than you did when you were young. You have developed a lot of skills. Before you had unbounded energy. Now you have sustainable energy. It's like being in the tenth mile of the marathon. That's where you finally feel comfortable. Now you're in your stride. So look at aging from a positive point of view.

You do start to show signs of aging, of course, but there is a lot you can do to slow it down. You start to get wrinkles. Your body starts to lose some of its elasticity. You start to lose your hair. Everyone in my family is bald. I would be too if it weren't for the fact that when I was thirty I began researching what men can do to keep their hair. Now my hair is so thick I have to get it cut once a week. It grows incredibly fast. My hair color is natural and I have no wrinkles. My skin looks younger today than it did twenty years ago.

The idea that we lose strength with age is also misleading. Athletes used to think that after twenty you could no longer be a swimmer. When you were thirty you could no longer be a boxer. At thirty-three you could not longer be a basketball player. At thirty-five you could no longer be a football player. What nonsense. How long you last as an athlete depends upon how well you condition yourself.

I'm an athlete. This year I won Track and Field Master Athlete in the Metropolitan Athletic Congress. I set six American age group records indoors and two outdoors. I won twenty-seven championships just this year, and I beat records that I set ten years ago. And I haven't even reached my peak yet. Why? Because I'm willing to go one step beyond my fear.

If you wake up in the morning with fear, you won't get very far. You may fear you're no longer attractive; that you don't have the same capacity you used to have; that you'll never win competing with people who are twenty.

It's only when you let go of fear that you have control of your day in a constructive way. That control allows you to go forward.

Our parents accepted the inevitability of the aging process. They thought they were old at thirty-five or forty. It was considered normal to eat the wrong foods and to end up with high blood pressure and diabetes. I'll never forget the day my mother decided to cut her hair and change her clothes because she had turned forty. I came home from school and said, "What's going on? Why do you have old people's hair?" She said she was acting her age. She would never think of going out to jog because she didn't want to seem out of place. It wouldn't look right.

When is the last time you saw a senior citizen in a gym pumping iron? Working out can help them to keep their bodies tight. It keeps their buttocks in, their jaws from falling, the wrinkles from appearing, the osteoarthritis and osteoporosis away. But most are not going to do it because of fear of failure.

Fear of the Consequences of Personal Neglect

I was talking with a friend of mine, the owner of a video store. He's gone through a lot of stress and has gained a lot of weight. Now he's having chest pains. I advised him to get the weight off and to deal with his stress. Otherwise, he might end up having a heart attack. He told me he was afraid this might happen. He's angry with himself about it. I said he should use his anger constructively and start taking care of his health. Tomorrow he is going to get a complete physical examination and cardiovascular stress test just to see what's going on.

Until you take care of yourself, you'll have fear and anger. Self-loathing occurs when you neglect yourself. And this applies not just to your physical needs; you must also tend to your emotional, intellectual, and creative needs. You need to stimulate your brain through reading, for example. And you must take care of interpersonal needs. People need to hug, to share, and to love.

How Do You Manifest Fear?

Your fear can emerge in many ways. Do you identify with any of these modes of manifesting fear?

Sickness

Getting sick keeps you from having to face your responsibilities and unpleasant situations. When you're sick, you don't get pressured. People tend to your needs and are kind and accepting.

Complaining and Blaming

Whenever I hear someone moan or complain, I know they're reacting from fear. They make excuses for not doing anything. "I'd get out there but it's too hot, too cold, too dry, too wet, too breezy."

Some people are always blaming someone else for their problems. "It's not my fault, it's yours." "You made me sick." "You gave me a headache." People who are always blaming others may think they're getting rid of their responsibilities; actually, they're just manifesting their fear of the responsibility.

Compulsive/Addictive Behaviors

Fearful people often engage in compulsive and addictive behaviors. They compulsively eat, drink, or gamble, for example. Instead of going out and doing something constructive with their lives, they will engage in acts that hurt themselves. Gamblers who risk everything are in effect saying, I hate myself so much that I'm willing to destroy everything I've accumulated, including the love for my family and my home. I'm going to give it all away because I don't know who in the hell I am and I don't know how to get in touch with my real needs. I'm not happy. If I was, I wouldn't be gambling.

Compulsive/addictive people are wrapped up in their fears. They act in ways that disguise their feelings of terror, as they try to convert their fear into something else.

Escapism

Our society is very escape-oriented. People find creative ways of displacing their real fears. They watch soap operas because they are afraid to confront their own feelings. No matter how bad their problems, they pale in comparison to those of make-believe people.

Chronic Tension

A chronically tense person is hypercritical. Their intensity is palpable. You never feel relaxed and spontaneous around such a person.

The tense person doesn't always understand why he's on red alert all the time. The fear that is breeding this energy is not apparent. But if you're a chronically tense person, until you get in touch with what underlies that tension and how it affects you, it will limit you.

Notice any unresolved fears that keep you chronically tense. Do you find yourself getting into fights? Are you afraid of losing control, of being less responsible than others expect you to be, or of showing your uncertainty to people? Your tension becomes a symptom of that.

Withdrawing and Hiding from Your Real Feelings

When a person hides his (or her) fear, he's afraid to let others know what he's really feeling. They might criticize him for it. If he's honest with them, they might come down on him like a ton of bricks.

Maybe he had an experience in the past that taught him not to be honest because it was too painful to be. Soon he is dishonest not only with others but with himself, not admitting even to himself that he is fearful. The problem is that now he is living a very limited life. Because of his hidden fear, he's never explored the options available to him.

Describe a Life Circumstance You Would Like To Change

Ideally, how would you like to respond to fear? Practically, how do you respond?

Think of a situation that you handled inappropriately. Afterward, you probably thought about what you could have said and done differently. You changed the scenario in your mind and came out the hero. You developed an ideal way of handling the situation that was different from the way you actually dealt with it.

Strive for the ideal. I would love to finish the marathon in under two hours. When I'm training I fantasize about having the strength and speed of a gazelle. I acknowledge my practical speed and work from there.

You don't have to live up to your ideal. And don't criticize yourself if you can't reach it; it may be outside your grasp. But you can at least try for it.

Which Attitudes and Behaviors Do You Need to Change?

List the attitudes and behaviors that don't work for you. Until you correct them, nothing will change. You will repeat the same old patterns of behavior and continue to manifest the identical problems. If you continue to eat the wrong foods, you will stay overweight. Until you take responsibility for your health, you can continue going to the doctor for vitamin drips and colonics but nothing will really change.

Sit quietly and write about what doesn't work for you. What are you doing that isn't healthy? Are you hurting other people? Are you disrespectful? Perhaps you're a strict parent. You order your children around and discourage them from asserting

themselves. You may not even realize how discouraging you
are. As a result, your children grow up hating you and probably everybody else. They take on your worst characteristics.

Start looking at your patterns of behavior. Until you do,
nothing will change. But once you can clearly see your own
behavior patterns, you can then find the courage to change
them.

Will You Choose Loss of Control or Positive Change?

Nothing changes on its own. You have to be the architect of
your life in order to direct the change. Otherwise, you lose
control and land in fear-provoking situations. If you neglect
your health then the doctors and the hospital are in charge.
Better to process wellness and maintain your autonomy.

If you become angry at someone for jumping ahead of you
in a movie line and start a fist fight, you also lose control. Now
the police, the insurance company, the lawyers, and the judge
control your fate.

Think of the times you lost control because you chose not
to be the architect of positive change.

Doubting Wastes Time

Think of a time you wanted to do something but were held
back by your doubts and fears. You may be fixated on that
scenario and replay it over and over in your mind. You think
about what you could have done and how your life would be
different. Were your doubts justified?

Doubting can be avoided when you let your intuition guide
you. I base every major life decision on intuition. I find that

following my feelings helps me to make a right decision, while relying only on my brain often leads me to a wrong one.

Everyone has intuition, but most people in our objectivity-oriented society need to pay more attention to it. When you are involved in a relationship, you know when someone is about to undermine you. You feel it. You know where you fit in. You travel to a country or a town and you just feel right being there. You also know when you don't feel right in a specific place. You know when you're with someone if you feel comfortable or not.

Learn to trust your intuition. Let it be your guide. Pay attention to it and use it. It's an important asset. Once you know what is right for you and act on it, you erase doubts and fears. Then you can go after what you want in life.

Do You Validate the Positive and Invalidate the Negative?

Life involves making choices. Each morning, you decide whether your day will be guided by fear or love. If you choose fear, you will be interfering with your happiness and growth. If you choose love, you re-empower yourself. Your health, for example, is dependent upon your state of mind. Health and disease are processes—not static entities. Your daily thoughts, feelings, and actions affirm well-being or sickness.

You need to get beyond blaming other people, such as your parents, and take responsibility for your life. You can spend your entire life justifying being unfulfilled, or take charge and make your life work. When part of your life is dysfunctional, recognize that you created the pattern and that only you can change it. People play games when they say, I can't do that. They really can. If your life is working in one area, it can be equally positive in another.

Notice negative thoughts and actions and weed them out. It

is the weak link in any situation that causes failure. It is what you don't pay attention to that brings you down.

Reclaim your values and emphasize what is important. Identify your real needs. Write down what you need to be happy in your career, at home, and with friends. If you need loyalty then be with people who are loyal friends. If you need honesty in your relationship, don't accept anything less. Break old, destructive patterns of behavior. If others can't honor your needs, they shouldn't be in your life.

An example of someone who validated the positive is Dr. Martin Feldman. He graduated from Yale Medical School, magna cum laude. He is a professor of neurology at Mt. Sinai. After all his education he saw that he was not helping his patients and decided to incorporate nutrition into his protocol. As a result, he shifted his practice. But he made a choice. He saw that his methods were not constructive and he changed them so that now they are. He gave up making rationalizations and excuses about why patients weren't getting better. Now he doesn't have to make those rationalizations or excuses.

Don't Filter Reality

Let reality be what it is. We're always trying to filter what we see and hear to make it into something else. But by seeing reality for what it is, we can deal with it. If there is corruption, we should see it for what it is. Then we can respond to it instead of pretending it isn't there.

Of course it's hard to change the world around us. Sometimes it's impossible. But I've learned that even if I can't change the world, I can change my response to it. I don't have to get crazy, fearful, and angry because other people act that way. I can maintain balance even if others are imbalanced. I can remain peaceful even if others are belligerent. It takes two clashing egos to fight.

I have learned how to remain free of someone else's negativity. I can have negative people around me, but I don't need to be a part of the negativity.

You can learn all these things, too.

Starting Over:
New Beginnings

❖

Do you ever wish you could go to sleep and wake to find your problems gone? Unfortunately, it's not that simple. Change requires an active role on your part. This section is designed to guide you through change.

You've already decided that you're sick and tired of being sick and tired. Perhaps relationships repeatedly fail. You're stuck in the same old boring job. You desperately want your life to work and are open to a new perspective on living. It's time to start over.

I believe that every person has the capacity to change who he or she is. I do not accept the notions of twelve-step programs, ongoing therapy, and the kind of self-help books that keep you reliving past traumas. You can engage in all these and still stay the same by using the past as an excuse not to actualize the present. You define who you are by what you've done and, in the process, lose sight of your potential.

You need to suspend judgment and become vulnerable in

order to accept that there is another way of perceiving life. If you're not open to that possibility then you have no future.

For example, let's say you act in dysfunctional ways because you were a battered child, or your father was an alcoholic. As a child you responded as best you could. As a young person of five or six, you may have had to adapt to an unhealthy situation in order to survive. You didn't yet have the intellectual capacity to deal with these issues. All you understood was that you needed to be loved and accepted.

Many people are influenced by those impressionable years for the rest of their lives. Authority figures, such as superiors at work, may represent your mother or father in your mind. You carefully watch what they do, how they look at you, and what their body language says. You acquiesce to their demands by never speaking up for yourself. When they talk to you, you look down.

Although you appear normal to the world, inside you may be filled with rage. You may sublimate that anger by working compulsively or engaging in other addictive behavior. There are a thousand ways to manifest self-contempt.

Why not change these unproductive patterns of behavior? Don't cling to them your whole life. The key is in acknowledging the present and letting go of the past. Realize that at any moment you can choose between living in the present, or in your memories. Let's begin the process by taking an honest look at the following questions. As you reflect on them, see what answers feel right to you.

What Are the Internal and External Limiting Factors in Your Life?

Answering this question helps you prepare for a new beginning. Make a list of your limits. Note the restrictions others place on you, such as those involved in being a woman or a member of a minority group, and those that you impose upon yourself, such as an assumption that you can't learn a particular skill.

Reviewing your list helps you see what restraints you need to overcome. If you hold yourself back because you are a woman, for instance, explore that issue. As a woman you need to know what you're up against. Until recently, women were barred from racing in marathons. Men wanted women to believe that their bodies couldn't handle the physiological stress. The truth is that women are better suited to racing. Today, according to Fred Lebow (director, New York City Marathon) more women run marathons than men and, some finish ahead of them.

Rampant sexism still prevails throughout society. Some men feel intimidated by women moving into the work force. As a result, male policymakers generally don't offer women the same opportunities or equal pay for identical responsibilities. Most sexual harassment occurs when a man feels threatened by a woman's presence. He suspects that she might be better at the job and replace him. Instead of competing fairly, he demeans her and makes her feel uncomfortable about being there.

Look at your list and ask yourself, where do my limitations come from? Then set your mind on overcoming them. Two dramatic examples come to mind here. The first is provided by a sixty-seven-year-old woman, named Queenie Thompson, who showed up one day a few years ago at my running and walking club in Central Park. She had three elements working against her: she was a woman, African-American, and a senior citizen. During the running clinic, I said to the group that I didn't care how slow anyone was. Today we start a process, I said. Don't expect immediate results; plan long-term goals. I promised them that if they would stick with this and believe in themselves as much as I believed in them, they would reach their goals and become models for others.

We started racing and Queenie was last in a group of a couple of hundred. I thought that everyone was finished when someone told me that one person was still way down the road. I went to meet her. Queenie was just barely moving. She was overweight and had some physical problems. I asked her how she was feeling and she told me that she didn't think racing was going to be for her. Her friends thought her coming to the club was a stupid idea and she should listen to them. She ought to act her age and spend Sunday mornings sitting on the boardwalk with the other old people, discussing her aches and pains.

I asked her then where she wanted to be. She told me she wanted to be here. "I only care where your mind wants to be," I said. "I'm not concerned about your body, because it will improve over time. But you need a strong mind to make the transition possible. Each week, as you get stronger, people are going to become more adamant about your stopping. The better you feel about yourself, the worse they'll feel about themselves. They'll project that onto you. You're holding up a mirror to these people and making them see that they don't have their lives together. You're going to get a lot of negative feedback. If you can handle that, everything else will fall into place."

Queenie kept on coming back. For the longest time she was the slowest person there, but she never lost sight of her goal. We kept encouraging her. Sometimes a voice would come into her head telling her to give up and act her age. She learned to pay it no mind. Instead she replaced her limiting thoughts with positive ones. She would say to herself, I'm getting younger. I'm having fun. I'm feeling great.

Her persistence paid off. Queenie Thompson no longer comes in last, but first. She has mounted the podium to take the gold medal for the twenty-third time in three years. Right now, at seventy, Queenie is a world champion. She won two gold medals at the international games. That means she is one of the best athletes, not just in America, but in the whole world.

Queenie Thompson is a completely different person from the woman at that first club meeting. She has a vivacious personality with a positive disposition. Her body is lean and muscular. Her wrinkles have disappeared and she looks like a young person. Her health is dramatically improved as well.

The second illustration is about a friend who overcame limiting beliefs about her work. Brenda Baskin used to be close to 275 pounds. She was very angry and bitter, even though she was financially successful as an art director for one of America's largest advertising agencies.

People expected a lot from her, and she never let them down. As a result, Brenda had no life outside of work. I'd call her at eight in the morning and she was at her job. At eleven at night she was still there. It wasn't her work she was doing, but work for other people. She often felt uncomfortable but thought she was powerless to change her situation. You can't tell a client you don't want to promote their product because the product's unhealthy. As a result, she became angry.

Finally, she decided that she had had enough. She started preparing for a new direction. That took six months. Then she quit her job and went back to school to become a chiropractor.

Now she's a different human being. She lost the excess weight and is light and happy. The child in her is out and playing. She's creating her own art and openly taking care of her own needs. She is becoming the healer she always wanted to be, and as a result feels empowered. She understands that this is her life to live, and no one else's.

These are just two examples among many I could give of why I believe there is a champion inside every human being.

Start by setting new limits. See yourself where you want to be. Visualize yourself as successful, a winner, crossing the finish line, practicing a new career, or completing whatever it is you want to do. Forget the rules you've been taught. They're for the conditioned self, not the new you.

Do You Consider Your Problems More Important than Your Ideals?

When you focus on your problems, you never get around to living your ideals. People tell me, "Gary, I'll develop spiritual and emotional growth later. In the future, I'll learn to be loving and nurturing and to develop bonds. I'll get around to doing service for society after I resolve my problems. Then I'll have time to help other human beings."

The trouble is, that time never comes. When you focus on problems, the moment you get rid of one, you replace it with another. You've got to let the problem mentality go.

When your mind is centered on difficulties you tend to compromise your ideals. Notice which problems and concerns you think about. When you need something so badly that you think you can't live without it, ask yourself, what am I giving up? I spoke to a man this morning who told me he resorted to stealing to maintain a lifestyle he and his family are used to living. Of course, something is terribly wrong when you lie, cheat, and steal to get money.

I advised him to let his house go. After all, it's just so much square footage. "Your ideals are more important than 1,600 or 2,000 square feet," I said. "You've got a whole world to explore. There are millions of people to relate to and myriad experiences to have. Who says that you've got to spend every ounce of your energy protecting that square footage? Think of how much of your life is wasted guarding that investment. Where is the higher ideal?"

He confided in me that he worried about his family not perceiving him as a provider. To this, I suggested that he and his family become co-providers. In other words, they needed to change their priorities and work together. They needed to work on their lives, not just be concerned with income. In the process, they would experience new people, cultures, and places instead of being prisoners of their own lifestyle. Giving things up can be freeing.

You can't just say, I'll change once I'm free of debt. That never works. The time to focus on your ideals is now.

Fooling Ourselves with Illusions

Before you can change you need to investigate the illusions under which you living.

Health

Have you been living with our society's common illusion about health? Our paradigm in this country lets people think they are healthy as long as they aren't dying in a hospital. People are never told that disease is a process that takes years to manifest and that they contribute to this process. As a result, the average person doesn't think that he or she has anything to do with creating diseases such as cancer or arthritis. Being passively healthy is a false illusion, and it's one we're not encouraged to challenge.

Could you imagine waking up each day and saying, "I only process wellness?" You would allow only healthful foods into your body and positive thoughts into your mind. You would associate only with cheerful people. Well, that's how I live my life. I view every day as a new beginning. I start each morning with a guided visualization in which I tell myself, "This day, the only things coming into my mind are positive, life-affirming thoughts. I assert that nothing but good comes to me and nothing but good comes from me."

Each day I allow nothing into my body that can cause me harm. I had lunch today with some people. As we were eating, one man said to me that nobody can be perfect. Everyone cheats sometimes. I said to him, "It's not a matter of perfection. I never cheat and I don't consider myself special. I think of myself as what should be normal." I continued, "Why would I eat something that is going to hurt me? You may think that you are getting away with something but I know better." I believe that if we make ourselves aware of the effects of our actions, we will never dishonor the body or the mind.

You have choices. True self-empowerment means you're using those choices to engage in thoughts and actions that sustain health. Make time each day for intellectual, emotional, and spiritual growth. Honor your heart and spirit. Every day reaffirm a new beginning. Start and end each day looking at your ideal. Don't read headlines or listen to the news. That's negative. It reminds you how bad things are. When you focus on the possibilities, you can let in the new.

Happiness

Many people live under the illusion that they are happy when in reality they are only complacent. For example, two people who are together a long time may learn to adapt to each other even though the feelings of bliss and excitement are long gone.

Be with people who excite you. I've had many of the same friends for twenty and thirty years, and I'm still excited about being with them. There is joy in our time together.

Love

Love is the most abused word in the vocabulary. People say they are making love when they're not. They're having sex. They say they're falling out of love. In reality, their codependent relationship is ending.

People confuse love with need. They think they're nobody unless somebody loves them because they need someone other than themselves to make them feel worthwhile. People do all kinds of things that compromise their basic values to gain someone else's attention and respect.

In its essence, love is something that comes from inside the self. You need to love yourself first. The more you love yourself, the more love you can give—and receive. You radiate a light that draws people.

Love should be manifested every day, in every way, and it can be. When you're starting over, begin with the idea that you can love yourself unconditionally. Every time you start to get down on yourself, stop and remind yourself that you choose to love yourself.

Job Security

There was, until recently, an illusion that as long as you put in your time and worked without complaining, you would have job security for life. Our society has learned a hard lesson about that illusion in the past decade.

The only way to become secure is to become self-sufficient. Those who wait for someone to take care of them end up disappointed, hostile, and self-abusive. They sit in front of the television set growing fat, or chain-smoking. Frequently they abuse their families. They deprive others of their love because their company betrayed them.

These people are terrified of change. They want things to be the way they were told they always would be. They're living by the control and power others have imposed on them. So when they no longer have a job, they have nothing to rely on because they've never trusted themselves.

You betray yourself by stopping your own growth. As long as you're growing you always land on your feet. You adapt.

Friends

How many of your friends are real friends? Are they there to share something? Or are they there because they want something? Or only *when* they want something? Did you ever think you had real friends only to discover you did not?

Home

People think that they are being cheated out of the American dream if they don't own a home; many perceive owning a home as the most important thing in life. One of the biggest sources of anxiety in America is the fear people have of losing their homes.

In reality, home is your heart. It's where you feel you belong. If we belong to ourselves then wherever we are, we're at home.

Have you ever been with people or in romances where you didn't care if you had a home? You just loved being with the person. Your whole day was centered around looking forward to what you could share together. Then after awhile, maybe you started focusing on the security of a home. The home became more important than the person. No home should ever be more important than love or sharing with another human being.

Make Dreams Come True

You must trust and believe in yourself. You must get excited by your own dreams and capabilities. Every day I look at the projects that I want to do. Then I write them down. They don't have to be done that day, but I want to keep my mind centered on my plans. I get excited by my ideas. I work on one idea at a time. I'm always examining my potential so I can make something happen.

Write down your ideas in order to keep your excitement level up. Put your ideas in front of you every day and just keep working on them. There is no one better than you to be your cheerleader and coach.

What else can you do to make your dreams come true?

Don't Welcome Your Old Self Back

The moment your old self starts to reappear—you start whining, complaining, moaning, feeling guilty, and feeling bad—stop and say, "Old self, you are not allowed in. Good-bye. Hello again, new self." You've got to keep bringing yourself back to where you want to be.

Don't Empower Boredom, Emptiness, and Fear

The moment you entertain fear, you don't try anything new. If you feel empty, it is because you are not allowing in all the wonderful things that can fill your life. Think of the beauty of the wilderness, of how wonderful human nature is when it's honest and open.

Don't allow a moment of your life to be empty. Put joy into each second. You can do this because you have choices. You can choose to spend a moment thinking, I'm not with someone, I'm alone. I'm lonely. Or you can think, I'm going to use this alone time to meditate, to reflect, to work on myself. Then you never have emptiness in your life.

No one who is excited by his or her own capacity is ever bored. How in the world can anyone be bored with the wonderful world we have and all the beautiful people we have in it? There are great places everywhere and amazing things being done by people every day. There's no way you can be bored once you engage in life. You can't engage in one billionth of what is out there to do. Anyone who is bored is saying, in effect, I'm closing myself off to life. Open yourself up.

Rediscover Your Childlike Aspects

If you're going to engage in new beginnings, this is the most important thing. This is where you get down to what really counts. I believe that in every human being there is a child, and that that child is the most beautiful part of the person's nature. Staying in touch with that part of your nature allows you to be vulnerable and grow.

Unfortunately, most people learn to tame that part of themselves. First your parents tell you to grow up and act your age. Then your teachers make you sit still and be quiet and obedient. You start to feel guilty and learn to follow their rules and expectations.

To start over in a healthy way, get in touch with the child you've buried inside. Allow the rebirth of that child. Every day find one new quality of childhood and manifest that trait all day. Let it come out at work, during play, and in your relationships. Keep using it. Bring it to the fore.

Look at the following qualities that children often display. Consider how you can use these qualities to enhance your life.

Innocence

As children, we were innocent about everything. As we advance through life, though, we lose touch with our innocence. We abuse the truth again and again, and in time become jaded. We believe the only way of communicating is through deception and half-truths. We let our real needs and feelings be neglected because we don't admit to them.

At this point we need more than ever to recreate the part of childhood that embodies innocence. We need to recall how we once acknowledged the wonder of learning, and how every single discovery was an exhilarating experience that redefined us and our environment. We need to appreciate people for who they are and not judge them by what society and our preconceived notions tell us to think.

By allowing the innocence of our childlike aspect to manifest itself, we are renewing our lives. We can have a fresh perspective once we clean the slate and allow each day to be brand new. Innocence is the quality at the heart of forgiveness and human growth.

Curiosity

Babies have amazing curiosity. Watch a baby monkey, a kitten, a puppy, a lion cub, or a human baby. They all have one thing in common. They find that everything is worth exploring. Every nook and cranny, and everything that moves, engages them in exploration. Life is a puzzle that they are actively trying to solve. They want to explore for the sake of exploring; they're not looking for some reward. They will taste things without knowing whether or not they will like them. They have the curiosity to try.

Curiosity allows people to grow. Without curiosity they repeat fixed patterns of behavior and every day becomes the same. I have always wondered how people could not be curious about things like ballet or folk dances, how a fiddle is made, or how a small engine gets a big plane off the ground. I'm curious about how a heart pumps, how an acorn becomes a tree, and what happens to the spirit after the body dies. All these wonderings stem from a childlike curiosity.

By bringing curiosity back into your life, you renew your passion for living. To do this, you must first eliminate the need for certainty, predictable outcomes, and control over your environment. The need for control smothers curiosity, destroys spontaneity, and extinguishes vitality.

Wouldn't you like to go out and explore people, events, places, experiences? Don't tame your curiosity. That makes you cynical and judgmental. Curiosity allows you to explore and grow.

Energy

If there's one thing that characterizes children, it's energy! If we want to get in better touch with the child within us, perhaps we can attune ourselves to the energy that is everywhere, and tap into it.

There are many forms of energy at work in your body. Electrical energy allows the central nervous system to transmit nerve impulses so that you can move. Chemical energy permits hormones and enzyme systems to synthesize. Thermal energy lets the internal body core temperature stay at ninety-eight degrees no matter how cold or hot your surroundings. Osmotic energy allows lymph and blood to flow through your system. Mechanical energy lets muscle movements occur.

All of these energies are part of a larger system, the life energy, which directs all other energies. Although energy is needed for motion, thought is needed even before that. Therefore, energy is consciousness. I don't tell the trillions of cells in my body what to do. I don't even know all the things they do. Yet they do what they're supposed to do twenty-four hours a day. How is that possible unless there is a grand system focusing all these energies?

Conscious energy always exists. It cannot be created or destroyed. Only its form can be altered. Your life, therefore, is merely a continuum of some energy that is immortal. Your body is a vehicle that, for a period of years, has the opportunity to use the energy you've been given. You may not be the wisest or most saintly person who has ever lived, but you can do something with your life energy if you understand that the first rule of life is to honor it.

By honoring the energy that life represents, you are becoming aware of your connection to nature. You're a part of it, because all energies are connected. George Leonard said that there is a silent thread that weaves its way through all people and connects us.

At some point, you must reconcile the difference between learned consciousness and universal consciousness. What you are conditioned to believe comprises your learned consciousness. That could be wrong. You could learn to be a racist. You could learn that your culture is better or worse than another. You could learn the art of self-denial and avoidance. You could learn insensitivity or subjugation. Then you are living your life as if your beliefs comprise the only reality there is.

It is the vanity and insecurity people feel in their everyday lives that force them to believe that they must continually prove themselves in order to protect what little they have. People constantly struggle to prove that they are worthy of love, respect, or social position. When a person becomes accepted on some level, efficient at doing something, or recognized for something, generally all their time and energy go into maintaining that image.

Universal consciousness, on the other hand, is the ultimate reality. When you connect with it, you intuitively know right from wrong. It permits you to love unconditionally, to respect all life, to honor others no matter what differences exist between you.

You can develop a deeper spiritual awareness by listening to your inner voice. It will connect you to a higher consciousness, which makes you aware that regardless of social position or financial wealth, you are still equal in all respects to any king or sage that has ever lived. The dynamics of a spiritual life balance all other things.

Fortunately, many people have connected to their inner voice and have allowed it to guide them. That's why we have humaneness. That's why we care about suffering, and why we have not lost our empathy and our motivation to be the best we can be.

Capacity to Learn

Children learn as naturally as sponges soak up water. Even when we are adults, there is no limit to what we can learn. But we should always remember that learning is not merely the ability to retain and retrieve facts. The most important lessons involve our capacity to surrender the need to be right and allow a natural process of cause and effect to occur. I've seen people who were taught the right way to racewalk and found it cumbersome and mechanically inappropriate for their bodies. When these people were allowed to modify the form so it was less technically correct but better adapted to their own bodies, they did much better. In our society we should begin to realize that our capacity to learn is directly related to our capacity to adjust and adapt to our own unique psychological, emotional, creative, and physiological requirements. No two people are the same. Yet people try to create standards as if all people were alike.

The capacity to learn also means that we can unlearn. The hardest thing to give up is knowledge, especially if that knowledge has served us well in some respects. But what serves us well in certain respects is not always the right thing to hold onto. Much of the knowledge that we have prided ourselves on maintaining is neither useful nor universally true.

A reality should be universal. Kindness, sensitivity, passion, and honesty are universal realities. Yet we alter universal realities to meet our own individual needs. That's not always wise, because we start bringing in our conditioning, which tells us to learn only what will benefit us.

As a result, people don't generally do things unless it gives them an immediate reward, either in terms of recognition, monetary value, or social position. So learning for the joy of learning and for the broadening of our consciousness, and giving up old ideas and replacing them with new ones, are not considered desirable activities.

Tolerance of Imperfection

Children don't examine their imperfections. They don't say, "I can't do this because . . . I can't do that because . . ." They don't particularly care about perfection as a virtue. Adults, on the other hand, like the idea of a flawless work of art, a flawless concerto, or a flawless poem. What is ignored is the process that leads to perfection. What we often don't understand is how many drafts go into writing the poem, how many lessons precede the masterpiece, and how many rehearsals go into the great performance.

I believe that your goal should not be perfection, which is impossible to achieve. Your goal should be, rather, the process that allows you to continue to grow your entire life, and to continue striving to enhance, renew, broaden, and deepen your awareness of what you're doing, but never to the point at which you feel you are flawless in what you do. That state—flawlessness—should always be just beyond your grasp.

Once we understand that nothing that we do in life will ever be perfect, striving for perfection is no longer our focus. We must continue to stretch beyond our comfort zone, and force our mind, body, and ideas into an area where there are no certainties. It's in the area of uncertainties, where we go further than we ever thought we were capable of going, that new inspiration occurs. Though we don't know how we create it, we do. Answers occur even to questions that we never thought to ask. The process allows that to occur.

Be like a child. Don't look at your flaws. Look at what works.

Fearlessness

Do you ever notice little children acting like little heroes? They're not afraid.

We look up to people who have overcome insurmountable challenges. They become our heroes. And we recognize the struggle of the heroic effort even if the goal is not always achieved. We become inspired by strength and focus in the face of an uncertain outcome. The effort itself is heroic.

Movies are great at capturing the essence of real-life heroism and depicting it for us. In the movie *Chariots of Fire*, the main character, a runner, falls on a track and seems to be out of the race. The film goes into slow motion as he gets back up, so that you can see the agony on his face when he is unsure that he can go forward. Then you see his determination as he pushes himself to catch up to the pack. He must let go of all of his fear, and trust that there is, within him, a strength that he has never tapped. It is that heroic strength that allows him to finally pass the others. In another movie, *Iron Will*, a boy in a dogsled race takes on a 500-mile trek from Canada to St. Paul, Minnesota. The boy has to endure everything that can go wrong, yet he never loses his spirit. He never says he's going to stop, even when his body can barely move. At the very end he wins the race with just a second to go, and clearly becomes a hero. People who make such sacrifices and are willing to go through such pain inspire others.

Heroes engage in life. Each day, in their own quiet way, without grandstanding, they go out to push just a little further beyond their comfort zone. That is what strengthens them. I believe that every person is a hero. You don't have to be a racer or engage in an activity that would be the subject of a movie. But you are a hero when you take a journey to challenge that which seems insurmountable. Start your hero's journey. Find one cause and commit yourself to an ideal.

Honesty

Children have no problem saying what they feel. Most adults have lost that ability. Think of what it would be like if you said what you felt. Start doing it. I do. It scares people because they are used to other people telling them what they would like to hear, not what you need to tell them. They want you to edit what you say so they can accept it.

When I do a radio show and tell things as they are, I'm not concerned about whether or not you can handle honesty. I must honor the sanctity of my inner being. You may say, "Gary, I don't like what you're saying. It hurts. I don't want to hear it." Or you may say, "Gary, thank you." The point is, I'm not going to tailor what I say in order to produce only the positive response.

Of course, you have to practice social decorum and be sensitive toward others' feelings. But that doesn't mean you should lie. I'd much rather be with someone who is honest with me than with someone who says what he thinks I want to hear but doesn't mean it.

Wonder

Look at life and be filled with all that is there. Don't restrict yourself to a narrow range of living, with the same repetitive actions and motions each day.

Look for the enchantment of discovery. Have you ever noticed how children do things for the sake of doing them? They don't need to be rewarded; the exploration and discovery are reward enough. A child plays with something, finds it exciting, and then is able to let it go and move on.

Adults tend to engage in activities for the reward. Then, once they get it, they try to guard and control the reward. They accumulate and are afraid of letting things go, because what they accrue becomes part of their identity. They become afraid to let go of their title, success, and money. Adults forget how to explore life for the joy of it. They become prisoners trapped by what they've accumulated.

The person who is happy with life is the person who achieves something but then moves on. That person will also be able to share the fruits of his or her experiences with other people.

Creativity

Children love to create. They create without the need to obtain something from it. You should too.

I write books, but don't allow myself to be called an author.

When you call yourself an author you establish an identity. You're an intellectual snob. For me, writing is a creative method of communicating, not a status-generator.

If you create for the joy of it, you become creative in everything you do. You redecorate your apartment, change your work space, or dress differently. Have fun and be creative in all things.

Adaptability

Children will adapt to any environment. You should learn from that. No matter where you find yourself, look for pleasure and joy there.

Forgiveness

Children always forgive. They can't hold a grudge. That's one of their most inspired qualities. Children are able to let go and get on with their lives.

Tomorrow, make a new beginning by forgiving people in your life. Forgive them and let go of the anger.

Happiness

Watch children. They find happiness in little things. In the middle of a wretched environment they still find happiness. As adults we lose that. We may have so much and not appreciate any of it. Sometimes we can't find happiness when we've been given every opportunity to be happy.

Start having happy times and feeling happy. Respect what you do have.

Love and Sharing

Every human being has the capacity to love; all of us certainly used that capacity daily as children, if given any opportunity at all to do so. I think we should start making a point every day, now, to show love.

The eighties were a time of me, me, me. Everything seemed to be geared to the self. But we're well past that decade. Isn't it time you started sharing with other people? Give something back and share with others.

Trust

A child trusts everyone. Until you hurt a child by betraying her trust, she will trust you. I believe in trust. Until you show me you can't be trusted, I will trust you. I believe trust is essential for growth. You need to trust other cultures, races, beliefs, and religions, and learn from them.

I trust there is good in all things if I look for it. While there is positive and negative in all things, I trust that I can separate the two.

Spontaneity

Children are naturally spontaneous, but as they grow up, people eventually become conditioned to plan everything they do. They start to think, do I want to or not? about every possible activity.

Why not just do stuff? It will give you freedom. I don't always think about what I do. I just do stuff all the time. For instance, the other night, a friend who had just come from a boring party, and was all dressed up, called me. She said, "What do you want to do?" I said, "Let's go down to the Bowery." We did, and as cars pulled up we washed people's windows for about an hour. People would say, "God, that looked like Gary Null!" They'd roll down the window and I'd give them a quarter. I'm sure their analysts are thinking they're absolutely psychotic. "Some guy in a tuxedo washed my window and gave me a quarter." That was fun.

What you remember about a lot of the experiences you share in life are the fun and spontaneity of them. You talk about what is different, interesting, and exciting. Get out of your own way and live.

Dream the Impossible

I love it when people tell me what they are dreaming about because they're creating new possibilities. That's exactly what they should be dreaming about.

It doesn't matter if you actually achieve your dreams. The important thing is the idea that you're not afraid of them. You're not scared of what is in your heart. How many times have you chased a rainbow even though you never found the end of it? As a child, I used to run all over the place looking for the end of a rainbow. I'd be gone for a whole afternoon. I'd get lost and not know where I was. I'd ask people, "Do you know where the end of the rainbow is?" I would just keep walking for miles and miles. I never found the end, but it was a wonderful adventure. The adventure was in seeking the dream.

Remember to dream and to follow your aspirations.

Ask for Help

When a child can't do something, he or she will come and ask you for help. That seems simple and sensible, but have you ever noticed how rarely adults do that? They won't admit that anything in their life is not working. Ask for help if you need help. There's nothing wrong with that.

Respect for the Self

Most people don't realize how worthy they are. Don't victimize yourself; there's no point to it. Be kind to yourself. List your worthy qualities. If you're like most people, you don't focus often enough on your good points. You have many wonderful qualities. Actually write them down and study the list. Then honor and use your wonderful qualities each day, as a child does.

Stop. Have You Played Today?

No? Then you're still too serious. Every day should include playtime. You work every day and need play to balance yourself.

A lot of people won't acknowledge their emotional needs. They'll justify not playing by thinking, "adults shouldn't do things like that." It doesn't go with their image. They're supposed to be serious in their enjoyments. They'll think to themselves, I'm supposed to enjoy poetry readings, books, and French movies I don't understand. I'm only supposed to laugh at politically appropriate things.

I believe that every man and woman has a desire to play just as children do. Play is interesting and fun. I want to be around people who are able to acknowledge this part of themselves; I don't want to be around serious people all the time. That's no fun.

Think of the people in your life. Are they able to find time for play, or is the relationship overly serious and predictable? Are you able to play wherever you're at, or do you reserve playtime just for vacations? You've got to be able to play without caring if anyone criticizes you for it.

Stop. Don't Bash Yourself

Whatever you do is okay. Don't look for perfection. Don't look for everything to be perfect or complete. Whatever you do, it's enough. Pat yourself on the back. Be kind to yourself. You're alright.

Stop. Problems Are Not About Blame

Problems help you learn and grow. We all have problems, but unless we look at the solutions we're going to perpetuate our problems. I don't blame anyone for what goes down and what comes around. I simply say, it's a part of life.

Stop Listening to What Doesn't Work

If you're putting your energy in one direction and not finding fulfillment, then change perspectives. Stop asking for advice from the same old tired voices. Get a different opinion. Get your own opinion. Whose life is it? Yours or someone else's?

Seek Until You Find

You may not know what is right for you in certain areas of your life. Continue searching for what feels right—no matter how many efforts you have to make. Don't stop because you've been conditioned to stop. If it isn't right, then it doesn't fit. It doesn't mean you or the other person is wrong. It doesn't mean that the job is wrong. It means that what you are doing doesn't meet your real needs.

For instance, working at a hundred jobs and quitting each one is better than working in one place and being unhappy. I'd much rather have someone say, "Gary, I can't work with you in this place," than to have the person work for me and be unhappy about it. If you are honest, there are no hard feelings. I don't consider that irresponsible. Likewise, I don't see anything wrong with going out with a hundred people—or a thousand people—or a million people—rather than settling for someone who isn't suited to you. Let's face it. With all the dysfunctional people in this world, or functional people who don't share your energy, you have a right to continue your search.

How many people do you know who are really fulfilled with their lives? Very few. But most people compromise their potential for fulfillment because of self-imposed limitations.

I believe we don't have to make that kind of compromise— not if we empower ourselves, each day, with the strength to renew our search.

Choosing Joy

Change Your Life for the Better

One day, when Gary Null was five years old, he set out with his lunch in his hand, on a journey to find the end of the rainbow. In the ten miles he traveled, he saw more of the world than he would have if he'd lacked an imagination of life's possibilities.

Our personal quests begin in the imagination. Only in an honest confrontation with the self, however—recognizing its strengths and candidly scrutinizing its limitations in terms of our energy types—can we realize our potential to journey to greater emotional comfort, spiritual enlightenment, intellectual growth, and bodily health. In Choosing Joy, *Null places such exhilarating possibilities within the reader's easy reach, not by providing glib answers but by simply asking a series of searching, carefully orchestrated questions. While your answers may not bring you to the end of your personal rainbow, they will show you where you're going and how to get there.*

Contents

Introduction

The day of my high school graduation was one of the saddest days of my life. After hats were thrown into the air, I came to the somber realization that nothing would ever be the same again. I had been friends with many of these people for most of my 18 years, and we were supposed to be friends for life. But in spite of childhood promises, I knew my friendships would suddenly evaporate after graduation day.

That night we all made the rounds, as in the movie *American Graffiti*, driving past our old haunts. I committed each smiling face that I encountered to memory. Despite the party atmosphere, my underlying feeling was morbid, as if I were looking into a casket and saying good-bye for the very last time. It was not a happy night.

When I arrived home, it was four o'clock in the morning. I was surprised to see my dad sitting on the steps waiting for me. He was a man who had a bittersweet existence, a brilliant man who, to my mind, was more innovative and progressive than it was comfortable for his friends and associates to acknowledge. Instead of receiving encouragement, he got negative feedback from the important people in his life. He tried to fit into society by acquiescing to its demands and expectations, and in the process suppressed his true spirit. Eventually he began to drink as a way of drowning out the creative part of his psyche. He never fell down drunk, but all my life he was belligerent, angry, and blaming.

On this night, however, he was not drinking. He was sitting there waiting for me, something he had never done before.

I asked, "What are you doing up, Dad? It's four o'clock in the morning."

He replied, "I realize there were many times in your life I should have helped you to understand how life changes, but I didn't and I'm sorry." He paused for a moment, then looked me square in the eye and went on, "My graduation from high school was one of the saddest days of my life because I knew things would never be the same again. I knew that everyone who had accepted me and supported my ideas would be gone. Childhood friendships would be over, along with feelings of being able to master anything. Even though we had different economic and cultural backgrounds, we all believed in our equal ability to do anything we set our minds to. But once we left school, everything changed."

I told him that was very strange because all day I had been having similar feelings. I had been acknowledged all these years for expressing myself through poetry, essays, and athletics, and for standing up to things I felt were unjust in society—but now I wasn't going to have anyone else's support.

He agreed that my perceptions were correct. Then he gave me some important advice.

"I want to share something with you that may give you a completely different view of life," my father said. "I want you to do something that I didn't do, Gary Michael. I want you to leave this community. This was a wonderful place to spend your childhood. There is innocence and honesty here, as well as the spirit of adventure and exploration. You were never told you couldn't do things. You were always encouraged, even when you climbed out your window at night and slid down the drainpipe right past your mother and me in the kitchen. We knew you were going out to build your tree house, but we didn't stop you.

"Another time you took your lunch box and went out for five hours to see if you could find the end of the rainbow. You were only five years old, but determined to find it. We let you walk all the way to the end of town, cross the bridge that separates West Virginia from Ohio, and go into the countryside ten miles away. We wanted you to know that you might not find the end of the rainbow, but it was worth looking for. You should always believe that you could. We felt it was important for you to have the sense that there is something out there for you, something more than the eye can see."

Before that talk, I never thought of all the positive values my parents had instilled in me. By allowing me the opportunity to explore life early, they encouraged me to be idealistic. I learned that honest people can be powerful and that systems are there to help, not to limit us.

As a child, I was allowed to see, hear, and speak to imaginary friends, and this taught me to be open to myriad possibilities in life. Had I been discouraged from believing in gods and goddesses, inner guides and inner spirits, it would have quickly stilled my childlike innocence. It would have taught me to accept only the materialistic processes of life and to distrust natural ones.

My father taught me to believe that I was connected to something larger than life and to question convention. Although I was raised as a Baptist, I was not afraid to challenge tradition. I was the only young person in church, for example, ever to stand up in front of the entire congregation and ask the embarrassed minister how we ended up with blacks and Chinese and other people in the world if Adam and Eve were the only two people ever created.

If my parents hadn't let me have those experiences, and if my father hadn't summed it up for me that night, I might have felt limited by the things I had not been allowed to do. Perhaps I would have broken away from them rebelliously so that I could do all the things they had prevented me from doing. Instead of learning that I could challenge old systems or make new ones, I might have fallen into line with everyone else.

My father then gave me his car keys for the first time. He wanted me to use the car to visit my friends and see that something had changed. I appreciated that and I gave him a hug. I told him how I was touched by his sharing this transition I was going through because it was lonely and terrifying. I had no idea what tomorrow would bring, but I knew it would be different.

"Leave this town as soon as you can and start your journey in life," my father repeated. He told me that my upbringing had been a preparation for my journey. He believed that it prepared me to leave home with a sense of integrity; it gave me patience and a work ethic. It gave me the confidence to make a life for myself, not just a living. It taught me to share, rather than manipulate, others, and helped me avoid competing for the wrong reasons—just to win, to prove myself right, or to engage in personal power plays. It kept me from being argumentative just to keep control of a conversation. Most importantly, it kept me from denigrating women. My dad had tried to keep any of those negative qualities from being instilled in me.

"Don't ever let anyone tell you that your values are implausible, naïve, stupid, or impractical," Dad warned. "And believe me, they'll try, because they have lost their vision and have become cynics. I don't want you to end up like me, Gary Michael," he went on. "When I was 17 years old, I was just like you. But I did not hold to my principles. No matter what happens, hold on to your principles."

The next day I took my father's car and went around to see all my friends. Just 24 hours earlier, we had been talking about things we wanted to do together. Now they were all too busy for me.

"Hi, Tim, want to go swimming?"

"I can't, Gary. Got to work in Dad's shop."

"Do you know when you can get free? Do you want to go fishing this weekend?"

"I can't, Gary."

"We've got a whole summer ahead."

"I'm going to be working all summer. Playtime's over. Got to grow up now. Got to take things seriously."

Every single person I visited said almost the same thing. I was faced with something I'd never seen before—the death of passion and desire. It was as if I had entered a town of Stepford wives. At the end of the day, I realized my father was right. To stay in town would mean conforming and surrendering all of my high aspirations. A new journey was about to begin.

I went to New York City with nothing but $53 in my billfold, and it was stolen the first day. Luckily I had another $12 in my pocket for emergencies. That and a positive attitude kept me going. I remembered that no matter what environment I was in, I should look for things that allowed me to feel good about myself. I refused to acknowledge the fact that I had no money. I slept sitting up in the bus station for three nights before finding work as a short-order cook. At least that gave me a place to eat. Then I found a YMCA that cost only $2.50 a night, and moved in.

That was my introduction to my new life. The beginnings were difficult and frightening but the results have been very rewarding. I now appreciate more than ever those lessons of growth and change. I understand that we are here on this earth to manifest a higher character and consciousness by continuing to use every event, crisis, and problem as another lesson of how to make better choices, and how to respond to them when we realize we've made the wrong ones. I cannot always create my own reality but I can choose how I want to respond to it.

I struggled to succeed many times in my life. I never stopped, even when my first book was rejected 130 times in two years and my income was less than $5000 a year. I never lost faith that one day I would succeed because I continued to seek the end of the rainbow. Sometimes I wonder what would have happened had I stopped at the second rejection or the eighth, when the editor added a little letter to the standard rejection form that read, "You'd best find another profession. Clearly writing is not your forte." That, coupled with the fact that I was so poor I couldn't even mail my manuscripts to publishers, could easily have discouraged me. But I never got angry. I never felt deprived. I took advantage of everything worthwhile that was free—outdoor concerts and plays, book forums and poetry readings, wonderful walks in the park, nice company and stimulating conversations, and especially the old New Yorker bookstore, a landmark in New York City, where I could read a book a day without having to buy one. Then one day a publisher liked my ideas and published my first book.

When I first decided to racewalk I was determined to succeed even though I was less than promising at the start. In the first race I entered there were more than 75 racewalkers, and of everyone racing I was dead last. People in their 70s walked faster than I did. In fact, I was so slow that no one realized I was still on the course. By the time I finished, the winners had received their awards and gone home. Someone came over to me and said, "What are you doing in this race?" I replied, "I'm learning." Winning wasn't important. I did it to learn, and anything I learned was going to be to my advantage.

It would be almost a year before I would understand enough about form, style, and proper training to be able to improve substantially, but my determination paid off. Recently, I was given an award for my achievements—Outstanding Track and Field MAC Master Champion Athlete of the Year. I've also won the indoor grand prix series for all athletes of all ages and all categories. That's the first time in history that a racewalker has won either of those two coveted prizes. I now hold many personal meet, course, and national records and have won more than 100 championships. What if I had thought of quitting in my first, fifth, or twentieth race when I came in last?

When I first started in broadcasting I worked from a tiny radio station where the listenership couldn't have been more than 100 or 200 people. The owner of the station openly discouraged me from doing more shows. He told me, "You don't have a radio voice."

To this I replied, "Why, because I have a soft voice and don't yell?"

"That's right," he said. "You have to have a hyperkinetic voice that excites and interests people."

"What if I share something of interest?" I questioned. "Does the announcer always have to be the main focus? Why not the message he's delivering?"

He didn't understand this and told me that I shouldn't be on the radio because I was talking about health and no one was interested.

But I didn't quit. I kept on. I was told that I couldn't syndicate a show, but I did. And I ended up in the top markets in prime time. Then I was told that I couldn't succeed on a non-commercial radio station, WBAI—The Pacifica Foundation. Not only have I succeeded, I've been there 20 years with one of the longest-running daily talk shows on noncommercial radio, uninterrupted, in American history.

The same story holds true for my other achievements—writing articles, doing scientific research, earning two doctorates. I always began in last place. I started with many disadvantages and a lot of negative feedback from all the naysayers.

I learned from these experiences to surround myself with positive people who have kind hearts and who are spiritually and emotionally healthy. There was a time I didn't do that. I thought that people would change if you were kind to them. But people who are negative are determined to bring you down with them and can only hurt your progress. Learning when to let go of such people is very important to your personal growth.

A few years ago I attended my twentieth high school reunion. It was a disturbing experience. My old classmates all looked older than their years to me as I went from table to table and asked them what they had been doing for the past 20 years. I was surprised at their answers. "Not a whole lot." "Nothing." "Just working." I didn't hear anyone talk about having fulfilled their dreams or even having looked for the rainbow. Many had been divorced two or three times and were angry and unfulfilled, almost bitter, about life.

I was surprised, however, that many of them had kept track of my career and had occasionally seen me on television. But none of them had read any of my books or had actually followed a health program. None had traveled to Europe or other far-off places. Most had stayed close to home their entire lives. Some said they were happy, but not many.

I felt very sorry for my old classmates and sad that the next time I would see most of them would be at their funerals. These people had gone from the bright horizons of childhood, when they believed everything was possible, to the narrow and limiting concepts of an adulthood in which they believed they could do only what they were told to do. They had lived their lives without ever having fulfilled any of their dreams. Even those who had gone to college fell back into the old routines when they returned, joining the family business and living in the old hometown.

I found the whole event depressing. But several months afterward, my perception of what I had seen at the reunion began to change. That was because I was starting to develop the concept of natural life energies, the idea that a person is driven predominantly by one of seven different types of energy. For instance, a Dynamic Aggressive is someone driven to organizing enterprises, thinking on a grand scale, and, in the process, delegating the day-to-day details to other people. The Adaptive Assertive, on the other hand, can be a detail person par excellence. The Creative Assertive is by innermost nature an artist of some sort, and the Adaptive Supportive, by contrast, is generally not impelled to create something new but rather to follow others' leads and enjoy a routine. Other energy types are the Adaptive Aggressive, the Dynamic Assertive, and the Dynamic Supportive. These are all described in depth in my book *Who Are You Really?: Understanding Your Life's Energy*, but the point here is that I hadn't been taking the differences in people's energy types into account.

As a result, my expectations about how my old high school friends should have been living their lives had been based too much on how I was conducting mine. As a Dynamic Assertive, I had been driven all my life by a love of ideas, specifically, of new ideas, ones that I could develop and explain to others, and then develop some more. I liked to push the envelope of what was generally accepted or even imagined, and, as an energy type that could get pushy and radical and be seen as a pain in the neck by more conventional folks, there was a good chance I would not have been happy staying in a small town after high school. My father was a Dynamic Assertive too, I now saw. That was why he'd been so adamant about my leaving town on graduation night. He himself had been constrained by the town's limited range of vision, and he didn't want me to experience the same life of feeling held in at every turn. I hadn't understood his foresight so clearly before.

I also hadn't seen that there is an energy type that actually thrives staying in the old neighborhood for a lifetime, and that's the Adaptive Supportive. People whose hearts are centered on their extended family, and who appreciate knowing what to expect each day in the workplace, have no need to emigrate from their home base, nor seek exciting jobs. Creative Assertives can do well in small towns too, as can Dynamic Supportives, especially after people with these energies have spent some years away in the big city. Then they can return and happily continue doing what matters to them—honing their craft or helping people, respectively. In short, I had to revise my conclusion that most everyone I'd seen at that reunion was miserable. Maybe the majority who'd insisted that they were happy really *were*. Maybe many who looked utterly defeated were just tired. Not that I accept looking totally spent in one's 40's, but there's a difference there, and I had to revise my judgment about my old classmates.

A strange point for a writer of a book like this to be making—that he'd had to revise his opinion, and recently too! But it's an important point. I'm not the authority. I'm not any smarter or more infallible than you are. This book is written mostly in a question-and-answer format, and there's a reason for that: Although I give my personal answers to the questions, you're supposed to come up with your own too, and if they're different from mine, or go beyond mine, so much the better. I'm a Dynamic Assertive, I can handle it! And seriously, the whole idea behind the book is to get you to think about important life issues, not to accept what I believe, necessarily.

All that said, I do still feel that many people at my high school reunion, and many that I encounter every day, are capable of having more joy in their lives than they have at present. That's why I wrote this book. In counseling people I get frustrated because I believe that most people don't realize how very close they are to fulfillment. So many fall into the trap of thinking their life would be better if their circumstances were different. They wonder what would happen if they had been born wealthy instead of middle-class or poor, if they had inherited greater athletic skills or more intellect. They think about what it would be like to have been born male instead of female or vice versa, or to have been born in Manhattan instead of Minnesota, or vice versa there too. They also look to others to save them. Politicians will give them a better quality of life, they believe. Doctors will keep them healthy. Teachers will make them smarter. Psychologists will make them feel better. Spiritual gurus will show them the way. Or so they think.

In this book I want to share a different perspective, one that may require you to rethink your assumptions about life, just as I have. Consider the following: *What if the things you thought were causing your problems really weren't? What if the problems didn't exist out there, but rather in you?*

Suddenly, with this perspective, life gets simpler, easier. Outside obstacles to doing what you want to do and being what you want to be begin to fall away, and you see that you have more choices—positive ones.

That's what this book is about—the positive things that you can start doing—right now. The chapter titles tell it all: becoming the hero in your own life, creating contentment, beating self-defeating habits, choosing joy. All of these are positive choices you can make if you drop the blaming-others, blaming-circumstances strategy and concentrate on your own strengths and sense of purpose. The idea behind this book is to help you find these, and, if you already have, to join with you in celebrating life's potential.

Choosing Joy

Making Life Simple Again

❖

Most of us can remember simpler times. Life was less complex, filled with fewer responsibilities, and seemed to contain more time. Many baby boomers today are examining their lives and finding themselves materially affluent but seemingly time-poor. After years of focusing on careers, families, and the accumulation of the "right" things, they're beginning to ask themselves what all the striving and rushing around are about. Many are now seeking ways to live less stressful lives, and not just on vacation or during a weekend. They want to live with a consistent sense of peace. This can be hard, though, after many years of daily turmoil.

In fact, most Americans have difficulty relaxing. They don't know how to unwind, and even find the process of unraveling on a vacation or a retreat to be stressful. I can tell you that from my experiences with people who have come down to my ranch in Texas. The first three days I have to give lots of workshops. I keep my guests busy all day because if there's a free moment, they panic and wonder, "Where should I go now?" "What should I do?"

By the end of the week, people are finally able to relax, and they don't need all the workshops. Instead, they want to spend more time by themselves, with the animals, with nature.

People could relax sooner if they could learn how to leave their problems and anxieties behind, to live in the moment. Living in the moment has become a cliché associated with the New Age movement. But what does it really mean, and how can we get there? First of all, what keeps us from being in the moment and how does that affect us?

Are You Aware of the Factors That Keep You from Fully Experiencing the Present?

Avoidance

How can you be in the moment if you are avoiding what you need to do? When you distract yourself from the task at hand, you are not allowing the moment to happen. When two things compete for your attention, neither one has it fully. You avoid going to the dentist, for example, because you have an abscess and are afraid. You distract yourself from the pain by watching television. You focus all your energy away from the problem. That keeps you out of the moment.

Rushing

Do you rush to avoid being late, even if you have plenty of time? In the process of worrying about being prompt, you create stress that prevents you from enjoying the moment. You lose touch with your natural rhythm. Going someplace in a hurry is a forced, highly aggressive state. You become hyper.

The moment is lost because you have allowed your mind to be someplace that your body is not. You are not comfortable with where your body is; you want it to be someplace else.

You feel that you are going to be judged. Why else would you be concerned about being someplace on time? Or you are judging yourself so that someone else won't judge you. Being harsh on yourself is a defense mechanism in that you hope by judging yourself, you'll avoid the criticism of others. After all, it's hard to beat up on someone emotionally if they've already beaten up on themselves! So we make sure we do a pretty good job of it.

Anticipating Others' Anger

What would happen if you decided to change how you dealt with other people's anger? What if you decided their anger was their business and not yours? What if you decided not to process it? Even if there is value and legitimacy in what they are angry about, the emotion is theirs to process. You don't have to clutter up your life with it. The moment you take on someone else's anger, you take on all of the negativity that comes with it.

Being Angry Ourselves

When we ourselves are angry, the emotion often prevents us from dealing with important issues. Frequently, it's borne of frustration. We feel that systems are too insensitive and corrupt to change. Anger, then, is used as a substitute for action. In effect, we are saying, "I am too powerless to do anything." If we give up at that point, we deprive ourselves from affecting the moment. Then our time to be constructive is gone.

Is What You Do Guided by What You Believe?

When I get up in the morning, I know that whatever I'm going to do that day will honor my life and my basic beliefs. It's the same every single day, which in a sense makes life extremely simple. My personal morality is a constant.

Never do I compromise on my principles. I was once offered a deal in which I was to receive $50,000 for endorsing a junk food product filled with sugar. I refused to do it even though I didn't have any money at the time. They tried hard to convince me to do the endorsement. They pointed out, "If you don't do this, Gary, another nutritionist will." They were right. Another nutritionist did.

I called that other nutritionist, and I asked, "You're not going to endorse this product, are you?"

He replied, "Why shouldn't I? It's $50,000."

"But it's not a good product," I said.

"There's a lot of not good products around," he retorted. "It's all relative. People can take some vitamins along with the stuff, so what's the big deal?"

I said, "That's like beating someone up and apologizing at the same time. Why beat them up to begin with?"

He pretended he didn't understand.

Then I started looking around, and I saw people everywhere making major compromises. Sometimes people do this to make money. And sometimes they do it to avoid feeling alienated. When you stand up and say how you feel, there's a chance others are not going to like you. Particularly if you're the one bringing unhappy tidings about wrongdoings, you're not going to be liked, and you're certainly not going to be accepted.

On the other hand, if you get into the habit of living honestly, you're going to like yourself. You'll be relieved of the burden of self-doubt and of the vague but ever-present unease that's the result of abandoning your principles. Choices will be clearer, and take less time to make.

So an important part of the process of making our lives less complicated—of uncluttering our lives—is learning to be honest, if we aren't already. That's really essential.

How Do You Perceive Time?

A more tangible step in simplifying your life is actually uncluttering your calendar by limiting or rearranging your obligations. First, think about the meaning of time for you. Is time an enemy or a friend? Do you assume there is too little time? Do you never have enough time to do the things you need to do? Lately our culture has made it seem like this is a desirable state of affairs, and that you're not a success if you don't have a time problem. But being in a constant time crunch is not a desirable state; it's frustrating and mentally constraining, and it prevents you from being in the moment.

Unlike money, time is something we all have the same amount of, in the sense that we all have 24 hours in each day. I believe, then, that it's simple: If you do not have enough time, it is because you are not using it wisely. Or you're planning your schedule unrealistically.

For example, if I tell a publisher that I can write an outstanding book in six months, but know in my heart that I need a year, then I am not going to give him the quality book I promised. In addition, I am placing myself under unnecessary stress, and I will be unhappy with the book I turn in. Likewise, if I plan to take part in ten organized activities during a weekend, I'm not going to be able to relax and fully participate in ar of them. My mind will always be jumping forward to w' I'll have to be in an hour, and how I'm going to get the' whether I'll have time to change clothes for that ne' and where I can buy what I'm expected to bring miliar?

Not only do we overschedule our own lives, ' eration of parents is notorious for oversch' dren's as well. Many middle-class chil' down to the preschool level—have appointment books as full of obligations as those of CEOs. They have to rush from school to dance class to playoff game to playdate, with scarcely a second to take a breath. Where's the time to be a child and just sit and look at the sky? Where's the time to—as I did—bounce around on a chenille-covered bed for the pure, silly joy of it, or to just be with a favorite animal for hours, and "talk" together, in your own ways?

These children didn't take their heavy loads of responsibilities on themselves. Their parents did it for them. People over-schedule their own and their children's lives for a number of reasons. The perceived need to keep up with the Joneses is one. Fear of idleness is another. Yet another is the idea that we've absorbed from our advertising culture that if you don't pay for something, it's not of value. That's why people will sign up for an expensive exercise class rather than walk for free in the park, or why parents feel that to spend quality time with their one-year-olds they have to enroll in a structured parent-and-toddler program rather than play peek-a-boo at their leisure, at home.

The Puritan ethic is part of this picture too. Many people have been brought up to believe that if the activity they're engaged in isn't strenuous, demanding, and at least a little bit unpleasant, they're doing something wrong.

With these attitudes, you can easily spend your whole life doing things you don't want to do, things that will never mean much to you or anyone else, except perhaps the people making money from them, and—here's the pitiable part—things you absolutely *don't have to do*. It's scary how much time you can waste. At some point you really ought to ask, "Why am I cluttering my life with all these less than rewarding activities, if I don't have time to relax, or to do what I really enjoy?"

At What Point in Life Do You Start Including That Which Is Essential to Your Real Nature?

Write down what is essential to your real nature. Are you, deep down, really a writer? An artist? A people-helper? Maybe you love to garden. Or are drawn to cities. Or have always wanted to be an athlete. Or a chef. Maybe you adore dogs. Maybe baseball is truly your passion. Are the things and activities to which you're drawn actually a part of your life right now? Or have you been putting them off for some future time that keeps receding?

Look at the way you live your life. Ask yourself, "Is this what I really want to be doing with my days?" If it is—then great. If it is not, what do you really want to do? If you are working in an institution, for example, would you rather be someplace where you could help people without bureaucratic limitations? Would you rather be someplace where people are not fighting against your efforts to help them? There are places in this world where you will be appreciated for your efforts. Allow yourself to be there.

Do You Love Your Work?

Okay, maybe you can't quit your boring day job to become a renowned musician. But there are ways you can work toward that goal each day. You can take lessons, practice at home, take out books from the library on your facet of the art.

Here's the goal I would set for every human being: Do the work you love to do. Follow your passion. Do work that gives your life meaning. Do not just work to make a living. Then you are only working to support a lifestyle cluttered with things that may give you a measure of status but that ultimately rob your life of purpose. Ask yourself, "What purpose do I have?" We all have one. Your purpose in life is what gives your life direction and meaning. Declare what is yours.

Do the "Little" Things in Your Life Work?

You need to examine every part of your life to assess whether or not it is working for you. This means not just the big issues, like where you work and how you relate to your family and friends, but the little things as well, such as whether you've painted your walls colors that you really like, or whether you've ever gotten around to buying good-quality pots and pans to cook your meals in. It always amazes me how people will go their whole lives with less than optimal living and eating and sleeping arrangements, when they can well afford to have them. It's the "better-keep-the-walls-beige-in-case-we-have-to-sell-the-house" mentality. Whose house is it anyway—the people's who'll be living in it after you're dead?

Make a list of everything in your life you feel is important to you as a physically aware creature. Include small details, the things you don't consider essential but that nevertheless matter to you. For instance, in addition to wall color and kitchenware, think about this: Do you sleep in the kind of bed that you really want to be in, on the kind of sheets that you want next to your body? Do you have a nice, warm comforter? These things can be more important than you think.

Growing up, I spent a lot of time at my aunt's house. My mother worked a lot, and my aunt took care of me and my brothers after school. Whenever we were there, she would insist that we have a nap. She said it would make us healthier. Of course, napping was the last thing we wanted to do. We were full of energy. So we'd go into the room, bounce up and down on the beds, play, sing, and wrestle. Still, I remember the smell in the room, and the feel of being there. The bed had a white chenille bedspread, the kind with little balls all over it.

It felt so good and warm that I've spent my whole adult life looking for chenille bed covers, unfashionable though they may be.

Everything about my aunt's house was warm. It was so unlike many of the uncomfortable homes of today. Today, you sit on the furniture and think, "What am I sitting here for? I don't feel good on this. I'm not going to sit on the floor; I'm not going to sit on the window sill; and I can't sit on the radiator because I'll burn myself. But the couch doesn't feel comfortable." You wonder why people ever buy some of the furniture they do.

One reason is that people equate "good" furniture with money and status. They'll say, "What do you think of it? It cost me $3000. I bought it at Bloomingdale's." And remember when we went through that whole phase of putting plastic on everything? The furniture was not only uncomfortable, it made us sweat. Nothing felt like you could nestle into it. The best you could do was melt into it—literally!

I never went in for plastic, or for status furniture. I wanted furniture that was comfortable. I didn't care how it looked, whether it matched or not. I found some big, super-soft couches and sofas. When you sat on them, you felt as if you were sitting on a fluffed-up featherbed. You felt that comfortable. Many times, people would sit on my couch and fall asleep. You should feel totally at ease on a couch.

It's the same with a bed. When you lie on a bed, it shouldn't feel like a board. The idea that a bed should be as hard as a board is a remnant of the Puritan ethic that makes no sense. And forget futons. A lot of people started lying on futons in the 70s because it was the hip thing to do. But sleep on a futon for a night, and you'll see why people go to chiropractors! You get up with aches and bumps and nothing working.

We hate to be honest about what we really want because what we really want is almost never given social approval. Even the color and shape of our clothes is dictated by others. Take a look at your clothes. Do you feel good about what you're wearing? Do you even *feel good* in your clothes, or are they constricting your body and your breathing? Think of how many times you dressed so as not to stand out. You had to look conservative, you felt, in order to fit in.

Imagine if your choices about what to wear, how to furnish your house, how to spend weekends, and even—or especially— how to spend your life—were dictated not by what you thought others would approve of, but by what *you* really wanted to choose. Life would be so much simpler then because there would be less speculation, guesswork, and self-doubt.

How Did You Learn What You Know?

School

The town I grew up in was less than cosmopolitan. At school, everyone knew everyone else. Some teachers were like fixtures; they had been there for ages. And certain teachers were noteworthy because they taught by the textbook only. Whatever the text said was God's word. They wouldn't deviate from the book. If the textbook was biased, then you learned a biased lesson.

In the South, there were a lot of biases. I always wondered how people could become lawyers, doctors, and judges and still be racist. In the process of becoming more educated, shouldn't they also be able to understand racism and give it up? I found it didn't work that way, and I couldn't figure that out. For the longest time I couldn't figure out how many so-called smart people in our country acted in such irresponsible ways.

I still see highly educated people, like scientists, acting dumb. Many of these Yale- and Harvard-educated people are brilliant in the laboratory. They could regale you with stories related to their field for days. But talk about anything other than what they do and they're no different than anyone else.

People keep themselves very narrowly defined in what they know. Generally, what they know is what they do. What they don't do they don't know about. They don't have balanced lives.

How do we get this way? Well, first, as I've mentioned, there are our teachers. And then there is the curriculum, which can be unbalanced for a variety of reasons, including economic ones. When my friend, holistic physician Dr. Marty Feldman, was in Yale Medical School and the Columbia School of Physicians and Surgeons, he was taught very little about nutrition. Instead, he learned that drugs are a primary source of healing. He was taught that because of the influence of pharmaceutical companies on medical schools. Drug companies are wise enough to endow medical school chairs, which are occupied by people they know will be supporting their particular line of drugs. In the 1950s, there was a mad scramble for pharmaceutical companies to dump tax-exempt money into foundations that would then support these schools. No one was funding research on meditation, biofeedback, alternative lifestyles, behavior modification, or exercise. There was no money in these things.

As a result of these influences, the whole medical field of 650,000 physicians is taught a one-sided approach to healing. They learn methods that often have no science behind them. For example, in the case of breast cancer, taking lymph nodes out of a woman's armpit was standard practice for years, even though there was never any research proving that doing this would increase lifespan. No one considered that the lymphatic system serves the purpose of supporting the body's immune response and aiding detoxification. No one thought that removing a part of this filtration system could result in the person succumbing to the cancer or to something else. So, everything was cut out and removed.

Only now is this beginning to change. But no one has ever apologized to all of the women needlessly mutilated.

When your basic belief system is wrong, then everything you learn and exponentially extend beyond that is also flawed. Wrong knowledge gets passed on.

A woman wrote a book about how to cure cancer with grapes, and everyone thought she was a nut. No one wanted to research what she had said. Well, recently it was proven that grapes help prevent cancer in laboratory animals.

Now, you can bet your bottom dollar that they're going to find a chemical within the grape that they can synthesize and make into a patented drug. You won't be told to eat grapes; you'll be told to take that drug. Unfortunately (for you) the drug will be expensive. Grapes aren't. And since the drug will be artificially synthesized, it will have the potential of being toxic. Grapes aren't. But it will be the drug that will be pushed. The paradigm doctors have been taught, of "drugs cure, and *only* drugs cure" is going to be pretty hard to overcome.

Family

Another way people learn is by being given information by their families. Some of this is helpful, but much of it can be biased as well.

I met a young Algerian fellow, named Ali. When I had a restaurant, I hired Ali as a chef there. One night I walked into the restaurant unexpectedly, as I had forgotten something. It was late and Ali was on his way out with two shopping bags full of food. I wasn't going to ask about the bags because I had no suspicion. But Ali volunteered, "You caught me." When I asked him what was in the bags he told me he had taken food. Then, when I asked him where he was going with the food he said, "Home." At this point, I was still thinking that he was taking food that we didn't sell or need. Then I learned that Ali had taken whole blocks of cheese. Since the restaurant was not a profit-making venture, the last thing I needed was someone stealing from it.

Ali and I had a long conversation about what happened. I didn't fire him because I learned that he had been taught at home that stealing was necessary. He came from a poor family, and poor families routinely went out each day to steal food. Stealing was almost like a job. Ali believed it was ethical to steal from someone richer. His family had taught him that.

Self-Exploration

Another mode of learning is through self-exploration. This is how we can learn most of our important lessons. Unfortunately, self-exploration is rare. People are reluctant to give credence to their own perceptions. Even if their own experience gives them pleasure, joy, happiness, and excitement, they will not trust their own judgment, if the authorities haven't validated it. Many times I see people experience something real. They love it. But instead of going forward with it, they say, "No, that's not me. I've got to go back here and play it safe. I'd better stick with what's traditional and regular."

"No," I always, in essence, try to say, "you ventured into life. You opened the door, and there you were. You were looking at yourself, beckoning yourself to come forward. You did. You took a step. It was real."

"Uh-uh. I can't rely upon me. I feel too uncomfortable. I'd rather follow the experts. I need my psychologist. My social worker. My 12-step program. I have to go every day and say I'm an addict. They tell me I am. They tell me I've got to live one day at a time and I'm an addict for life. And if I ever try anything again I'll become an addict again. I live with fear, nothing but fear. I'm afraid that if I don't do exactly what I'm supposed to do—come to these meetings, say stupid things, and be with people who smoke and drink coffee, I'm going to be an addict again. Now I'm a passive addict, but I might become an active addict again."

People are so ready to accept others' truths about them.

As a teacher and counselor, I encourage others to go forward. But if the only time a person does something meaningful is under my guidance, then that person is merely being a follower. The person is merely a parasite to my life process. If I do something, they do something. I stop doing something; they stop doing it. I do it again; they do it. That's not a life. That's being a shadow to someone else.

When people go forward through self-exploration, they don't look for teachers. They accept the inner teacher. The inner teacher resonates as true. Support, yes; indoctrination, no.

Life is just about passages, and all we have are moments of conscious attention in our passages. That's all we have. The wise person self-explores during each passage to get the most out of the journey—and the moment.

Have You Ever Challenged Your Formal Learning Experiences?

Seeing the danger of conformity, I grew up challenging my teachers all the time. I was not impolite, but I challenged them. Growing up in a small town, my teachers were often the same people who had taught my father and my older brother. I had a reputation for saying irreverent or wrong things. So, my challenges weren't taken seriously and I never influenced anybody. But at least I was very honest.

I still don't influence very many people. For years, I thought I was making a difference, not realizing that the people sitting across from me had not committed themselves to real, meaningful change. Desperate when they came to me, these people only showed up after all their experts or doctors said there was nothing more they could do. Still, they were not open to looking at another way of approaching their problems. They came because there was nothing else to do and their families told them that they had to do something so they should go see Gary Null. They would show up at my door as skeptical as ever. No matter what I would suggest for them to do, they would not listen. Oh, they would talk to me, and act like they were considering my words. But then they would go right back to the person who had offered them no help, for instance, a doctor who had told them they had just three months to live.

They would go back and tell the doctor, "Gary Null said I should try ozone therapy."

"That's quackery. Don't do that," the doctor would say.

"Okay, I won't."

To that I would say, "If they're giving you no chance to live, and I give you a suggestion, shouldn't you at least try it?"

Their response: "I don't want to get my doctor angry at me." I've seen this happen hundreds of times.

You should be adopting new ways of approaching problems before the point of desperation. You should be eating right, exercising, and taking chelation therapy before you get a heart attack. That takes self-exploration. But conditioning makes it very hard for most people to change. It prevents them from allowing anything new in. The person is filled with the principles given to them by their mother, father, brother, sister, aunt, uncle, rabbi, priest, and nun. It's all those people inside that someone has to convince before a new experience is allowed in. That's why people have so much guilt, fear and loathing about doing something differently. It's not because of the self that change is not happening; it's because of everyone else's early admonitions and conditioning.

Does Curiosity Motivate You to Learn?

How curious are you? What are you curious about? And what are you willing to do about it? Are you willing to engage your curiosity? Are you willing to transgress boundaries set up by others in order to explore?

Kids are naturally curious in an innocent way. We allow kids to say and do things that we, as adults, do not allow ourselves to do out of fear. What if we were curious about everything and willing to explore completely?

I believe we have the right to explore anything that helps us to discover who we are. I don't believe in drugs or in anything else that is self-destructive. But I do believe in doing anything positive that allows us to grow. Doing this pushes us up against social norms, religious norms, familial norms, political norms, and professional norms.

Most of us adapt to the world's expectations. But we lose ourselves in the process. And the world, in truth, loses something too.

Think of how many surgeons do unnecessary operations knowing they shouldn't do them. What would happen if, out of curiosity, a physician decided to take another route? People would wonder why. Picture the doctor defending his point: "With prostate cancer, it's been shown that whether or not you receive surgery you live equally long. Therefore, I'm not going to do surgery."

"You can't do that, you're a surgeon."

"I know I'm a surgeon, but I'm also a doctor. A doctor is supposed to be a healer. Therefore, I'm going to broaden my approach."

"You can't broaden. You're board-certified!"

Isn't it amazing that the more prestigious you become, the more narrow becomes the scope of what you are supposed to do, say, and be?

Are You Willing to Look Foolish Until You Get It Right?

Have you not done something because you didn't know how to do it? Have you never gone skiing, ice skating, roller blading? What else haven't you done that you would like to do? Have you avoided bicycle riding, dancing, swimming? There are so many great activities you can miss out on if you're afraid you'll look silly trying.

You will, you know. You'll look silly for quite some time until you get these skills right. But so what? Looking silly doing them is so much better than feeling unsatisfied not doing them. Besides, you'll get the skills right sooner or later.

Here's another problem: Perhaps you don't know the "proper" way to respond to certain new things. Have you not seen some interesting foreign language films because you thought you wouldn't know how to react to them? Have you not gone to the ballet or the opera because you might make an "inappropriate" comment about the performance while you were there? And what about saying the "wrong" thing to the waiter at a fancy restaurant? Has that prospect prevented you from ever going to one?

A friend tells me an interesting story about just such a scenario. She had gone to an upscale eatery with several co-workers. It was the kind of New York restaurant where the waiters have their noses in the air and the menu has a lot of expensive dishes with fancy foreign names on it. Everyone chose something to order. But one of her colleagues wanted something that was not on the menu.

"Have you got spaghetti and meatballs?" he asked the waiter.

The waiter was aghast. "Sir, we do not serve spaghetti and meatballs here," were his words, but his meaning was clearly, "Sir, you have said a totally wrong thing, one that marks you as the lowest-class idiot that has ever entered this restaurant!"

Many people would have practically sunk under the table after such an exchange, but not this man. "You mean you don't have spaghetti and meatballs here?" he said. "You have all this other stuff on the menu and you don't have spaghetti and meatballs? What kind of a place *is* this?"

My friend had to laugh. Her colleague had just turned the tables on the waiter and made it seem like *he* had said the wrong thing. It was then that she realized that if you have a strong sense of self and know what you want and believe, you're never going to say the wrong thing, because there is no wrong thing to say.

Do You Rationalize So You Can Keep on Accepting Things as They Are?

Think of a time when something wasn't working in your life, and yet you tried to rationalize in order to justify holding on to the situation. The list of common rationalizations is practically endless.

"The pay's good."

"I get medical benefits."

"If I stay another six months, I'll get a bonus."

"You can't beat this rent."

"It's too much trouble to move."

"It's not that bad a relationship. So, we have arguments. Everyone does."

"He doesn't lie all the time."

"He's going through a bad period."

"So, he beats me once in awhile. He has a good side too."

Think of all the times you've made excuses for a situation in order to keep from changing it. How could you improve your life if you stopped rationalizing?

Just accept something or reject it. If it's not right for you, simply let it go.

Do You Recognize That Your Thoughts, Feelings, and Actions Have a Physical Correlation?

There is cause and effect. You eat something that you shouldn't eat and your body reacts unfavorably. Your body reacts because you have done something to disrupt the body's natural flow. If at the same time you are worried, you create further disharmony. On top of that, expressing yourself negatively creates spiritual disharmony. Now you've caused disharmony on multiple levels. What if we do hundreds of things per day that create perpetual disharmony? We're creating an environment conducive to disease. Then, we get surprised when we wake up one day and we have a disease.

There's a natural order to life. When you go against it, you always pay a price. The wise person connects with the natural order and does that which is mentally, spiritually, and physically uplifting. Anything that creates an imbalance creates a disharmony that dishonors the consciousness within every cell of our bodies. Following the natural order of life is what gives us our meaning, direction, and purpose in life. People who are just working for a living, who are just living for a relationship—all are in disharmony. All the excuses and rationalizations in the world will not change that.

At What Pace Do You Function Best? Fast? Slow? In Between?

Part of the natural order of your own life is your pace. We've all heard about how different people have different rates of internal metabolism; that's why some people have a harder time burning off calories than others. Likewise, when we interact with the external world, each person has a natural speed. Some people naturally function faster than others. That's normal for them, and they'd be frustrated if they had to restrain themselves to others' seemingly snail-like pace. Not that speed is necessarily better than a slow, deliberate course through life. Those who function slowly may consider that the speedsters are missing a lot along the way.

If you can help it, never artificially speed up or slow down to fit into the mold of what society seems to expect. Right now, as we've mentioned, a fast and frenzied pace is in vogue, but not everyone is comfortable with that. In fact, it's making a lot of people sick. So feel what is optimal for you. At what level do you function best? That's the level at which you should maintain your lifestyle. Don't look around for examples from friends, because they are not you. I can do a lot, and it's normal for me. And I can do very little and it would still be all right, but it wouldn't be normal for me. Pace yourself at a comfortable rate. Either speed it up or slow it down so it's perfect for you.

Life is a journey, but just as we don't all take it along the same road, we don't all have to travel at the same speed.

Staying Positive in a Negative World

❖

Everything in life is about choices. And often we make the wrong ones. At the time, we may even suspect that we are making a mistake, but fear, anger, bitterness, and other negative feelings influence our judgment. Only later, when we must face the consequences of our decision, do we truly understand our mistake.

A simple karmic rule states that once something is done, it can never be undone. This is not to suggest that we should avoid making errors. After all, we're only human. What I am suggesting is that we learn from our mistakes and avoid repeating them. In this way we can learn lessons, grow from the experience, and move forward. We can take a negative experience and transform it into a positive one. An example of such a turnaround would be when you get into a conflict with someone—perhaps as a result of something you said but shouldn't have—and then you resolve the conflict by apologizing, ending up with an even stronger relationship than you had in the first place.

This is not all that common an occurrence, unfortunately. How many times in life did you mutter to yourself, after you said or did something, "I shouldn't have said that. I shouldn't have done that. It was stupid. I got my ego in there. I closed a door I shouldn't have closed"? But you didn't go back and apologize.

When is the last time you did apologize about anything? You may not even be able to remember, which is a shame because apologies that come from the heart can clear a lot of negativity. They show that you value your relationship and honesty above your ego.

Are You Honest?

I grew up in an area of the country where people were honest about things. It was one of the virtues of small-town West Virginia, and of my family in particular. When you grow up in a family where you have to be honest—because if you're not, they call you on it right away—you get used to saying what you feel. That's why now I'll say a thing without thinking about what I say, if I know it's honest. I just say it. And I assume, if there's going to be a consequence, so be it. Anyway, if I started editing everything I said so that no one would be offended by anything I said, I'd never say anything. I'd be a mute. So to me, honesty is not only the best policy—it's the only policy I know how to operate with.

I call honesty a big component of positive energy and of the positive life. Although there are others—like friendliness.

How Does Positive, Friendly Energy
Make You Feel?

Recently, while traveling in Florida, it was wonderful to meet strangers who would greet me with, "Hi, how are you?" What a contrast to the way I had been treated in New York! On my way to the airport there, a bicycle messenger had screamed at my cab driver and spit on the window. When my plane landed in Florida, I was approached by a person who said, "It's awfully hot. Let me give you a ride." A total stranger rode me over to the car rental booth for free.

Such friendly behavior proved to be the norm. In a sporting goods store, a salesman spent an hour and a half talking about equipment, even though he knew I wasn't ready to buy anything. In fact, he told me about another store where I could get what I needed at a cheaper price. Such consideration is unheard of in New York. When you walk into a store you're urged to buy what you see now because what you need is about to be discontinued.

Humane treatment continued as I walked into a food store, trying to hurry my orders so as not to anger the five or six people waiting in line behind me. My sense of uneasiness must have been apparent because the clerk said I should slow down, that nobody was in a rush for anything.

Everybody was so nice. Nobody honked their horn the instant the light turned green, as if your delaying to put your foot to the gas for one nanosecond was a mortal affront to those behind you. Nobody in lobbies or elevators avoided eye contact, as if they suspected you of being a recently escaped psychopathic felon who was somehow carrying concealed weapons in your jogging shorts. (In New York, you can encounter the same person on the elevator every morning for three years, and they'll still get nervous and pretend to be reading their mail!) The friendliness in Florida took some getting used to. But after a couple of days there, I felt really good from all the positive energy. And it all comes from people being considerate of other people.

Do You Surround Yourself with Positive People?

We can't all move to friendlier locales. Nor can we ensure that everyone in our lives has a positive attitude. But we can aim for a life filled with those kind of people.

Think of the people around you now, and ask yourself, are we sharing positive energy? Can I trust this person? Do they have my best interests at heart? You'll know when positive energy is there because you'll feel it. Your guard will be down because there will be no need for it. You can be who you naturally are.

Surrounding yourself with positive energy is especially important when you need healing. Unfortunately, lots of relationships are filled with negativity. People express anger and bitterness toward each other, which drains good energy and creates sickness. How can you possibly heal when that much negativity is being thrown at you? To heal, you need to be surrounded by joy, love, compassion, understanding, and acceptance.

There is, of course, another side to the coin here, which is that *you* want to be a positive influence on those whose lives *you* touch. You don't want to drag others down with defeatist attitudes, or by holding a grudge. I consider holding a grudge to be one of the most emotionally corrosive things you can do, both to yourself and to others.

Let Go, Already!

If you're a perpetual grudge-holder, there comes a time when you simply have to let go. Train yourself to say, "What am I gaining by carrying on with my negative energy toward someone? What's the purpose of it?" The ability to change that, to forgive, to let go, is crucial to the healing process. It's so healthy to just clear away bad feeling, instead of dragging it around like a dead animal. You begin to smell after awhile if you do that.

It's never healthy when people hold on to negative energy. Have you had this experience in a relationship? Someone brings something up to you, something that happened a long time ago that you thought was a dead issue. It's over, but all of a sudden they'll say, in essence, "It's not over. We're happy now, for the past nine-and-a-half years of a ten-year relationship, but two months into that relationship, you said this to me. And I've been holding onto this the whole time. It's eating my guts out."

"Oh, really? Why didn't you tell me? What else are you holding in?"

"Well, get me angry again, and I'll bring out a whole laundry list!"

Soon the person's got you bringing out your laundry list in retaliation, and you've gotten into a mutually destructive pattern more appropriate to kindergarten than to an adult relationship.

Do You Value the Simple and Authentic?

Positive means simple. When I travel, I spend time talking with people. I'll go out for a run in the morning, and speak with folks I meet. Often I ask them, "Why do you live here?" Many times, I meet people who leave their small town for the big city, only to return. A big metropolis looks glamorous at first, but after awhile, all the crises and turmoil get to them. They get to a point where they decide that they have had enough, that there is something more essential and important in life: the positive simplicity of a more authentic existence.

When you have authenticity in your life, what more do you need? By contrast, when you lead an artificial existence, you never have enough. You can eat lots of junk food and never feel satiated, but all you need is one real food and you're sat-isfied. It's the same way with junk love, junk relationships, junk jobs, junk friends. They don't fill you up. They may stimulate you, titillate you, excite you, but it's all temporary. In the morning you wake up and realize that it wasn't the experience you had hoped for.

Do You Value What You Have?

Most people in our society today don't have to work for a living. We work for a certain *standard* of living. Do you realize that people in the poorest strata of American society today, on public assistance, have more than the kings and queens of Europe did 300 years ago? If you get up today, and you're in the poorest town in America, you can still pop something in the oven and immediately have something to eat; they couldn't. You have a toilet; they didn't. You've got running water; they didn't. You've got electricity; they didn't. In the winter, you've got heat; they didn't. They didn't even have kitchens in their castles.

What has happened is that we've forgotten to appreciate and respect what we have. Now we all want something more.

We want a junk life. We want superfluous and value-less toys, food, clothes, gadgets, amusements, spectacles, diversions. Look at our affluent suburbs. Everyone has at least ten times more food, shelter, and clothing than they really need, not to mention countless entertainment options, and they're still complaining.

Are You a Complainer, Blamer, Whiner, Moaner?

Complainers never see anything as being right. Perfectionists are the biggest complainers. You never can do anything right enough for them. Nothing is ever good enough. If you feed them a 12-course gourmet meal, and you forget the toothpick at the end, they'll condemn the meal. If you take them on a vacation to paradise, and it rains one day, they'll moan about the rotten weather. The negative always takes precedence.

Recently, I was in a man's house. He was showing me his art collection. When he was halfway through, he started complaining about things he didn't have. I said that I thought he already had an awful lot there. But he insisted that what he had was nothing.

"Don't say it's nothing," I said. "Unless you're living in a Biafran hut, where someone can kill you tonight, and where you're starving to death, you have no right to complain that you have nothing. Don't you think you ought to be a little more positive?"

I won't let someone like this complain negatively to me. I just won't listen. I've seen real suffering, and when you've got a perspective like that, you can't help but think that we are a nation of babies.

Now I'm not saying that people living above the African poverty level do not have a right to share their troubles with others as a way of seeking support, help, and suggestions for positive change. I don't believe people have to be stoic or secretive about their problems, and it's certainly okay to vent your emotions when you're feeling frustrated, angry, or scared. But vent once. Vent twice. Don't keep venting, and venting, and venting, making dissatisfaction a way of life. Chronic complainers have absolutely no intention of making any positive changes; you could hand them a foolproof plan for improving their life on a silver platter, and they still wouldn't take it.

When you hear someone like this begin to complain, or to blame someone or something, stop them before they get going. Let them know that you don't want them sharing that negative energy with you.

Stop the moaners too. Stop them, and say, "Hold on. Is there something else you can do besides moan?" When you tell someone they're moaning, they'll stop. If they start again, remind them. Say to them, "Don't share this with me. You can moan to those who want to hear it, but I don't. I'm in my sanctuary. If you want to come into my house, into my heart, and into my mind, respect who I am. Don't dump your emotional garbage on me. It dishonors me."

Also recognize when you do it to yourself.

Do You Blame the World When You Feel Bad, Angry, or Helpless?

People blame the world for how they feel all the time. What if you were to stop blaming others for how you feel? What if you changed how you felt instead?

Before reacting to your feelings, find a quiet place, and take a moment to sit down and ask yourself if you can make yourself feel any different. For example, if someone says something about you that you don't like, and that's not true, instead of getting angry, you could have an inner dialogue that goes something like this: "It's just some words. That's all it is. I'm more than some words. And I'm certainly more than what someone thinks of me. It's what I think of me that counts. If everyone thinks I'm bad, and I know that I'm good, I have to accept that I'm good. I'm not going to accept what other people assume that I am. Therefore, I'm not going to allow myself to be angry with anyone or with myself."

We can change the way we deal with something that's thrown at us. We don't have to become victimized by it.

Do You Express Who You Really Are?

When we are in touch with who we really are, we are positive and light because we let the spiritual part of ourselves emerge. This is the part of us that wants to proclaim itself, to come out and speak. Sometimes it's easy to get in touch with this part of our nature because we've had good parents and friends, and a supportive environment.

At the other extreme, we may be completely out of touch with who we really are. Everything we do is influenced by the conditioned mind. We look for the rewards we can gain, and aren't motivated by the sheer joy of doing something. This often stems from being raised in a family where we weren't accepted for who we really were. Perhaps our parents only accepted us if we brought home a perfect report card: "If you don't get an A, you're grounded." We were made to feel that something we do is the key to acceptance and love. Getting a B or worse made us no longer lovable. Thus we learned to believe that we're not a good person for who we naturally are. That becomes our reality, and it can manifest all through life in self-doubt, low self-esteem, and the inability to try anything where we risk not succeeding.

Show me a child who was given unconditional love, and I'll show you a child who is not afraid to do anything because they know they'll be accepted, no matter how many times they fail at something. Failure is not equated with a character fault. It's merely a learning experience. These fortunate children are allowed to grow through their mistakes.

Is How You Spend Your Time Reflective of Who You Are?

Being in or out of touch with who we are is reflected in the work we do. Many people work hard, but do so because they are addicted to their work, meaning they use work as a way to escape from themselves. Others work hard but do so for the love of it. Picasso slept in front of his paintings because he loved his work. To him, work was not an addiction, but a passion.

Take a moment to assess how you spend your time. Pull back from your daily routine and really look at it to see if it expresses who you are. Is your day so filled with appointments that you never have quality time for yourself and others? Is your work fulfilling in itself? Does it allow you to express a part of yourself? Or is it just a job? What things do you really love to do? Are you doing them?

Are You Trustworthy?

I counsel a lot of well-known people. And I can't tell you how many times journalists have asked me about different celebrities. But I would never talk about them. I never even keep records because I don't want information getting into the wrong hands.

You never see successful people betraying anyone. Positive, happy, balanced people don't need to live through someone else's pain and suffering.

Are You a Taker Without Being a Giver?

I have a daily radio program on a noncommercial radio station that depends on audience support for its existence. Many of my listeners tune in every day, and have done so for years. From the show, they get valuable information, not just from me but from a variety of top-rate sources on health, nutrition, and more. But only five percent of my radio audience supports WBAI. Now what does that tell you? It tells me that most people are selfish. Who, but an absolutely negative person, would take so much positive, life-enhancing, even lifesaving information and never give back anything in return? It seems awfully selfish to me.

When one of my unsupportive listeners says they're not selfish, I ask him or her, "How much do you have to get before you can give?" Suddenly, they're challenged. "What do you mean by that?" they ask. "Well," I reply, "if someone gives you 1000 hours of knowledge for free, how much is that worth? What would you pay for that if you went to college? Wouldn't you think that a small pledge to the station might be appropriate in return?"

When a person is unwilling to give, and only takes, it shows something about their character. I'm willing to bet that the WBAI "takers" deal with everyone similarly. I believe they take advantage of everyone, whenever they can.

Are You Flexible Enough to Go with the Flow? Or Are You Stuck with Rigid Ideas, Patterns, and Images?

Nearly 25 million Americans have lost their jobs in the past 20 years. Now, many people who are being laid off are not minimum-wage earners. They're people who were coming home with $75,000, $100,000, and $200,000 a year.

Do you know what some of these people don't do? They don't make any changes. They're afraid to change their lifestyle because they're afraid it will change their image, and their image is more important than anything else. So they keep holding on to their previous standard of living. In the process they go through their savings, cash in their insurance policies, sell their furnishings, and so on, until all the money is gone. Then they blame the world for not giving them another job like the one they left. Their egos won't let them change.

What does it say when someone wants to have what they had, and is not willing to transform any part of their life? It means they're rigid and stuck. These affluent people who have lost their jobs could be looking on their circumstance as an opportunity—to try out new skills, to take stock of their lives, to develop parts of themselves that were previously dormant. I'm not trying to sugarcoat their situation, but they could be using it as an opportunity for learning.

One of the things they could be learning is that *you* don't change because something is lost. The essential *you* is the same after the loss as before. It's just that now you can't hide behind your high-status job and salary.

When Making Changes, Do You Surround Yourself with Positive People?

At no time is it more important to have positive people around you than when you are making changes in your life. So you might want to reconsider who you have in your life at those times. I only want positive people in mine, people who believe very much in what they're doing. Those are the ones who are going to believe in what *I'm* doing.

Negative people can drain you. They will try to thwart your plans before you begin acting on them. Fortunately, there are enough positive people in this world to make being around negative ones unnecessary.

Down at my ranch, I advise people to separate from others who are negative. People are there to heal, to contemplate new directions, and they need quiet, peaceful time. There will usually be a small group of negative people who criticize everything going on. I have to send people home because of that. Often they don't understand why they were sent home. They don't see it because being negative is such a part of them.

Do You Pay More Attention to the Prophets of Doom or the Prophets of Happiness?

Doom usually gets the attention, while happiness is usually ignored. Impending doom creates the need for urgency, and it gives negative people something to blame for their lives not working. Each day is the same for negative people. There's never anything new and bright to look forward to.

Have you ever noticed how negative people get together and share negative energy? And it strengthens them. They can go on forever. They don't get tired.

"Give it a break! Give it up for a moment!"

"No, we're happy, we're trashing, we're gossiping. Leave the room; we'll gossip about you."

Positive people are too busy living meaningful lives to talk about others. They're too excited about living each moment. Each day is another day to live, another experience, another adventure.

What Happens When You Anticipate the Worst-Case Scenario?

When you believe something will happen, it probably will. By anticipating the worst-case scenario, you are focusing your thoughts in a negative direction. Since action and emotions follow thought, your expectations have a good chance of being manifested.

People think negatively because on some level it benefits them. They may not like the consequences of their thoughts, but it helps them to identify who they think they are.

Do You Sabotage Yourself by Creating Unachievable Expectations?

Think of the things that you want to achieve. How realistic are they? When you don't achieve what you set out to do, do you blame everyone else for your not having accomplished your goals? Many people set expectations far in excess of what they need. There is a big gray area between what they need and what they try to achieve.

Set realistic expectations. Accept that you are capable of being more than you currently are. But don't make what you want impossible to attain.

Ask For What You Want or Need

Are there things you need, but don't ask for? Do you feel undeserving or that you will not get them? I suggest that you ask for what you need. Otherwise, you will continue to live without your essential wants and needs being met.

Are You the Epicenter of Your Own Experience, or Do You Seek Validation From Friends and Family?

When you experience something, do you look at it, realize what it is, and then let it go? Or do you immediately get on the phone and talk to people about it? Most people seek validation from someone else. Most people don't even know what they've experienced. They can't even trust their own experience.

Imagine what it would be like if we didn't have to have anyone else validate our experience. We could do it ourselves. Do you realize how much you could let go of in a hurry? Do you realize how much time you would have that you would otherwise be wasting with endless talking that never gets you anywhere?

Describe Your Negative Self-Talk, and You'll Be Able to Start the Process of Change

Negative patterns of behavior repeat themselves all day long. Let's say there's something that you cannot handle, or there's something not happening that you wish would happen, or there is a situation in your life that you're not able to be in control of and you wish you were—if you're negative you're going to talk out the problem all day long. But you will always be defeatist about it. When people feel overwhelmed, used, hurt, unable to control the outcome of events, or betrayed, they tend to look at themselves as victims.

What would happen if, instead of all this negative self-talk, you started positive self-talk, and stopped yourself every time you started in with the negative? Say, "Hold on. This is going nowhere. I'm not going to feel good after this. What can I do in place of the negative?"

That's how the process of change begins. First, identify when you're engaged in negative self-talk. Second, don't let the negative go beyond you. Don't allow the negative self-talk to generate the emotion that causes the action. Then you get the reaction that you don't like the consequences of. Stemming this negative pattern keeps you from unnecessary arguments, accusations, condemning, blaming, and complaining, and allows you, then, to be at the epicenter of your own life.

Third, replace the negative with the positive. Look at the positive options for solving your problem or improving your situation. Select the one or several that seem the best. And then start implementing them, not in a panicked, desperate way, but with resolve and balance.

Happy People Are Balanced

Look at people who are happy. They're always balanced in their life. There are never excesses there. There's never an extreme. There's always a positive energy, but it's often a subtle energy.

The negative, by contrast, is spastic, volatile, and highly excitable. It exaggerates and draws attention to itself. It's insecure.

Have you ever noticed the following? When someone attains a success they don't deserve, they don't know how to deal with it. They almost always promote their success, as if they have to prove that they deserve it. They're insecure about what they have because they know they can lose it at any time, and often they do.

When people are legitimately happy and successful, they're understated; they're quieter. You don't see them parading their success around. They don't have to because what they have is well-deserved; it's theirs and no one can take it away from them.

Happiness Isn't a State; It's a Skill

Advertising and other aspects of popular culture have led us to believe that happiness is a state you achieve after you've managed to accumulate the right set of possessions. Nothing could be further from the truth.

Happiness isn't a state; it's a skill. It's the skill of knowing how to take what life throws your way and make the most of it. It's the skill of intuiting what you should be doing during your time on the planet, and then of making choices so that you can actually be doing it.

Some of those choices may not be popular ones. And ironically, having the "right" set of possessions may get in the way of your making them. But they're your choices, your chances at happiness. Make them boldly, and your world will be transformed.

Creating Contentment

Where can happiness be found? It's an age-old question, answered differently in different cultures. In America, people tend to look for something outside themselves to bring them happiness. They spend a lot of time and energy to get something to make them feel better inwardly. They strive for a better job, for instance, or a bigger house, or a larger family. People are always saying, "If only I had more money, I wouldn't have all of these problems." It's assumed that the lack of money or things is the cause of their inner discord.

This idea is contrary to experience. When most people are first dating, for example, they generally don't have a lot of money. Still, they're happy and excited. They've got each other, they've got passion, and they've got boundless energy and joy.

Later on, they often have everything that money can buy—but they've lost that happiness. Eventually, they wake up and experience a crisis. Suddenly they're 30 or 40 or 50, and they have many things, but no happiness. Something is wrong inside. They have feelings of irritation, emptiness, and loneliness. Their lives are not working.

Many people react by doing what they've always done. They get new and more possessions, such as fancier cars and computers. Some people replace the people in their lives. They find a new boyfriend, girlfriend, husband, or wife. Others lose themselves in their work. Men, in particular, tend to become overly responsible and work longer hours than necessary. Such actions, though, are merely momentary distractions that never address the root cause of the problem.

It's difficult for us in the U.S. to comprehend people of other cultures who choose not to chase these illusory dreams. But such an attitude exists in many cultures, such as in India or Tibet, where people commonly lead happy lives without needing to have things. And even in countries that are closer to us, culturally, than India, there are differences in attitude. England comes to mind. Personal possessions there are fewer, smaller, and older than in the U.S. Homes and other buildings are generally smaller and older too. But these differences are in no way negatives, and the English people don't seem any the worse for them.

Visiting London, you have to downsize your expectations if your eyes are focused to an American's typical perspective. It took me a little while to do that when I was there. For instance, I'll never forget the time I couldn't find the Palladium. The Palladium is a world-famous London concert hall, sort of like New York's Radio City or Carnegie Hall. I'd consulted a map, so I knew the location of this attraction. But walking up and down the street, I couldn't find the place. It was nowhere to be seen. Concluding that the map was wrong, I was about to move on, but I figured I'd consult a cab driver first.

"It's right there," he said, pointing to a spot just behind me. And sure enough, there it was. I'd overlooked it because the renowned Palladium was—well—little. We have Gap stores larger than this.

My experience with theater in London was similar. As on Broadway, tickets for plays were offered at various prices, depending on the section of the theater you sat in. Figuring that, as on Broadway, if you got the cheapest ticket you'd need binoculars to see the play, I opted for a costlier seat. But at showtime I discovered that wasn't necessary. The theater was tiny! Compared to New York theaters, there were a ridiculously small number of rows in each section, and I could have had an intimate theater experience from any seat in the house.

In fact, that was a big part of the appeal of England—everything was intimate and personal because it was small in scale. Monuments, castles, restaurants, and inns were practically miniature by American standards, but there was a charm and intimacy in that, that made visiting them a delightful experience. There was also a factor of age that added to the charm. It's not unusual for an English inn to be several hundred years old, and to still be served by its original wood plank floors and stone walls. Homes too, are hundreds of years old; it's nothing out of the ordinary for an English family to be living in a centuries-old house that here would have landmark plaques nailed up all over it and be featured in magazines. Of course, here, most such buildings have been razed long ago, as have many of their replacements. We're always looking for something new.

I talk to people when I travel because I like to get a sense of how people live, day to day. I found out that in England prices for necessities are similar to what they are here, for a whole range of things, like houses and cars and haircuts and food. But the English, on average, earn less than people here do—20 to 50 percent less. How do they manage, especially when gas, food, rent, clothes, and entertainment are about the same cost?

Their expectations are different. The English do it by having realistic standards for what one should possess, by valuing what they do possess, and by taking care of their assets.

And not just of their own personal assets, by the way, but of their communities'. For instance, London's Hyde Park, comparable to New York's Central Park but a mile smaller, was a sparkling showpiece compared to it—graffiti-less, immaculate, and with lawn chairs left out and left standing. Another asset of the English is their pretty countryside. It's not spectacular in the sense of a Yosemite National Park, but you can see that they value their landscape in the way they maintain footpaths throughout it. You can walk through that whole country.

On a personal level, the English are not into waste. They buy clothes with an eye toward quality and years of use. "I don't have a thing to wear!" people here wail, even when they've got wardrobes stuffed with clothes. But consider an English closet. It's not unusual for a husband and wife to share one small one. That's all they need. Each member of the couple may have only one work outfit, one formal outfit, and one casual one. Their footwear collection would be along those lines too.

Some English austerity is a proud holdover from the spartan lifestyle that kept the country going during World War Two. Some of it just stems from necessity. I don't mean to glamorize the English, because no people have a corner on virtue. But I do understand the pull of England and other "quaint" countries, for Americans. I felt that pull myself. It's not just an "isn't that cute?" thing. It's a sense that life's more intimate and nurturing, more manageable in scale. It's Main Street versus a mega-mall; the corner store versus Wal-Mart; a cozy old house with a little garden versus a colossus of a residence with a killer lawn. For many people it's a re-connection to what had existed at one time, perhaps in their own childhoods.

Do the different values of the English mean that they're happier than we are? I wouldn't presume to say for sure, although I'd guess yes. At any rate, they didn't seem *less* happy, even though they generally had less than we do in terms of possessions, and what they had was smaller. Touring that country, I couldn't help but think about whether we Americans are too busy trying to create contentment the wrong way—with things. I thought about how the English didn't seem to feel that they had to *have* enough in order to *be* enough. There wasn't this constant acquisition and discarding of things, including clothes, houses, and even values, for that matter. Rather, there seemed to be a respect for what you already had, in its purity. There was a pervading sense that some things were not meant to be changed, but rather nurtured and enjoyed, for a long, long time.

Do You Try to Possess Things as if You Can Find Your Happiness Within Them?

In our culture people don't usually want things for survival reasons. Rather, they think that things will make them feel good. So they work to maintain or elevate their standard of living. This makes them feel more accepted, and they use this acceptance as a basis for self-esteem. They need someone else's acknowledgment to make them feel okay. And that's the way it has to be if you carry around a projection of who you should be based on the expectations of parents, friends, schoolteachers from the past, or even commercial advertisements.

Much of this process is subconscious. People live like robots, accumulating lots of material possessions, achievements, and responsibilities. But if they're not doing it for themselves, sooner or later they may begin to realize that they have no real life. They're living in a dream.

There comes a time when you need to wake up. You've got to awaken and ask yourself, "Who am I?" Because until you look within, you won't have the opportunity for lasting happiness and fulfillment.

In What Do You Find Pleasure and Beauty? And How Often Do You Allow Yourself These Moments?

Everyone finds beauty in waterfalls, sunsets, and other natural wonders. How often do you give yourself time for these things?

If you are like most people, the answer is once in a while. You might watch the sunset while on vacation. But there is a sunset every night.

If you take the beauty and pleasure out of life, you're left with a functional existence. You pay the rent, the mortgage, the car payments. You hope one day to become rich and powerful enough to enjoy your leisure. In reality, though, people busy making money often become busier than ever once they've made it. I know people who could go anywhere but choose to remain in their Wall Street offices and make more money.

At what point do they have enough to feel that they can enjoy the beauty and pleasure of life? Generally, they never do, unless they have a stroke or some other life-threatening illness. At that point, they may suddenly realize the importance of beauty and pleasure. I'm suggesting we re-prioritize our lives so that what is most important comes first.

What is the Message of a Crisis?

We all experience crises. A loved one dies, we lose a job, or we have to move. During these times, it's important to ask ourselves the following questions: "What's the message here?" "What can I learn from this experience?" The Chinese interpret a crisis as an opportunity as well as a danger. We must appreciate the occasion for what it can teach us, as well as dealing with situations as they arise.

Many times a crisis can be avoided by attuning ourselves to our inner needs and taking action before an emergency arises. An example of this can be seen in the person who eats healthfully and meditates, thereby avoiding an otherwise imminent heart attack. The opposite situation can be seen in the experience of a friend of mine who had a stroke after refusing to pay attention to the warning signs.

I had attempted to convince this friend to go to my ranch to detoxify his system and meditate on his life. He refused to listen. In his mind, everything else was more important than health.

As I predicted, he had a stroke. Now he's in bad shape—bedridden and, in fact, totally immobile—and has no choice but to slow down and think about taking care of himself. He has to put his life into perspective and examine what is really important to him. It's a sad situation, but the point is, he himself created this crisis state by ignoring the warning signs that were leading up to it. By attending to his real needs beforehand, he could have prevented the crisis from occurring.

Sometimes a crisis forces us to speed up and take immediate action for change. I lecture a lot in Santa Fe and Albuquerque, where the audience is comprised largely of former New Yorkers. These people generally don't live in the $800,000 homes in the hills but choose to live moderately in an environment that sustains them. Two people who attend my lectures demonstrate how difficult but necessary this transition sometimes is.

This couple comes from a burnt-out neighborhood in Brooklyn where drugs, street gangs, and crime are rampant. They found it difficult to leave the neighborhood they had known their whole lives, but the seriousness of the situation finally forced them to do so. By the time they decided to leave New York, the police weren't able to do enough to stop crime. The highlight, or rather, nadir, of their crisis occurred after the woman was beaten up in the school where she taught.

This event propelled them to ask themselves, "Is there any place in this world that we can call home? Is there a place where we can work and enjoy life without feeling that we're in a combat zone? Is there a place where people will appreciate the lessons we're trying to share?"

With these questions in mind, they took action to change their situation. They bought a trailer and traveled around the United States. They found the answers they were looking for in Albuquerque, where they have since settled down.

We can do the same if we question the situation surrounding our crisis and search for the answers, trusting that a solution is there. Note: Sometimes the solution involves being unpredictable and doing something that no one expects from us. Often it involves changing the way we've been living up to this point. But it's imperative at these times that we pay attention to our own inner needs, because only then can we regain homeostasis, or balance.

When We Feel Discomfort, What Is Our First Response?

We all experience discomfort. We feel it when we take the kids out of one school and put them into another, when we start a new job, or when we end a relationship. Most of us try to escape this feeling. We overeat, drink, go for a drive, panic, or withdraw.

What if, instead of avoiding the experience, we take the opposite approach and immerse ourselves in it? We can take this attitude: "I don't feel good right now, but I'm going to learn something from what is happening." Immersing ourselves in what we're feeling, no matter how uncomfortable, and learning from it, is the only way we can ultimately resolve our problems. Otherwise, we repeat the experience over and over.

One situation that exemplifies this point is in athletics. I see lots of people jogging and racewalking in the park. Yet many of them never show much real physical improvement. They don't lose a whole lot of extra weight. This is because they're only working at their comfort level. When they feel discomfort, they hold themselves back from going any further. They don't push through their discomfort. They view any uneasiness as a barrier to further change. The mind acknowledges these limits and says, "I can't go any further."

If we never allow ourselves to experience feelings of discomfort, we never learn, change, or grow. We begin to feel helpless. If we face our feelings of discomfort, on the other hand, we learn, we grow, we pick ourselves up, and we forgive ourselves. We get through every crisis and create a new sense of exhilaration in our life.

How Do We Stop Ourselves From Being Happy?

While we don't consciously try to subvert our own happiness, there are habitual attitudes we sometimes adopt that have the same effect.

Needing to Have Others Validate Us

I went back to school only to realize later that I needn't have done so. I did it because I was trying to conform to the expectations of society, which acknowledges academic credentials as measures of your intellectual worth.

I now realize that when people reject you, often nothing in the world that you do will change their opinion of you. For instance, when people spurn others because of their culture, color, gender, or beliefs, there is, many times, nothing that can be done to change that attitude, because their minds are closed—and they long ago threw away the key.

This was an important lesson for me to learn. I now know that we needn't go through life achieving things to prove to others that we're okay.

Fear of Loss

Frequently, we hold on to things we don't need because they are associated with an image we have of ourselves. The things are merely part of a picture we've created to conform to the expectations of others.

When we're no longer afraid of losing what we have, we are

free. We're no longer concerned about someone else's perception because we know who we are.

Fear of Failure

Because many of us are preoccupied with how others see us, we can't be comfortable with ourselves unless we feel perfect. But think of all our bad hair days, how many times a day our breath smells, all the times we look in the mirror and don't like the way we look. Think of how many times we do something that doesn't turn out exactly right. If we can't be comfortable with ourselves during all these times, we're spending an awful lot of our lives in a state of unease.

We shouldn't expect ourselves to be perfect. People in sports achieve proficiency only with practice. Actors who seem so flawless on the movie screen do so only after many rehearsals. Perfection is an illusion. When you see Frank Sinatra singing, Nancy Kerrigan skating, or Joe Namath throwing a football, there are moments when it all seems so effortless. In reality, there was a great deal of trial and error involved in getting to that point. That's what we don't see. We don't see the outtakes, the mistakes, or the confusion, just the final performance.

We judge ourselves too harshly, acting as if everything we say and do were the final product. We need to focus on being honest about who we are rather than worry about being right all the time. Don't look at your life as a performance.

Loss of Spontaneity

When we are not in control of our life, but living according to the expectations of others, we lose our spontaneity. Why is spontaneity so important? It allows us to be who we are and to be in the moment. It allows us to feel. Children are always spontaneous. That's why they're honest and unpredictable; we never quite know what they're going to do or say. It's also why they're happy.

Children know how to live in the moment, which is something we often forget as adults. Imagine if we had to pay for each day. How differently we would live! But life's free and we generally take it for granted. Then one day we wake up and realize it's almost over, and that we've wasted a lot of it. If we lived in the moment, we would never feel our time was wasted.

Being spontaneous allows us to live life to the fullest. People ask me how I'm able to write several books, produce a number of full-length documentaries, go to movies and plays each week, maintain meaningful friendships, spend connected time with my family, and travel extensively—all within a year. I can do so because I never waste a moment. Also, I'm fully present in each moment. When I'm physically present, I'm emotionally present as well. I listen to the person I'm with, not just to myself.

The Constant Desire for More

I grew up around older people. I'll never forget one woman, Hattie, who lived on my corner. She was always happy and singing in her backyard. Hattie would make me sassafras tea and tell me stories.

I saw her again after college, when I was in my early twenties. I asked, "Hattie, why have you always been so happy?" She said, "Whatever I have, I consider a gift, and I cherish every gift I've been given."

Hattie wasn't talking about the things that money can buy. She didn't have too many of those. But she enjoyed the flowers, the sun, reading, and what she could do. She had shelves filled with books, all of which she read. Hattie would say, "I've got eyes. Why do I need to watch television when I can learn from the richness of these literary minds?" Television was too passive for her. "I don't want to just be entertained," she would say. "I want to engage my mind." The most beautiful garden on the entire block belonged to Hattie. Everybody admired it.

Other people in my home town could have had beautiful gardens too, but they didn't feel it was important. They could have read books, but they didn't find the time. They could have enjoyed the day, but they didn't make the time. They always thought that something else was more important than being in the moment. They would often complain about what they didn't have. "If only I had this I would be happy," they would say, or "I wouldn't have ulcers if I had this." The truth was that people like Hattie, who didn't have very many things, but who knew how to appreciate life, were the ones without the ulcers and with the greatest happiness.

Trying to Re-create Enjoyable Moments

Sometimes we do understand that it's how we spend our time—not what we have—that can make us happy. But we fall into this particular trap: we try to recreate enjoyable moments from the past. Think of how much of our life is based upon repetition. We tend to want to have the same fun in the same way. We think that just because something happened once it can happen a hundred times. In actuality, though, we limit our lives by trying to re-grasp something that we enjoyed. We can't have a moment unless we're spontaneous and let it be what it is. We should never try to re-create it; it can't be re-created. Nothing can ever be the same again. It can be different—even better—but it can't be the same.

Inability to Appreciate What We Have

Often we appreciate something only once we no longer have it. The friend I talked about earlier, who is lying helplessly in bed, now appreciates what his legs and arms can do. I'm sure he'd give anything in the world to have that ability back now.

Think of people whom we've had in our lives whom we never made an effort to spend quality time with, people who have since died. If only they could come back for a short time, how different we would be. Suddenly, we'd know that we had a period of time to share what was meaningful.

Why wait until we don't have something any longer? Why not appreciate what we have today? Take an inventory of what you have in the way of friends, family, and assets, that you can enjoy. Your list may not be as long, materially, as that of a Trump or a Rockefeller, but on the other hand, your inventory will contain people, opportunities, and assets that are unique to you and so truly priceless that you wouldn't trade them with anyone in the world, for anything.

When you take inventory this way, you may realize how much you've learned and experienced in your life. Look at what you've done that has given you happiness. Start to make a list in your diary of the things that have given you great joy in your life. You will begin to see that good feelings stem from you, and that you can renew that joy.

Working Toward
Self-Sufficiency

❖

Have you ever spent time in the Italian countryside?

Picture an evergreen-sprinkled hill. Eight to fifteen stone and wood houses are nestled on the side of this hill, flanked by low stone walls and hand-tilled fields beyond. In fact, every house, fence, and field in this village has to be hand-built or tended because this is not the kind of hill that you can get machinery on.

During a recent visit to the Italian countryside, I would run 10 to 20 miles daily, going from one tiny village like this to another and enjoying the picturesqueness of it all. But what I really marveled at was how much the people in these areas had done with their own hands, and were doing. For instance, in the early morning hours, when I ran, they'd be baking. And I'd see chickens, sheep, and goats, suppliers of eggs, wool, and milk for the villagers. I'd see horses, helpers with the farm labor. I did get to meet many people in the countryside—there aren't more hospitable people anywhere—so I got to enter homes and see how people lived and the extent of their self-sufficiency. It was impressive.

These people could just about do it all! They were their own builders, masons, plumbers, and carpenters. They were their own farmers and gardeners and vintners too—in addition to its own garden, each house had its own vineyard and pressed its own grapes for wine. Plus they had herb gardens and grew an astonishing number of herbs that they used medicinally, as well is in cooking. Some of their home apothecaries would be unmatchable in variety by any store here. So you could say that, in many cases, they were their own doctors and pharmacists too.

With all these things to do, basically to maintain their lives, the people in these Italian villages were busy. I noticed, though, that there was a pacing to their busyness; there was no frenetic quality to it but rather a constancy, interrupted by needed relaxation periods. The key to their scheduling success: They didn't waste time on what I call make-work stress. They stuck to the essentials.

Some people in the U.S. are returning, or making a first-time transition, to this kind of simpler, more self-sufficient life. They're moving out to the Santa Fe, or Tucson, or Salt Lake City, and setting up a back-to-basics type of existence. Interestingly, this is happening in Italy as well. I was told that many Italians who'd grown up in small villages, and were now in their 40s and 50s, were making a move back to rural areas after having enjoyed successful careers in the cities. It seems that the appeal of the self-sufficient life is universal.

I've always valued the concept of self-sufficiency myself. But when I think of this ideal I broaden the concept, because I see self-sufficiency not just as a matter of whether you can bake your own bread or build your own furniture, although these are wonderful skills to have. The way I see it, being self-sufficient also involves mental and emotional components. So it's a matter of whether you can form your own opinions and plans, and stick with them. It's a matter of directing your own life and supporting yourself emotionally, even during those times when no one else is, as they say, "there for you."

Self-sufficiency in the physical and emotional areas may be related; that is, to the extent that you're self-sufficient physically, you have more chance of being emotionally balanced. Of course that doesn't mean that we who live in the cities should all pack up and move to farms so that we can grow our own food. But perhaps there are things that we could be doing for ourselves that we aren't. Examples include: baking our own bread, growing our own herbs in kitchen flowerpots, entertaining ourselves with conversation rather than electronically, taking charge of our own health, and becoming involved in our local governments or school systems, so that we can affect what happens in our communities.

Being self-sufficient is not an easy thing. It's not a total thing either—nor should it be. But I do see it as a valuable principle and a goal worth working toward. That's why I believe we should all periodically examine our lives to take stock of our own strengths. We should look at ways to develop them, too.

Have You Ever Correctly Assessed Your Own Potential? Or Are You Habitually Selling Yourself Short?

People can generally achieve a lot more on their own than they think they can. I believe you can achieve independence, confidence, self-control, and self-esteem, taking responsibility that's appropriate for yourself and, where necessary, for others. You can achieve just about anything. Of course if you feel that you are limited in what you can achieve on your own, then to the degree that you believe you can't do something, you absolutely will not try. You will stop yourself. You will gridlock and block. Then what you want won't happen, because you won't believe that you can do it. You'll blame not having the right teacher, parents, or financier.

Being self-sufficient requires effort, and it does not come naturally to everyone. I had a clear example of that a few years ago when I took some people from New York who wanted to learn about alternative lifestyles to my ranch. Dr. Martin Feldman and I started a project. We set aside ten acres and offered people half of everything that they grew. We bought them seeds, books, and machinery. We spent about $30,000 on this project. Five New Yorkers went down there with varying backgrounds. We told them that the plan of action was to remain positive, to read and learn, and to garden, grow, and market. They loved the idea.

Within two months, the New Yorkers had squandered everything. Weeds were growing. Nothing had been planted. They were into interpersonal politics and relationships to the exclusion of doing anything productive. In fact, they were doing nothing but staying up all night and watching television. They were running up $500 a week bills for organic produce that they were buying in a store to eat. I finally had to send them on their way because they were unappreciative of the opportunity they had been given.

I then brought in a Mexican family, and within three weeks everything got done. The gardens were perfectly manicured and food was growing. It was amazing; they had that place blooming. In one of my conversations with the father, he said, "We come from a very poor area in Mexico where we have to do everything for ourselves. We don't work fast but we work consistently. We think about what has to be done and then use all of our resources to do it. If you ever watch Mexicans work, you will notice that we work at a constant pace and always get the job done. We don't work fast and then burn out." He was absolutely correct, and his words were actually a great capsule description of how to master the art of self-sufficiency. By the way, the slow and steady work pace he described was the same one I later observed in those Italian villages.

Here in urban America we have services to do everything for

us. Yes, this is convenient and time-saving, and can help us concentrate on our careers. But the down side of having all these services is that it can lead us to feel helpless in many areas of life, so that in the face of any problem, we focus only on the problem. We step away and say, "I can't do anything."

I hired a friend of mine a while back, someone who had run a big, successful advertising agency. At first I thought that his having been an executive would be a plus. Soon, though, I noticed that week in and week out he would only focus on the problems. He would stop working and nothing would get done. Finally, I asked him if it had ever occurred to him to be positive and look for solutions. It seemed that the experience of running an agency had gotten him so used to looking at the negative and to blaming others or having others do things for him that he was incapable of coping with problems on his own. All he could do was delegate responsibility to other people.

In our society, you see too many people living like that. Then you see why, from a certain perspective, it's good that American corporations are shaking out all that middle management. These are often the people who have lost the art of doing anything for themselves. If you want to get something done, give it to someone who is used to doing things for himself—especially someone who's had to for reasons of survival.

What Don't You Need or Want From Others?

I Can Do It Myself, Thank You

This is a phrase I like to keep in mind because I think we generally take too much from others, sometimes in the guise of help. But to give a new spin to an old phrase, with help like this, who needs hindrance? Sometimes you're better off going it alone.

Let's look at a few examples of what you don't need or want from others. This is important in helping you identify what not to allow into your life. It can help you break the pattern of letting something unhealthy into your life over and over again. Stop accepting what you don't want and don't need by being honest and saying, *This is something I don't want and don't need. Thank you but no. I'd rather do it myself.*

Dishonesty

No one should live with dishonesty. Take a survey of all the places in your life where dishonesty is part of the relationship. Look at your interactions with coworkers, friends, and family. Do you engage in dishonest relationships, or are you able to say, "This is no good. I don't want this"? Once you assert what you won't accept from others, you'll stop dishonesty from entering your life.

I only maintain honest relationships. Once people dishonor me in some way, they are out of my life forever. I don't care what we've shared in the past. A person has to reaffirm today, and people who continue to work with me year in and year out understand that. Those who think that just because they've been with me for a month or two they can drift into not being on time, or not paying attention to the quality of their work because they've been accepted, are wrong. Those people are out. I won't give people a second chance at honesty. They're either honest or they're dishonest, and if they're dishonest, they're not in my life.

This sounds pretty harsh. But I feel that since there is no shortage of people who will honor you, why even bother with those who don't? So I refuse to lower my expectations of others, even when I see this going on all around me. Human relationships are too important to dishonor.

Lack of Trustworthiness

Related to honesty is trustworthiness. Why is this important? Trust allows you a solid foundation to stand on and to build on. You can be yourself around someone you trust. But how seldom is trust maintained! Look at how intimates of the famous turn around and run to the tabloids to sell stories about their "friends." If you were the person being betrayed, how would you feel?

What does this type of situation tell us? It doesn't tell us a thing about the betrayers. They never really disguised who they were. We shouldn't have those kind of people in our life to begin with. They give us a thousand signals not to trust them and we continue to let them stay. The lesson, then, is not for them. It's for you.

I was thinking recently about Princess Diana having an affair with a man who ran off and sold the story for four million dollars. He's not the problem, though, because he could not have disguised himself. Energy cannot lie. I've never met a person who could tell me a lie where I didn't know they were lying. Nor did you. That's because there's a universal consciousness. Tap into it and all the knowledge you need is there. It's called intuition. When you trust your intuition you're always right.

Constant Supervision

Are you in a supervised relationship? Supervision means that the other person in the relationship is always controlling you. They ask questions such as, where are you going? Where were you? Who were you with? The supervised person in the relationship adapts to that. Not adapting becomes equated with challenge, and rather than being challenging, with the resultant hassle, the supervised party acquiesces. Basically, you've got a dominant/submissive situation with supervision.

But being dominated violates a person's very essence. The

real part of the person starts to burn up inside, thinking, I'm a mature person. I don't need to be supervised. I don't need someone to tell me what to do and when and how to do it.

Remember this: You're an adult. An adult relationship is about two individuals sharing what they find most compatible about each other, without loss of autonomy. Supervision is for children, prison inmates, and certain pets.

Others' Opinions About You

Sure, you should be interested in what other people think about you—to an extent, a very limited one. You see, everybody has an opinion about you, and if you pay too much attention to what others think about you, you start taking a lot of your cues from them. You decide to do or not do something, say or not say something, share or not share. What you do, say, and share can all become based on other people's opinions when you want them to have a good opinion of you.

No matter what you do, though, you're never going to please everybody. And by the time you get around to having enough people liking you, you're not going to like yourself anymore because of all the compromises you have had to make to meet their standards. I'd rather be hated by everybody but loved by myself than be loved by everybody and hate myself.

Manipulative Criticism

Well-thought-out criticism can be a good thing. A problem comes in, though, when criticism is self-serving, and when people add a twist of control in to it. You hear talk of constructive criticism, but there's often a question of exactly what's being constructed, and why. For instance, you're a young artist, happy in what you're doing but struggling financially. Your father tells you you're lazy and lack ambition, that you ought to go to school to get an MBA, and then get a "real" job. Just what is he constructing? A more fulfilling life for you? Or the realization of his image of what a child of his should be?

No one knows you the way you know yourself. No one can know what you're feeling. Many times, others' judgments of you are merely projections of themselves and have nothing to do with who you are. Always question others' judgments about you. Always.

Pain

The Upper West Side of Manhattan seems to attract the intellectual, long-suffering, cloistered minds of the world. You see them in bookstores. You see them in restaurants. You see them in very intense conversation with furrowed brow, leaning forward, pointing in someone's face, pounding on tables, frothing at the mouth. This is where the heart of activism and social commentary is located. There's a lot of pain here.

I'm all for social activism—as one facet of life. But many people take their identity more from their pain than from their pleasure. They believe that their lives are justified by the pain that they feel and exhibit. In fact, they are terrified by the idea that there can be pleasure in life without pain.

We're not comfortable when people enjoy pleasure. If a woman engages in pleasure, we have derogatory names for her. A woman doctor was on my show the other day. She is a gynecologist/obstetrician and a very angry woman. She said that the men in the hospitals where she worked put her down because she displayed pleasure, passion, and creativity in her work. They couldn't handle it.

We're very limited in the amount of pleasure we allow. Pleasure has to be of very short duration and it has to be socially constructed. So it's acceptable to take pleasure in going to church to pray. Or in going on a family vacation—provided that we've truly earned it by working like crazy beforehand, and that it's not too long.

Caretaking

A caretaker is an okay thing to have—on an estate. But not in my adult relationship, please! By caretaking I mean when a person feels that their purpose is to serve you. Everything they do involves making your life better. Implied in their caretaker role is that they don't think you're adult enough to take care of yourself. You're being treated like a child. As in the supervised relationship, you can never be completely independent.

A lot of people base relationships on how much caretaking they do for their partner. Often it's the woman who assumes or gets assigned this role. Even in the 90s, many women are expected to do all the household chores. So they wash all the dishes, cook all the food, iron all the clothes, sometimes willingly, at least for a while. What would happen if the man were to share those chores? You might have a truly adult relationship.

What Do Others Do for You That You Could Do for Yourself?

Do you look to others too much? List all the things you expect from other people that you could easily do yourself. Think carefully; you may be surprised at the length of your list. Doing this exercise and acting on it will give you more freedom to be who you are. It will improve your relationships too.

Yes, it's sometimes wonderful to have people do things for us when we don't strictly need them to. The trouble is, we can develop rigid expectations when we ought to be flexible. For instance, husbands often expect wives to do the cooking, and as we just discussed in the previous section, caretaker-oriented wives may be happy to. This is all okay, during those times when it's mutually acceptable. But what if one day you, as the husband, come home and see that your wife has had a hard day, and she's tired? She may not feel well. Will you expect her to fulfill her customary role, or will you take some responsibility for those chores yourself? Or what would happen if you said, "Let's change this. I'll cook one day, you cook the next"? Suddenly, it increases the respect each person has for the other. It acknowledges the other in that moment. It acknowledges the importance of the moment.

If, on the other hand, you say, "Nope; this is the way it is. The woman does this, I do that, period." Then there's no respect, no moment, only something old that's based upon the past that you're living with as if it's unchangeable law. It's fine to live with antiques, but not when they're ideas.

Think of all the women who pick up the clothes and do the laundry just because it's expected of them. Are you one of them? What if you started to say to those you live with, there's no reason why you can't do the laundry, why you can't clean the dishes, why you can't vacuum? I'm a fervent believer in the idea that we should never allow permanency in the way we live. We should have so much flexibility in our life arrangements that we can adjust and change without it seeming like a major trauma in which people start accusing one another. Respect the moment. Things change. Nothing is ever the same.

Do You Need or Seek Approval?

Have you ever been a stamp collector, getting sets of stamps sent to you monthly, "on approval"? If you liked the stamps you could accept and pay for them; if not, you could send them back. The on-approval mode is fine in the hobbyist's world, but some people live their lives like this, offering up their every action for scrutiny by others before they commit themselves to it.

Do you live your life in this tentative, on-approval mode, not really finalizing anything until you've got someone else's go-ahead? For instance, do you dress for someone else? Do you do your hair for others? Or do you do these things for you? When you do things with an eye to approval from other people, you should at least ask yourself if what you are doing is authentic to your own spirit as well.

When you need someone else's approval, you set the stage for problems. You run the risk of not getting the approval you seek or of getting it for a while and then being cut off from it. If you are cut off, you internalize that by feeling a silent sense of betrayal. Then you start to resent the other person.

Sometimes people try to get approval for their pain. What happens if you don't acknowledge that? I'm the last person in the world you should ever complain to because I'll expect you to come up with a solution to your problem and act on it. I believe you can instantaneously tap into every answer you need to be absolutely content, positive, well, happy, balanced, and fulfilled in your life. Allow that in and it will immerse you. That energy is there to be used. Why seek someone else's approval when you already know everything you need to know?

Do You Focus on Learning or on Succeeding?

Learning is more important than succeeding, although not many people seem to think so. Think of all the people who get their MBAs and go out there to succeed without really learning anything. Many of these people spend more than what they earn, living beyond their means in order to show that they are somebody. Their educational, career, and monetary successes teach them nothing. As a result, when they lose any part of it, their whole self-image is diminished.

What if they went out to learn first? Then success would not be important and learning would be. If success occurred it would merely be as a side effect of learning. When I go out to race, it's not important that I win. I can feel just as good coming in last as first, because what I'm most interested in is what I can learn. Every time I train and every time I race, I'm learning. Yes, I have won a lot of races, hundreds of them. But I don't need to remind myself with trophies and plaques because the winning came as a result of what I learned, and it's the learning process that was the most important part of the experience. Another important aspect of it for me is that as a result of what I've learned, I've been able to teach other people. They in turn teach others, and everyone continues to grow.

Think of the mistakes you make because you are more interested in the goal of success than in the learning process. Try getting up in the morning with the attitude of wanting to learn. Ask yourself, what do I want to learn today? That will put your mind and emotions in a whole new stance vis-a-vis that day's activities. If you're only interested in succeeding, you may reach your goal, you may have a conquest of some type, but what will you have learned in the process? Nothing. It will be a hollow success, and you yourself will still feel empty. As a result you'll create more and more goals. You'll never have achieved enough. When you get into the learning mode, by contrast, you don't have to have constant success. You're fulfilled by the learning process.

What Messages Do You Carry With You?

Subconsciously, you carry with you the messages of your childhood. Your personality evolves from these messages. While for some people the messages of early life are positive, involving unconditional love and acceptance, if we've received negative ones they can hobble us later on, without our ever realizing it. Here are some examples of negative messages that children receive. Were some of these transmitted to you?

What You Believe Is Untrue

As an example, you're 10 years old. Your mother is speaking negatively about someone, and you overhear it. You say, "Mom, what are you talking about?" And she says, "Oh, nothing." Later, you ask, "Did you say something bad about someone?" And she says, "No." But you know that she has. She makes you feel as if what you're hearing and seeing is not true. She has denied your experience.

What You Perceive Is Irrelevant

Everything is relevant to a young child. Every new discovery becomes a new reality, hence, a new sensation and a new perception. The last thing you should do is tell a child that something is irrelevant. That teaches the child that nothing has importance. If nothing the child discovers has importance, then the only thing that is important is what the mother or father says. This becomes the focus of the child.

As a result, children grow up to become insensitive. They become uninterested in other people's realities. These become irrelevant.

Look at commuters who ride into Manhattan each day from the suburbs. Many go right through slums, not caring. These neighborhoods are irrelevant to them. Many are insensitive to the obviously unemployed around them. These people are irrelevant to them. *They're* not going to lose *their* job.

Do you fall into this pattern? If a friend or family member shares her feelings with you, do you realize that what that person is saying is important to her? Do you really pay attention, and try to understand that person's predicament? If you don't, you may be acting on internalized messages from long ago. If you do, though, you're empowering not just that friend or family member, but yourself.

You Can't Be Trusted

How many times have you been told that you couldn't be trusted? You weren't responsible? You let people down? Someone immediately corrected you and showed you the right way of doing or saying something. Every time someone did that, you began to feel a certain ineffectualness, an inability to do. That creates helplessness.

How often do you see men showing women how to do things? The woman says, "I don't know how to do this; please show me." This pattern, one that goes back to early training, plays both ways in reinforcing helplessness.

In Sweden, every citizen is required to know how to fix a car engine; otherwise, you could get stranded in the snow there and die. So men and women, young and old, have to master auto mechanics to get their driver's license. It's a matter of survival.

You Are Not Lovable

If you buy into this one, you keep people away. Or the people you do allow into your life are the ones who reinforce your self-concept of unlovableness. You find relationships that keep you in constant conflict. In that way, you continue to believe you are undeserving of affection.

You Are Stupid

Have you ever been told that you were stupid? Why in the world would someone say that? They must have been frustrated and impatient. They wanted something done immediately. They didn't recognize that we can have different solutions to one problem and all be right. They wanted you to see things their way and work in their time frame. They wanted you to come up with their solutions. In short, they wanted you to fit into their agenda.

All you need are a few of these "you are stupid" messages at a sensitive age and you start to pull back. You hold back all your vulnerability. You become completely isolated from any sense of a self that is going to be courageous enough to break through and actually do something on your own. Thus, you start to show that you *are* stupid. You won't take any risks or chances, and people believe that you are stupid simply because of what you refuse to do.

Why do you think so many people in our society never take any risks at all, living a passive spectator existence, watching safely from the sidelines as others take the risks? It's because they grew up believing they were stupid, and they are not going to do anything that will bring any more contempt upon them.

You Are Evil

Many of us were taught that curiosity about sex is evil, when it is natural. Other cultures explore their bodies without shame, embarrassment, or ridicule. For many children here, though, one of the first admonitions given is not to masturbate. Children are told it is evil, and if they're caught, they're reprimanded, smacked, punished, humiliated.

As a result of our grossly repressed sexuality, we become afraid to explore the depths of our sexual feelings. The moment we do, we have both guilt and fear. We even restrain our capacity to fantasize. We literally block it. Or if we do fantasize, we begin to feel evil and dirty. If, as a child, you were rejected, punished, and ridiculed for wanting to be in touch with your own sexuality, it may not be easy to be sexual as an adult.

Boys and Girls Don't Take Risks; Children Are Seen and Not Heard

Here are other messages that live deep within our subconscious. As a result of these, many people keep their true feelings inside. They only talk for utilitarian purposes or to express frustration, never as a way of freeing or empowering themselves. They are silent about the issues they should be discussing and the feelings they should be voicing.

If you feel strongly about something, you should find your voice and talk about the issue. Face it, confront it, and engage with it. I see people who will gossip about a situation but not face the issue head-on. To me, that shows they've learned the negative lessons of early childhood too well.

Are You Self-Empowered?

Being empowered means being in control of your life. When you recognize your own authority, you feel good about yourself. You move at your own pace. You feel full whether or not you are busy. When you are not in charge of your life, on the other hand, you look to other things or people to fill you up. These could be a cult, church, fraternity, sorority, spouse, girlfriend, club, or workplace. The problem here? If you're not self-empowered, their power is likely to supersede your own.

True self-empowerment is not mirrored in worldly power, success, wealth, or possessions. It's mirrored in your manner of living, because true empowerment is accompanied by a sense of inner peace. You know where you should be and what you should be doing. I've met truck drivers, farmers, schoolteachers, and other people in all areas of life who feel completely in balance. They are empowered and feel good about themselves. Empowerment gives them an inner direction; other people can't sway them.

Empowerment is the actualization of your potential. Most

people intellectualize about what they should be doing instead of living up to their abilities. When you are empowered, though, you live your life the way you need to live it—you don't just talk about it. You do what you know you essentially need to be doing.

The movie *Forrest Gump* showed a man who was self-empowered. He always did what he believed in. He ran back and forth across the country because he felt that was what he should be doing. Other people followed him for the wrong reasons. They thought that if Forrest did it, they should do it. They were copycats. Unlike the others, Forrest was always motivated from within himself. He acted out of his beliefs in everything he did, from playing ping-pong to running a shrimp boat to going to war.

Look at your own life. What don't you like about yourself? Think of the things you do that you are not happy about. Be aware of what you think, say, and do that disempowers you. In fact, write down what you think, say, and do in a day. How do these things make you feel? Are they empowering or disempowering? If you feel disempowered, what can you do to change the situation to enhance your well-being?

If You Were to Draw a Blueprint for a New Life, What Would It Look Like?

Let's say you were starting over today from scratch. What would a blueprint for your life look like?

You can start over at any point in your life. In my running and walking group I meet many people who are beginning to turn their lives around, and believe me, there is no right age to do this. Rather, there is no *wrong* age; they're all right! Harry, for instance, is 81 and he just started changing his life at 79. He gave up his friends because they were talking about death and disease and he didn't want to engage in that. He chose to re-engage in life and to start running marathons. Harry became the architect of his life.

I'm suggesting that you can start out fresh today. To do this you must be willing to change your perceptions about life. You must realize that you are in control. You make life happen; life is not something that happens to you.

There are three important stages in the process. Let's go through them.

Imagine Your Ideals

Visualize your new life as if it already exists. Ask yourself, what do I want in my life? See a picture of it in your mind. Write about it and look at what you've written. Don't edit your description. Believe that anything is possible, because it is. Recently, for the first time in American history, a 63-year-old woman won an award for being the outstanding athlete of the year for all age groups. The first time I met her, seven years before that, she could hardly lift a weight or run up stairs. She persevered toward her goal because she had a vivid dream in her mind of what she could do. What she saw allowed her to keep on going.

You need to start with an idealistic image. Don't be afraid of having ideals in a society that has so few.

Take Practical Steps

After you create an image of what you desire, determine the steps you will take to get there. Then, give yourself a timetable. As an example, I'm currently working on a new project, an organic farm in Florida. I visualize a cooperative venture with a lot of people participating. I see a 10- to 15-acre farm with lots of gardens. In the middle of this farm is a big, beautiful 1800s-style general store. There is a large organic health food store. People can walk through a kitchen behind glass and see food being freshly made, everything from Essene breads baking to sprouts being grown. There are also greenhouses where hydroponics are grown, gardens with exotic flowers from all over the Americas, a restaurant, and a crafts center. I see all this.

To make it happen, I must see this developing in stages. I have an architect drawing my plans. The project will take three years to complete.

You have to know how to stage your life. When you see what you ideally want, where you want to be, what you want to be doing, and whom you want to be with, plan it out in stages. Don't jump ahead of yourself. Don't expect big changes to occur too quickly. Take your time. Work on it gradually, and give yourself a lot of leeway. Don't overstress yourself.

Get Support

Share your plans with people who support you. Telling your story is like a rite of passage because making a transition is always significant and talking about it to others strengthens your commitment to change. Giving voice to your ideas makes them more real. They're no longer just a little secret in your head that nobody knows about.

Bring the significant people in your life together. Invite them to lunch or dinner. (Note: Don't invite the habitual naysayers to this particular meal. You know who they are!) Share with your supporters where you are at in your life. Telling your story is so important; never assume that it's not of interest. So tell it. Explain to people what works for you and what doesn't. Then show them where your life is going and how you are going to get there. Let them know what role you would like them to play in your life. You want people to celebrate your change. You are saying: I'm changing, here is what I'm doing, and here is what I need. People who really support you will love that! And you will love their response.

Note this too: If it should be the case that at this particular juncture in your life, you have no supporters, that happens sometimes. Don't abort your plans because of this circumstance. Remember that believing in yourself is really the most important thing by far.

In Order to Believe That You Can Do Anything, You Must First Believe in Your Completeness

A lot of people believe that they are going to change their lives. They want to change them, and they have good ideas about what they want to do. But nothing changes. Part of the reason that nothing really changes is that they don't see themselves as complete enough to engage in the change. You have to be complete to engage in change. It's the completeness that gives you the ability to go forward. In the absence of completeness, only fragmented parts of the self venture forward.

Only from your sense of completeness and the totality of your being do you go forward with meaning. When you allow the complete self out, everything becomes a point of excitement. Have you ever watched a child? They see something new and they become excited. They're so complete. It's the totality of the child that responds. They've involved themselves totally in the excitement of discovery because they have no fear.

I am complete enough to do anything at any time, anywhere that I choose. I can be what I want to be. I am whole and have everything I need. Every recipe I need to make my life work is here within me. And the same is true for you.

Becoming the Hero in Your
Own Life

Over the years, I've helped thousands of people prepare themselves for participation in marathons. And of course I've trained for numerous marathons myself. It's an amazing process, one that never ceases to inspire me, because it affects all aspects of one's being. In fact, I'd say that a marathon runner's training is more than the sum of all its individual parts. It's more than vitamins, diet, exercise, stress management, and guided visualization. All these components have a place, but none of them embody the heart of it. At the core of training, we learn what it means to live life as a hero.

We're living in a time plagued with dysfunction, much of which is self-inflicted. We hear people whine, moan, blame, and complain. We witness people who relish being victims when they don't have to be victims.

In running and racewalking you see the healthier side of the coin. You see a woman on crutches with multiple sclerosis making it to the finish line. Long after everyone else has finished the race she pushes onward, cold and fatigued, without the cheering fans and without the water stops.

Such a courageous accomplishment demonstrates that we can do amazing things when we are determined and when our hearts are in what we do. We start to realize that our pain and blisters are not so bad when we see others reaching seemingly insurmountable goals.

Over the years, I have had the opportunity to run and communicate with athletes from countries the world over. People explain to me their rationale for training and talk about what keeps them going. The theme that emerges is one of becoming the hero in your own life.

I have met many heroes. Such people are easy to identify. They do not feel the need to draw attention to themselves. Nor do they brag about their accomplishments or conquests. Heroes are often quiet people who engage in life rather than talking about it. They choose to work rather than to talk and they don't feel the need to engage in debates to convince you that their point of view is the right one.

Doing the marathon is an enormous challenge for many people, one that can be terrifying. Think of running or racewalking for 26 miles, alone. This is not a team sport. You do it with other people but it's a uniquely individual process. At times you feel that you can't do it but at the very same moment something in you says yes, I can. You go through the fear, absorb it, let it go, and then become transformed at the end of the process.

Heroics in this sport is well exemplified in the movie *On the Edge*, with Bruce Dern. This movie is about a great athlete, one of America's best, who tries out for the Olympics. Due to dirty politics on the part of some competitors, he becomes disqualified and is barred from ever competing again.

Almost ten years go by before he decides that yes, he will compete again. He chooses a famous run that takes place on a murderous course in San Francisco. The course is extremely hilly; it goes straight up a gigantic hill and then straight down.

I ran that course and found it to be the toughest course I ever ran in my life.

The athlete comes to town and trains every day. He has almost no money but rents a room in town and devotes all his time to his task. Each day he marks off the days until the race on his calendar, and each night he records his progress in a diary. The man seems to have no life outside of his training. His only purpose appears to be to redeem his reputation.

During this arduous process, he meets a wise, old athletic coach, who tells him that he is training all wrong; he is not training with his heart but with anger. The coach advises him not to run to prove people wrong but for the love of what he is doing. In effect, he is turning a negative situation into a positive one through a change in focus.

From that point on, Bruce Dern begins to train with full investment of his mind and heart. You can immediately see the transformation in him.

The day of the race is beset with obstacles. His nemesis, the person who disqualified him ten years earlier, is again one of the race's sponsors. At first Dern is able to hide from him but later on, in the middle of the race when he starts to gain, he is noticed. The sponsor does everything in his power to stop him. He calls the police and asks them to prevent Dern from getting over the top of the hill.

Just before that happens, the other runners realize what is going on and begin to protect him. Now no one is able to stop him. At the end of the course, Dern actually breaks free and is in the lead. Just before crossing the finish line, though, he pulls back and joins hands with the other runners. They all cross the finish line together.

An athlete immediately associates with the heroism in this movie. But anyone can. And let's broaden the picture to understand that not everyone has to run a marathon to be a hero. There are life experiences that are the character-proving equivalent of crossing the finish line. In fact, there's a good chance you already have gone through at least one. Maybe it was a risky job change that you made, or a relationship breakup that you struggled to get through. Maybe it was an academic degree that you worked years to attain, an illness that you overcame, or a move that you made to a strange city. Whatever it was, if you've gone out and met the challenge you know that you don't have to fear that kind of challenge any more. You've proved that you have the inner strength to deal with it. So you may already be a hero without realizing it.

Realize it.

What Do You Do When You Are Dissatisfied with Your Life?

If you are like many people, you try to compensate for your dissatisfaction by distracting yourself from it. Instead of thinking through your situation and working toward change, you distract yourself through escapist endeavors. You may watch TV excessively or overeat. You may gamble or take drugs. You may get into bad relationships or become overly responsible for others. In short, you do something that takes you away from yourself. So you become too busy to ever think about being a hero. You seem to sneak though the days, just managing to get by, instead of really living your life. Time goes by and you take no journey, you learn no lesson, you leave no legacy.

How does that change? It changes when you learn to be yourself. Being yourself will make you a hero in your own life.

Is There Something You Would Love to Do but Fear Trying?

For example, have you ever thought about writing a book or about engaging in some other form of creative expression? What stops you from doing that?

You Think It Would Take Too Much Time

Perhaps you think that writing a book takes too much time. What gives you this impression? An average book contains approximately between 20,000 to 100,000 words. That's about twice or three times the words than many people say in a day. When you put it into that perspective, writing a book is really not such a big deal, is it?

Learn to put whatever you're afraid of trying into a new perspective.

You're Not Focused on Personal Goals

Perhaps you're not accustomed to working for yourself. I talked to a typist who believed she could never write a book, yet every day she typed a hundred pages for other people. Working at that rate for herself she could have typed a major manuscript in a week's time. Of course she would have had to write original material as well, but the point is that she was not in the habit of choosing where to focus her energy.

You Fear Not Being Accepted

None of us is accepted by everyone. In fact, many of us are intimately acquainted with the experience of nonacceptance.

For example, artists aren't accepted by many people in mainstream society. Neither are gay people, African Americans, or liberals.

Worrying about who is going to accept you is a waste of time. You are who you are; why be unsure about yourself? Why look for validation out there instead of attuning yourself to your own values? Why aspire to society's values instead of asserting your own?

The moment you give over your power in that way, you lose control of your life. Now I'm not advocating acting irresponsibly. And I'm not condoning people's flaunting themselves or becoming exaggerated exhibitionists. That's not balanced. I'm talking about not being fearful that what you are is insufficient. I'm talking about not needing someone else to validate you before you believe you're okay.

Remember, no two people will have the same thoughts and perceptions of you. And no one will ever know you the way you know yourself. You can give away your power of self-validation or you can claim it. Two powers cannot share the same space with equal intensity at the same time—this is a dynamic law of physics. So to the degree that you need someone else to accept you, you have given away your own life. Taking back the power is how you regain the strength to become a hero.

In short, you can only be a hero once you stop being concerned about what everyone else thinks. Heroes don't do things for other people's adulation or respect. Being a hero is a quiet, essentially solitary process.

You Fear Failure

A person who fears failing is often a person who was told, especially early in life, that they are a failure. When people are repeatedly told things like, "You can't do it right; let me do it for you," that transgresses their intellectual sanctity and eventually distorts their perception of themselves.

The moment someone disempowers you that way, you begin to feel stupid. Soon you begin to believe that you can't accomplish anything. It takes effort then to turn your self-image around.

What Opportunities Did You Let Go Because You Doubted You Could Handle Them?

Chances are that beliefs you have accepted as real have kept you from doing things. As a result, opportunities came and went. You may have had many opportunities, but if you didn't have confidence at that moment, they disappeared. Then you have regrets. You think, "What if?" The other part of you says, "But you didn't."

Heroes greet opportunities head-on, and embrace them. So make this mental note to yourself:

Think before you let the next opportunity slip by, because the day will come when you won't have any more. Of course one way to increase the number of opportunities that present themselves is to have a positive outlook. Positive people have far more opportunities because they make them every day. A positive person's mind is constantly open, and the nice thing about being open and free is that there's no limit to the opportunities you create for yourself. I've never met a creative, open, healthy person who didn't have far more ideas than what they could achieve in four lifetimes.

The person who falls back on the predictable "I can't" mindset loses out. Every opportunity goes right by that individual. The person may flirt with an opportunity, be tempted by it, or even sample it, but not embrace it. There's a big difference there.

Can You Embrace Challenge?

Think of a time when you've embraced challenge, even though you were scared to death of it. Has there been such a time? If so, you'll probably long remember every detail of it. You may even savor those memories too.

I think back to a day in Maine a couple of years ago. That was when a group of friends and I went whitewater rafting, which is one great trip, if you're up for some cold water and a few adrenaline surges. Several of my friends had never shot rapids before. As they got settled into the raft, their bodies were stiff, and you could tell they were terrified.

I asked them if they wanted to do this.

Yes, we want to do this! they said. Even though we're scared to death, we want to do this!

There were only about three minutes of preparation, during which we learned how to position our bodies in the boat, what to do if we got thrown out of it, and how to get back in. It was like Survival 101—The Crash Course—condensed.

On calm water, you can't imagine how rough it might get just around the bend. You simply can't. However, preparing your mind for the eventuality does help; in fact, it makes all the difference. So, while you're still in calm water, you review mentally what you will have to do when turbulence hits: Lean forward—lean into the boat, and paddle like hell. Keep a complete sense of focus and keep your body relaxed enough so that your own rigidity doesn't throw you against somebody else or throw you out of the boat. We *had* been paying attention during those three minutes.

The calm was short-lived; it took only one turn and turbid water hit. Waves and swells that seemed 10 feet high assaulted us. Then, almost before we knew what was happening, we went into a kind of combination water hole and wave, and our raft was—for want of a more accurate term—underwater.

Why had we done this? This was really dangerous! Through

the little spaces of air that were somehow still around us came the words, "Paddle like hell!"

Yes, we knew what to do! We were already doing it—leaning forward, into the boat, paddling like hell. We kept a complete sense of focus and kept our bodies relaxed enough so that our own rigidity didn't throw us against somebody else or out of the boat. Thus we came up above the wave and out of the water hole.

Everybody clapped and cheered! We all high-fived each other, because clearly, we had discovered an exciting new level of potential in ourselves. Some of my friends' lives were profoundly changed then, and—I find this truly amazing—it had taken only 5 or 6 seconds for that to happen.

What these friends now understood was that the category of what they could experience and achieve was much more vast than they'd assumed. They'd delved deeper into the possibilities of their lives by overcoming fears and going out to meet a new challenge. Now they knew that they'd never find themselves walking along the river's edge, wondering if they could survive the rapids. They'd already mastered them.

My friends talked about "that big wave" for days. "What about that big wave!" was practically the only thing they could say for a long time after the trip. It was as if they were fascinated by that wave. But they knew it wasn't that particular wall of water itself that was so enchanting—it was their own strength in coming through it. Maybe they could even go on to become the heroes in their own lives.

We Complete Many Obstacle Courses in Life

People are usually open about what they can't do, but they're less willing to acknowledge, especially to themselves, what they *can* do. For instance, most people develop all kinds of coping skills over the years, albeit often out of necessity. I believe that practically everyone who's made it as far as adulthood has done things in life that are far more difficult than negotiating some rapids or running a marathon. Have you lost a loved one? Lost a job? Been in a good relationship that went bad and felt the pain of getting out of it? As we mentioned earlier, these are the kinds of situations that mold and reveal heroes.

But unlike whitewater rafting adventures or marathons, these situations don't get resolved in a few hours. They take months or years to get through. It takes an enormous amount of courage to get past them, but once you grieve and let go, you become stronger for it.

Give yourself credit, then, for what you have gone through. Acknowledge as many positive traits about yourself as you can. That will remind you that you're not just starting this journey toward heroism today; you've been engaged in it for a long time.

How Do You Respond to Ineptitude?

What's your most common response to ineptitude? You probably judge it. You're most likely critical, and condemn yourself or others for it. But what would happen if, instead of condemning ineptitude, you intervened in a nonjudgmental way to try to help the inept person? This is particularly important when that person is yourself!

Think of yourself as a coach instead of an athlete. The first thing a coach has to do is to empathize with what the athlete is going through. Isn't it more constructive to work with a person by saying, "Let's see if we can figure out a better way of doing this together?" Then, you engage the person in problem-solving instead of making the person feel as if they're the problem. Again, if *you're* the one you're coaching, this is particularly important.

Learn to turn off the critical mind that tends to have knee-jerk reactions to anything it doesn't want to deal with. Give yourself and others the benefit of the doubt. Try taking a step back, disengaging the ego, and dealing with the situation honestly and openly in a constructive way. With that attitude you are sure to find solutions.

What Would You Change if Every Act Was a Measure of Your Character?

Actually, every act is. But what if every act of yours was made known? Would you act in the same way as usual, or would you change? Imagine a screen above your head allowing the public to see everything you did. Everything about you would suddenly be known.

Examining your life as if that was how you had to live it is one way to keep yourself on a positive emotional and spiritual path.

Here's an even better way: Forget about the public viewing that screen. Imagine *yourself* viewing and critiquing it.

How Do You Respond to Conflict?

I'll always remember the time I was walking down the street with an accomplished martial arts master when we noticed a "wolf pack" of young toughs approaching in our direction. My first instinct was to meet the attack head-on, an approach to physical threat that had worked for me in the past. But my companion insisted that we do a meditation instead. I knew he could have stopped all of the guys single-handedly if he wanted to; he had that much energy. So I wondered, why use meditation at such a time?

I followed his lead, though, and sure enough, this gang walked around us as if we didn't exist. Never in my life had I experienced anything like that. I knew it wasn't because of me, because I was in fear and ready to fight. I knew it had to do with my companion's simple technique, which involved sending out energy.

I came out of that experience with the understanding that you needn't go head-to-head with anyone. I had learned something about the ego, about how surrendering it can sometimes be the heroic thing to do. Of course, such training takes years and years before it can successfully be put into practice. But knowing the method exists makes it worth striving for.

Learning to approach conflict—or anything else—in a new way necessitates giving up old ways of thinking and being. You have to give something up before you can take in something new.

Are You a Warrior Hero?

Historically, we've associated military warriors with heroes. There are nonviolent warriors too, though. The nonviolent warrior is the person who is determined, who fights for something significant, and who represents the best in humanity. Think of people who champion causes and challenge evils, inadequacies, and injustices. Think of the Ralph Naders and Mother Teresas of the world, and of all the people working for similar causes.

Ideally, you should seek your warrior energy while you are still young, healthy, and growing. But some people evolve into warriors only after going through a lot of pain, as a result of being hurt, disempowered, or made ill. At some point, their hurt, pain, and victimization become anger.

That's all right, but you don't want to let anger turn into rage, causing you to lash out. You want to become strong and grow from your experience, and then use your anger constructively to tap into the warrior hero, the part of you that will go out there and take action.

Can You Be a Warrior Hero Over the Long Haul?

If you are looking to improve the quality of your life, one of your highest aspirations is to become one with life. To be at peace allows you the balance to commit yourself to issues without becoming absorbed by them. When a group called Nader's Raiders started, it consisted of 500 young lawyers and activists. Within three months their numbers dwindled to 20. Today only a handful are left.

Why do people lose their initial drive? It happens when they don't have a sense of peace and balance. These qualities are needed before you can commit yourself to a cause over a long span of time.

Expending energy without being at peace causes you to become burned out. You get involved in ego conflicts and become overwhelmed by the challenges you take on. When you see that everything is not going to become righted by your activism, you manifest the opposite extreme by becoming apathetic and giving up.

Do You Hesitate to Engage in Your Dreams?

Do you dream about something all the time but fail to engage in it? What do you have that's so important that you're afraid of losing it? Why do you hold on to old habits? How do they serve you?

If you investigate these questions you'll probably find that many habits give you the illusion of stability and comfort, but not true satisfaction. They keep you limited and bored, but you hold on to them because they make your life predictable. If you value the known you probably fear challenge and the uncertainty of taking risks.

The hero has no certainties. Where he's going, what will happen, how he'll feel—these are unknowns. But that's how life should be lived. Life is always most exciting when you're on the edge, when you have absolutely no certainty that the next step is not going to throw you into an abyss, into darkness, chaos, and crisis. That's when you pay the most attention.

What if, on a day-to-day basis, you could live in such a way? You would always be challenging yourself, always taking risks. You would constantly engage yourself in something instead of always seeking safety behind the conformity of rituals, patterns, and dogmas. Living on the edge would help you to see more clearly. You wouldn't be involved in fantasy.

Reality is always richer than fantasy. But the average American lives more with illusion than with reality. I say this in the sense that we're very image-conscious. The clothes we wear, the jobs and houses and cars we have, where we live, and even our friends, are often components of illusions we're trying to project to tell people who we are. We're normal, we're trying to tell people through these things. We're regular folks.

What if you didn't do that? What if the only way that you could tell people who you were was by the good deeds that you did, the challenges you took, and the risks you faced? It takes no courage to be normal. Normal is not where heroes live.

Do You Have to Win at Sports, or in Other Aspects of Your Life?

Knowing how to exercise discipline, whether you win or lose, allows you to feel like a winner. Actually, I myself don't think in winner or loser terms anymore. That's why I no longer enter marathons to race them; I enter simply to run. My joy comes from running with other people and helping them to get through. It's so enjoyable when you don't have to prove something by racing.

The same holds true for other activities in life. Can you imagine how different the world would be if people believed they didn't have to compete with one another, and cooperated instead? What a difference that would make. We wouldn't be exploited. We wouldn't have the haves and have-nots. We wouldn't have the gross disparities in wealth.

"In Hoc Signo Vinces"
(In This Sign Thou Shalt Conquer)

Throughout history, groups of people from all walks of life have recognized those among them who have taken a step in a different direction. Most individuals, however, hide their differences. They're afraid to stand out in a crowd and even to project differences in a relationship with one other person. They are afraid they will be scorned for their differences, and therefore choose to hide vital parts of themselves.

But by compromising yourself in order to be accepted, you're paying a really high price. You've got to hide your passions, dreams, inspirations, and ideals. Is it worth doing all this just to be accepted?

The hero and the warrior never compromise, nor do they care if they're accepted.

Ten minutes before going to sleep, think about how you can be more of who you are. Think of how different your life could be if you stopped worrying about being accepted. What would you change? What ideals would you live by? What would it feel like to be the hero in your own life?

The next morning, you can find out.

Issues of Interest to Women

And the Feminine Side of Men

*Put aside your fears and create change
just for the joy of it. You can take action
from a positive stance.*

Are You Fulfilled in Life?

Evaluate the important areas of your life to determine if your needs are being met. These areas may include:

- Career
- Children
- Play

Career

Your career needs may include satisfaction, recognition, contribution, creativity, self-esteem, money, freedom, accomplishment, growth, connections, bonding and joy. Write these needs down. Above all, a career must honor your real needs and honor you as a human being.

Children

Do you and your children communicate your needs to each other? Perhaps your teenage children need a space that's exclusively their own, where you enter only by invitation. And you, as a parent, may need the same. Explain the concepts of private time and communal time to your children so that everyone's needs are met.

Also, recognize that you must make the transition from parent to friend if you are to have a lifelong relationship with your children. When your child begins to establish mature friendships, it's important that you be included as one of those friends. The parents who are friends with their teenagers are the ones who remain friends for life.

Play

Let's not forget that the serious side of life needs to be balanced by the lighter moments. The ability to play adds tremendous quality to our lives. We always remember the fun we have had and rarely remember the work we have done. So why should we have such little fun?

Do You Feel Empowered?

List the areas of your life in which you feel you are powerful. Do you make use of that power? If so, in what way? Also, consider the areas of your life in which you do not feel powerful. If you express power at work but not at home, write that down. What does this mean to you? To understand these distinctions, delve into your past to review how your patterns of power developed. When and where did you start to feel disempowered? By re-tracing these events, you can restore your power in all areas of your life.

What Lessons Can Your Inner Little Girl Teach You Now?

When little girls reach the age of seven, eight or nine, they have a natural desire to explore the world. They want to do things just for the sake of doing them. They want to explore the world just because it is there. The little girl is no different from the little boy in this respect. All children possess a natural assertiveness and a desire for self-expression.

Every little girl is also a magician, what Robert Bly refers to as a "mythical trickster." This quality allows the girl to change. She weaves fantasies, illusions and spells into her life that allow her to be absolutely anything. Then, as she is taught to follow cultural prescriptions for being a "nice girl," she starts to shut down. In our culture's training of males, curiosity is a positive value. Boys and men are encouraged to investigate the world around them. Curious females are often called "nosy" and are encouraged to stay close to home. They are trained not to ask impolite questions about what lies behind appearances. They begin to ignore and shut down the natural intuitive abilities that lead them to question.

If you were not valued for yourself during your early years, you were doubly discouraged. Was your parents' attention contingent upon your being or acting a particular way? Perhaps you were noticed only when you were intelligent, or when you made your parents laugh, and otherwise you were ignored. If so, some aspects of your personality will have become unduly exaggerated while others will have been ignored. You must recover the rejected parts of yourself.

Specific family pressures may have caused you to become overly attuned to others and underattuned to your own instincts. For example, a parent who was unavailable due to absence, depression or alcoholism may have been unable to enjoy your company or support your endeavors, giving you the impression that you are unlovable and ineffective. Perhaps you were forced into an adult role such as surrogate mother for younger siblings, which further required you to ignore your own feelings and fantasies. Regardless of how difficult your life circumstances have been, you can begin at any time to reignite your pleasure in being alive.

Right now, no matter what your age or circumstances, you can rekindle the dreams of your girlhood and learn to honor your instinctive self. If you can ignore your conditioning, you will discover that your curiosity is still alive and that you have inner guidance and resources that will show you how to feel alive. When you allow your thinking to be energized by your instincts and your intuitions, you can do anything in the world you want. Dream your dreams and your inner guides will show you how to accomplish the impossible.

How can you do this? Start by letting yourself imagine what would give you joy in your life (in work, relationships and other important areas). If you draw a blank, recall the times when you felt most excited and happy as a child. What were you doing? What were you thinking of doing? What would you have liked to be doing? Bring those dreams back. The child inside you will guide your fantasies and allow you to feel playful and spontaneous. Other archetypal inner figures—your trickster, your heroine, your wild woman—will give you clues about how to carry them out. They will suggest new directions for you to explore and tell you how your life is out of balance.

To make contact with your guides, pay attention to your dreams and practice listening to your intuition. Ignore inner voices that are critical, controlling or competitive—the voices that discourage intuition. Be curious. Find the courage to be conscious of what you see and hear.

How Important Is Autonomy to You?

Women, for the most part, have been conditioned to derive their identity from their relationships. While relationships are important, true inner identity must be maintained as well. You must nurture yourself before you can become part of a healthy relationship. Life is an inner journey that each of us must take alone. Establish boundaries for yourself that allow you to collect your thoughts and identify who you are.

In your journal, record your thoughts on the importance of having time and space to yourself. In what areas of your life are you fiercely autonomous? In what areas do you need to develop more autonomy?

What Are You Doing That Is Vital and Energizing?

Vitality is not something we occasionally need in our lives. Every single day should be life-affirming. List the aspects of your daily life that are vital.

What in Your Life Represents Gender Compliance?

You must begin to recognize patterns that affect your well-being. Examine each area of your life to determine if you are compliant because you are a woman, or if you are able to participate as an equal. Do you do things just because they are "required" of you in your role as a woman? Are you in a pattern of continual compliance merely because of your sex?

Avoid taking compliant, role-model positions in life that conflict with your inner feelings. When you do something, let it be because you get joy from it, not because it is a form of gender compliance. Does your husband expect you to perform household chores after work because it is your role? That doesn't make sense, and it may prevent you from actualizing who you really are.

Do You Trust Your Own Values, Perceptions and Needs?

Many people find it difficult to follow their personal calling because they feel pressured to fulfill the expectations of others. Should you venture off in a new direction and fail, you will be reminded over and over again of your failure. You may even be told that you are selfish because you disappointed others who depend on you.

Consider this example: A friend of mine gave up a secure job as an accountant after 22 years to start his own business, even though he wasn't sure that he would succeed. His family was terribly angry because his decision threatened their sense of security. They tried to undermine him and eventually succeeded. Within a year, their lack of confidence in him and his own uncertainty got him into serious trouble. He made some bad business decisions and finally had to sell his home. His family blamed him for being a failure.

I talked with his children one day. I asked them if their father had ever acted like a hero and they said no. I then asked them to define what a hero was. They said that a hero was a person who took risks. "Didn't your father take a risk?" I asked. They agreed that he had. "Isn't he a hero then?" I asked. They told me they had never thought of it in that way before. I reminded them that their father was willing to take a chance and start over again at the age of 50. I also pointed out that their father's experience gave them the chance to start over again and to learn that less is more. It gave them a chance to spend more time together as a family. Before, their father had always worked at night to earn extra money for the mortgage.

The children began to appreciate this concept. What changed was not the reality of their situation. They still didn't have any money. But their perception of not having money changed. No longer did they view themselves as failures.

Look at the times in your life when you took a chance. Acknowledge yourself for taking these risks and note the positive lessons that came from these experiences.

What Truths Have You Yet to Explore or Actualize?

You have truths in you that need to be explored and expressed. What are they? These feelings come from your heart, and you need to write them down. The key to your diary is not to think about what you plan to write, but just to begin writing. Don't let the conditioned part of yourself edit your original thoughts. Doubts will creep in and deter you from the truth you need to express. You may know inside that you want to change careers, for example, but your conditioned responses may tell you that you don't have the education or that you have too many responsibilities to meet and bills to pay.

Put your immediate thoughts down on paper. Look at them, feel them, let them ferment. That's how change starts. It's a difficult process, but you must allow yourself to face harsh truths about your life—what you have given up, the inadequacies of your relationships, the feelings of personal or spiritual emptiness. Perhaps you would rather not let yourself know about these things, but you will feel much stronger and more powerful when you become truthful with yourself and those around you.

Your hidden personal truth includes positive things about yourself, such as talents you've never acknowledged. Perhaps you have a good singing voice that you've been too self-conscious to develop.

What Goals Have You Achieved, and How Have They Affected You?

Don't look for change to happen all at once. Life is lived in small measures. Every day, small things come together that work. If you think you haven't achieved much in life, you may not be acknowledging all the little things you have done that add up to major accomplishments. Remember that small goals are the essence of life; they validate us.

Write down the small goals you have accomplished. How did you feel when you achieved them? What did they mean to you? If one of your goals was to exercise every day and you went out and did it, that's a goal accomplished. How do you feel? What patterns changed because you accomplished your goal? You may realize that after four months of daily exercise, you began to reprioritize your schedule and make more time for yourself. Perhaps you never realized how much time you were giving to others until you began to satisfy your need to exercise. Allotting time to yourself for exercising may make you feel better emotionally, physically and spiritually. Your confidence may improve, allowing you to gain control in other ways. So you see, one pattern leads to another pattern, which leads to the process of change.

What Goals Have You Set but Not Yet Reached?

Consider why you have failed to reach certain goals. In some cases, the reason may be that other people who want to maintain the status quo deter you from your goals. Maybe you become sidetracked by feelings of guilt. One woman came to my running club for two months, for example, and then stopped suddenly. It seemed that her family resented her absence, even though she was only gone three hours a week. They wanted her to be there exclusively for them, and they certainly didn't want her to take charge of any part of her life. They felt threatened by their loss of control over her every moment, even though she was losing weight, feeling good, having new insights and making positive changes. This woman felt tremendous guilt. If she allowed herself to change any further, she feared she might not know how to control her life and things might never be the same.

Well, of course things will never be the same. Yesterday is not like today, and you can't control tomorrow. But look at the reasons why you haven't fulfilled some of your goals. Don't be afraid to negotiate new arrangements when your needs count.

Female social conditioning, early family circumstances and genetic inheritance can make women extremely sensitive to other people's feelings. While your sensitivity can be a positive quality in some circumstances, it can also rule your life in a very negative way if you let it. To be fully alive, you must remain open to change. Women often feel that it is their job to maintain stability at home by never making changes or doing anything that would upset their families. That attitude doesn't help anyone. What you need to do is to remain emotionally connected and attached to your children while allowing change to happen. They will learn flexibility and joy in their own lives by watching you. It is your choice to emphasize your feelings of guilt or to tolerate the guilt you feel in the name of growth for yourself and, ultimately, for those close to you.

What Goals Have You Done Nothing About?

List the goals that you have not yet begun to pursue. What seems to be causing the delay? Acknowledging that you have these goals will begin the process of change. It also helps you to understand why you have avoided these goals until now.

Don't berate yourself for having trouble getting started, but stick with the effort. In particular, don't be frightened off by feelings such as depression that may turn up when you start to let go of old patterns. You are mourning the loss of your old self, but you know that the change must take place.

Are Your Needs Realistic, or Are They Dictated by Society?

Do you really desire the things that others expect you to pursue? If your needs stem from a traditional upbringing, rather than your real self, they will prove to be burdensome and unfulfilling. For example, you may think you need to own a home and all the trappings, including a mortgage, because your parents have instilled this desire in you. In reality, however, the economics of owning a home have changed in recent years. There are no guarantees that you will be able to make your mortgage payments in the present economy. Therefore, you must ask yourself if owning a home is a realistic need.

Evaluate all of your needs to determine whether they are realistic.

Are Your Needs Reasonable or Are They Conditional?

Define your real needs. Consider whether they are being compromised. If you earn an attractive salary but your work conditions are hazardous, your basic need for safety is not being met. In this society, we have been conditioned to believe that if the money is sufficient, then issues such as job safety and satisfaction don't count. Don't be afraid to assert your needs, and don't accept conditions that compromise them.

Are You Looking for Fulfillment from Your Relationships?

Do you look for partners who can make you feel more complete? Do you expect others to make you feel good about who you are? If so, you may be in a pattern of codependency. It's one thing to appreciate and be attracted to a person whose life "works." It's another to be drawn to such a person because your life does not work and you hope to fix it through your association with this person. That's the wrong reason to be drawn into a relationship.

In healthy relationships in which the partners share their energy, one accepts the other unconditionally. He does not try to change you, control you or manipulate you. When such conditions start to surface, it's time to say good-bye.

Evaluate your relationships honestly. In each instance, consider whether you have an unhealthy need to be with the other person. Are you there because of codependency, or are you there because you have something to share?

Is Your Time Spent Meeting Your Own or Other People's Needs?

Make a list of all the needs you meet on a given day. Determine which needs are your own and which are other people's. Beyond that, which needs are necessary and which are not? Use this list to identify any imbalances in your life. An honest evaluation will show you where your life isn't working and reveal which needs are most pertinent to your life.

Without this list, you may never know where you spend your time. Talking on the telephone and watching television, for example, may drain time and energy that would be better spent on yourself. Get right down to the nitty gritty; look at everything you do every day for yourself and others.

Are You a Caretaker?
How Does This Role Affect You?

Many people believe that others can't survive without them, and they spend an inordinate amount of time in a caretaking role. How much time do you devote to taking care of other people? With whom do you play this role, and under what conditions? If you spend too much time and energy taking care of others, it may be wise to reconsider your relationship with these people.

Do You Try to Manipulate the Feelings or Attitudes of Others?

Think of the ways you are dishonest and manipulative in your dealings with others. Do you perceive situations and relationships as they truly are, or, rather, the way you want to see them? If something's not right in your life, say so. Then determine how you will fix it. You must accept that some aspect of your life does not work before you can change it. If you deny that the situation exists, it will only get worse. It's manipulative to be dishonest about your attitudes and feelings and how they affect others. If I have a friend who is very sick, I'm going to tell him he's very sick. But I will also tell him I'm there for him if he wants my help.

Do You Alter Your Communications to Please Others?

In certain relationships, you may modify what you say to gain acceptance. Your words and feelings are at odds because you are withholding your true opinions. This makes you uncomfortable with yourself. Take note of the things you say that conflict with your true feelings. Ask yourself, am I communicating in this way to gain this person's approval? What is the worst that could happen if I expressed myself honestly and this person did not accept me? In the end, you do not want to be in relationship with someone who cannot accept a difference of opinion.

How Often Are You Overcome with Fear, Anxiety, Depression, or Guilt?

All of these emotions merely cover up our insecurities. They result from a lack of full empowerment in our lives. There was a time in America when most people took responsibility for their own lives. There was very little litigation because people generally didn't accuse others when their lives did not work.

In recent times, however, it has become fashionable to blame others for our own shortcomings—anything not to blame ourselves.

Examine all areas of your life to determine where you are blaming others for your failures. Stop the accusations and start looking to yourself for the answers. That's the only way you will find a solution to your problems. When you blame others, you give away your power to them. As a result, you never resolve the issues at hand and go forward with your life.

Are You Still Denying Your Real Needs?

Think about what you really want from yourself and your friendships. Are your expectations of yourself too low? Make a list of them. You will feel dissatisfied if you haven't allowed yourself to grow and reach your full potential. This could be the case if your sole intent in getting an education, for example, was to land a job that would provide you with material possessions and security. You may have pushed yourself in some areas of growth but overlooked others. You may be denying the virtue and benefit of things that can enhance life.

Do You Take Risks?
How Does It Feel When You Do?

What types of risks do you take in life? Are you willing to take risks that will make you feel uncomfortable? Write them down. Until you stretch past your comfort zone, you will not accelerate your growth. Many runners, for example, settle into a comfortable running pace even though they are capable of much more. I teach racers that they must push past this barrier if they are to excel.

Do You Play It Safe?

At work, do you let your boss hear only what he or she wants to hear? Do you under-actualize your potential so that no one feels threatened by your intelligence? Are you intimidated by authority or worried about acceptance from your peers? Make a list of the ways in which you play it safe. Think about how you feel in those situations. It is especially important that you examine any long-held beliefs that are making your life so safe and secure that you do not develop to the next level. Don't be overprotective of yourself.

How Do You Control Your Emotions?

You may restrain your emotions in a variety of ways. List them. For example, you may overeat, overexercise, drink, take drugs, sleep too much or get sick frequently. You also may deny your own emotions, or you may take responsibility for everyone else's so that you have no time for your own.

Do You Recognize the Cause-and-Effect Relationship in Your Actions?

When communicating with others, beware of the tendency to say things just to stimulate a certain reaction. If you argue with someone, recognize that what you say will cause the other person to react. Do you see how his or her reaction might have been different had you acted differently? In the same way, do you provoke your partner in order to stir things up?

You must learn to control your emotions before you speak and express yourself in a non-blaming way. Learn self-control by asking yourself what the likely results of your words or actions will be. Begin to anticipate what could happen, positively or negatively. If you can speak reasonably and rationally, that's great. But that is often difficult when you are upset.

On the other hand, don't avoid talking to another person because you can't be entirely logical and clear about your emotions. People often rationalize a decision not to communicate by telling themselves that their reactions are not reasonable. So what? Just avoid blaming others and be clear about what bothers you. The other person will give you another perspective. If you are being irrational, then you can get back to what it is in your life that made you so sensitive to begin with. Unreasonable reactions are clues to areas you need to work on.

Do Your Motivations Derive from Fear?

Reacting from fear is a dangerous way to live. When you make changes in your life, your motivation should be something other than fear. You can create change just for the joy of it. You can take action from a positive, not a negative, stance. Change is inevitable. It's our attitude toward it that makes all the difference. Once we accept that life is a process of change, we can be more positive about the events around us.

Make a list of the things you do, or don't do, which are motivated by fear. What would you like to change in your life? What is stopping you? Which changes do you accept and which do you not accept? Why do you resist change?

Are Your Expectations of Others Realistic?

When someone enters your life, ask yourself these simple questions: Why is this person here? What can we share? You must accept people for who they are, not for what you expect to come of the relationship. Identify what you really want from a relationship and see if the other person can fulfill those needs. By the same token, can you fulfill theirs? Is there a mutual basis for growth? Explain who you are, what you want and what you can give. Be honest about your real needs from the start and listen carefully to theirs. Don't waste your energy on counterproductive relationships.

How Do You Handle Daily Stress?

When you feel stressed and irritable, examine the events of the day to identify any unresolved issues. At what moment did your irritability start? Never dismiss any thought or feeling as irrational. It may be—but it may also have some personal significance to you. Look at any ongoing factors or attitudes that contribute to your stress. Sometimes you need to resolve psychological problems before the physical manifestations go away and your balance is restored.

The connection between mental and physical pain can express itself in many ways. If your back feels tight and sore, for example, you may sit down to work but feel overburdened by your responsibilities. You may appear calm on the outside but feel quite anxious on the inside. Your job is more than you can handle and you begin to feel incompetent. Your body processes these feelings as stress.

Are You Bored with Life?

When we are young, life seems to be full of new and exciting experiences. But as we age, we tend to establish well-worn patterns in our daily lives. Life becomes comfortable and routine. You eat the same breakfast cereal every day, watch the same television programs, and even get out of bed on the same side each morning. When life becomes too mundane, boredom sets in.

As an adult, you must fight this boredom and stretch beyond your comfort zone. Otherwise, you will never grow. Think of the things you do consistently that have come to bore you. What can you do to break those patterns?

Where Are You Growing?
Where Do You Need to Grow?

Make a chart with two columns. On one side, list the areas in your life where you need to grow. On the other, list the areas where you have grown. For example, if you would like to read more often or start an exercise program, write down these goals in the "need to grow" column.

Put the chart in a prominent place to remind yourself of these goals. Note any progress you make on the chart each day. By writing down your intentions and reading them to yourself daily, you will send a clear message to your subconscious that you are ready and willing to change. These simple lists can help keep you alive and vital.

Were You Ever Victimized?
How Did This Affect You?

Make a list of the ways in which you have been victimized. Are these incidents controlling your life today? If so, you must learn to forgive and let go of the past. It's time to move on with your life. Don't be a perpetual victim.

Were You Given Negative Messages as a Child?

As a child, you probably believed whatever your parents told you because they were authority figures. Their messages, positive or negative, were accepted at face value. The question is, how have you dealt with the negative messages they conveyed to you? To sort through this issue, make a list of your parents' attitudes, noting whether they are positive or negative. Then go back and note which attitudes you have adopted as your own, both toward yourself and regarding your expectations about the world.

Until you evaluate these messages and discard the negatives ones, they will remain a guiding force in your life. You now have an adult mind and adult ego strength. You have the ability to tolerate pain that you could not understand or handle as a child. You also have the opportunity to make important changes in yourself, provided you can find the courage to ask the hard questions about your past and present. When you stop blocking your awareness of your past hurts and current fears, you will gradually become energized. Your pain and fear will be less each time you make contact with them.

Are Your Choices Driven by Fear or Confidence?

Most people's lives are driven by fear. They avoid many of the things they want to say and do—such as confront their boss, their mate, their friends and perhaps their children—for fear of the consequences. They don't want to lose their job or to feel alone and unloved.

You must put aside your fears and build your confidence instead. Then you will be able to assert yourself in any situation. However, be careful not to confuse arrogance with confidence. Arrogant people act out of a need to feel superior. They, too, are motivated by fear and insecurity. When you are truly confident, you will feel good about your actions.

Do You Respect Boundaries?

In a relationship, do you communicate your boundaries to the other person and, in turn, respect his or hers? In an honest, healthy relationship a mutual respect of boundaries must exist. When these boundaries are overstepped, the process will distract from your time, joy and ability to utilize your love of life. Establish boundaries that feel comfortable and healthy to you.

Are You Trusting?

Do you accept a person's word until he or she proves otherwise, or do you immediately label certain types of people as untrustworthy? If you have had a bad experience with several men, for example, do you conclude that all men are untrustworthy? Or can you judge each one on his own merits? Examine your prejudices and work to eliminate them.

What Are Your Addictions?

Addictive behaviors mask reality. They allow you to disguise the areas of your life that are not working. List your addictions and their possible causes. You must identify the unfulfilled areas of your life that you have replaced with addictive behaviors and confront each one. Any behavior that you perform compulsively can be likened to an addiction in the sense that you use it to avoid feelings and maintain the illusion of control.

You may eat, drink, work, fantasize or seek relationships in an addictive fashion.

Do You Avoid Responsibility for Fear of Failure?

Our society measures success by what we have accomplished. We are deemed to be failures if we attempt something new and fail. This concept is reinforced when others praise us for our successes and reprimand us for our failures. We do not receive credit for having tried; rather, we are considered to be inadequate because we did not succeed.

A fear of failure prevents many people from taking on new responsibilities that would allow them to grow. In reality, however, most successes are preceded by many failures. Go back in your life and assess your own failures. What did you learn from these experiences? Acknowledge yourself for having tried and for the lessons learned.

Are You Looking to the Right People for Support?

You must share your dreams and goals with people who offer positive support. Some people will always find a hole in your plans, yet you may return to these unsupportive people time and again for support. Since their advice will only discourage you, be more aware of who you turn to for help. Watch your patterns and learn to interact with people who will be the most supportive and understanding of your needs and goals.

Are You a Motivator or an Instigator?

As an adult, you should be able to express yourself to friends without imposing your beliefs on them. Consider your communications: Do you say things that will enhance their lives? Are you insensitive to their feelings? If you respect other people's uniqueness, you will be sensitive in your approach to relating. Remember that what's important to you may not be important to them. Ask yourself, "Am I imposing my beliefs on this person? How would it feel to be on the receiving end of what I am sharing now?" If it doesn't feel right, then don't share it, at least not in that manner.

Are You On the Road to Burnout?

A variety of negative behavior patterns can lead to burnout, including compulsions, addictions, codependency, overintensity and a tendency to go beyond your limits. The baby-boomer generation is an example. Their compulsive need to become highly educated and make money has caused them to burn out at an alarming rate.

You can prevent burnout by taking time to relax and have fun. The child within—an integral part of your nature—will guide you in this area. Don't be concerned that others may perceive you to be childlike. Expressing this part of yourself will keep you sane and prevent you from burning out.

Does Self-Doubt Interfere with Your Life?

Many people undervalue themselves. They don't attach any value to their courage, intellect, creativity and other strengths. This mistaken perception can lead to self-doubt, as can poor reinforcement during your formative years. As a child, you may have been told that who and what you were was not good enough. But as an adult, you can recognize that you are more capable and lovable then you were led to believe. You can then replace self-doubt with self-confidence.

Do You Try to Force a Relationship?

People who have not been valued for themselves often try to force a bond with others. In many cases, they control their relationships by using whatever approach worked in their families of origin. They may act weak and helpless so that others feel responsible for them. They may use complaints and intimidation to gain control. Either way, they may believe they are strengthening the relationship when, in fact, they are undermining it. True bonds cannot be forced. They result when two people share and grow together.

Do You Have Hidden Agendas?

When forming a relationship, be sure to explore and identify your motivations for doing so. It's best to communicate these motivations from the start, because they will eventually surface anyway and undermine the relationship. For example, you may discover that one hidden agenda in a relationship is financial security. If both partners do not know this, the relationship is bound to fail.

Does Your Life Mimic Your Experiences or Reflect the Real You?

Along with negative cultural forces, early conditioning is the most common source of people's current life difficulties. Negative experiences will limit your life if you allow them to do so. You must become conscious of what has happened to you; otherwise, your life energy will be drawn to the same conditioned patterns until they are resolved. This repetition can make you feel limited, mistrusting, cynical or insecure. And it can keep you from reaching your full potential.

Consider this example: As a child, you became an extremely organized caretaker of others. Now, as a grown woman, you have no sense of your own needs because you are constantly trying to anticipate the needs of others and make things right for everyone around you. You have become overly active, controlling and detail-oriented—all attitudes that cut you off from your intuition. To grow and reconnect to your feminine side, you must look at the past experiences that have limited you.

Do You React from Reality or Conditioning?

Like most people, you probably express yourself based on past experiences, rather than by reasoning through each situation in which you find yourself. If you assume that a person who is shabbily dressed must be poor and uneducated, for example, your reaction is based upon conditioned beliefs.

In the same way, you may allow feelings from previous situations to influence the present. Suppose that you lose a job and then take it out on your family. You are reacting from pent-up emotions, not from the reality of the moment. And your children, of course, will not understand your behavior.

They may believe you are angry with them because they are bad. This can cause them to be confused in their relationships later on.

You need to examine your feelings and resolve them as they occur. Ask yourself if your emotions are related to the moment or if you are processing something from the past.

What Energizes You?

Most people live passively. They expect the world and worldly things to entertain and excite them. Eventually, they lose touch with spontaneous emotion and rely on recycled energy from outside sources. They turn on the television set and watch the same unfunny shows, reacting along with the canned laughter. And they require extreme intensity to feel anything. Hence, suspense movies have been replaced with grotesque horror films.

Society, for the most part, has lost its desire to self-energize. To foster the process of growth, you must be excited by your own potential and the many things you can do. You need to start each day with the influence of your inner self, not the outer world. You might decide to read more, engage in a hobby or learn a new skill. Or you might decide to spend the morning exercising instead of watching television passively.

Take control of your life. Do something constructive and you will become perpetually energized. When you get in tune with your inner self, you become more vital because you are engaging in uplifting activities that have personal meaning to you.

Do You Feel Hopeful or Hopeless About Important Issues in Your Life?

Make a list of the things you feel either hopeless or hopeful about. In your "hopeless" column, note the areas that make you feel consistently hopeless. You can never stick to a diet, for example, or you can't seem to stop smoking. These items can serve as a guide, revealing where you need to go deeper to understand why you have created these patterns. Consider what happened in your life to make you feel this way.

Evaluate your "hopeful" column in the same manner. No doubt you succeed at certain things and feel hopeful about them because you devote the necessary energy to them. If you devote the same type of energy to the items in your "hopeless" column, you can begin to turn them around.

Do You Let Your Emotions Flow Freely, or Do You Keep Up a Front?

Don't let problems accumulate and gnaw away at you from the inside. Resolve them as they occur. If something is bothering you, no one benefits if you smile on the outside and feel angry on the inside. Keeping up a false front has a negative influence on the expression of your true feelings. Let people know how you feel.

Do You Mimic the Example Set by Your Parents?

Are you your own person? Like many adults, you will reflect your parental examples by doing exactly as they did or by doing the exact opposite. Make a list of your personality traits and compare them to those of your parents. Then, think about whether your characteristics reflect your true self. For example, your mother may have been totally submissive to your father. As a reaction, you may have become the mirror image of her or the exact opposite, whereas your true nature is actually somewhere in between. Check each trait and think of ways to modify the extremes.

How Do the Roles You Play Affect Your Life?

List the roles you play in life, such as mother, daughter, sister, wife, lover and businesswoman.

Notice how your behavior may change depending on the role. For example, you may be a single parent who fills the roles of mother, father and friend to your children. At work you assume a subordinate role, and with your friends and acquaintances, you are dominant with some and passive with others. It's important to see how these roles interchange, and affect your feelings and behaviors.

How Do You Handle Your Thoughts and Feelings When They Go Against the Social Norm?

You must learn to live by your true feelings. If you suppress your beliefs for fear of scorn and ridicule, you will not contribute to the process of social change. Many people feel compassion toward cruelty and injustice, for example, but a part of them is afraid to rock the boat. They remain silent because they do not want to threaten their economic or social position or their political survival. When this silence occurs in the majority, important issues may never reach the forefront.

Indeed, change is generally brought about by a small group of people who are willing to speak out while the majority stands by. The lesson: If we do not use our power, somebody else will use theirs. And in the end, we lose control of our own lives.

How Do You React to Rejection?

Most people deny that rejection affects them. They pretend that it doesn't matter, adopting a "who wants to belong to their club anyhow" attitude. The truth is, nobody likes to be rejected. Rejection is a form of alienation that makes you feel you do not count. When you begin to feel isolated in this way, get in touch with your feelings and address the issue there and then. Reinforce the fact that you do count.

What Happens to Your Unresolved Feelings?

Unless you face your feelings and conflicts, a part of your energy will be consumed by the process of resolving them. And this, in turn, prevents you from living fully in the present. You also expend a huge amount of energy when you avoid situations that make you feel vulnerable. As a result, you feel listless and underenergized. Remember that your future is your past. You need to shift your focus from problems to solutions, using your ingenuity, creativity, and originality.

What Are the Socially Accepted Behaviors for Women?

Society tends to cast women as powerless, helpless and dependent. And we often behave in the way people expect us to behave, forgetting that we have a choice. The media and movies portray women as victims or helpless people who need a strong man to hold things together, for example. But does that mean you have to follow these narrowly defined roles? Think about the behaviors you exhibit that do not reflect the real you. These are the ones you need to eliminate from your life.

Do You Overlook Your Needs and Cater to Others?

Virtually everything we do is tempered by other people's feelings. When we do what others expect of us, we get good feelings and acceptance in return. The problem is, the actions that please others may not fulfill your inner needs. You must create space in your life for the things that make you feel like a whole person. While other people, such as your husband, may object to your pursuit of personal goals, ultimately both of you will benefit from a truer and more open relationship.

It takes courage to actualize your needs. Identify the essential parts of yourself and the real needs that were ignored, denied or misunderstood when you were growing up. Recognize them now and begin to deal with them. You must discover who you are and what you want to do. Then you must take action. Taking the views of others into consideration is fine; allowing them to intimidate or control you is not.

Do You Strive for Love and Acceptance
or Success?

Materialism does not necessarily have to negate love, but in our society it generally does. That's because so many people have sacrificed attention to self and others to achieve their goals. If you have sacrificed love for material success, think about what you can do to restore some balance in your life.

How Do You Define Love?

Love is the manifestation of life. It radiates joy, comfort, kindness and patience. You're drawn to its energy. You know when love is being shared—and when it isn't—by listening to your heart. If someone falsely claims to love you, or tries to prove his love with material possessions, you know it's not real because you do not feel it. You may have lost your ability to love if you are impatient with yourself and others. You will become busy outwardly to compensate for the coldness and lack of love you feel inside.

True love is given freely, with no expectations attached. If you are filled with love, you give it automatically. If you require a response, you are motivated by the need for acceptance or another ulterior motive. Why do you think Mother Teresa does more to help disadvantaged people than all the hospitals and welfare centers put together? It's because she accepts people for who they are and passes no judgment. No matter that they are petty thieves, muggers, itinerant farmers or lepers. She doesn't say, "I can't love you because of your faults." She just loves.

Every human being is capable of being loving. But you will not know how to open the love inside you until someone has given love to you. Think of something or someone you love.

Do you give that love unconditionally or do you expect something in return? Who are you really giving for? Be honest about your motives. It's important to understand why you do something. You need to feel good about what you do and recognize that love emanates from within.

Is Your Need for Love Fulfilled?

You've probably been conditioned to believe that you are undesirable until someone loves you. Parental and societal norms tell us that we will gain love by getting married, having a family and carrying on the traditions. This conditioning has caused most single people in our society to feel miserable. By these rules, love cannot exist outside a narrowly defined relationship. But what about a relationship with life, work and yourself? What about a relationship between friends? Most people overlook these valid expressions of love.

What Is the Difference Between Having Something with Love or Without Love?

Anything built from love is empowering because it derives from what is real. Conversely, anything created without love is disempowering and based on an illusion. Ultimately, it will collapse because illusions are held together by force. You may use illusions to force a relationship or fall prey to illusions in which others force their will on you.

In many cult movements, for example, the leaders will tell you that they alone love you. They may brainwash you to believe that your family should be feared instead of loved. Then when a family member calls, your heart pounds and you begin to sweat. Such incidents serve to reinforce the cult's power over you. But in time the illusion will dissipate and you will be back to nothing.

Love, on the other hand, empowers and strengthens us. If you love yourself and love life, diseases do not have the space to manifest. Make a list of the things you really love and those you are involved in that do not feel right to you. Do the same thing for the people in your life. With whom do you associate out of a genuine respect for that person? With whom do you feel uncomfortable? Do these people and situations give to you or take from you? Are they concerned for your well-being or for theirs alone?

Are You Seeking Love in the Wrong Way?

If the love you received as a child was conditional—based on your ability to please your parents—then as an adult you will seek love and acceptance through the same actions that gained you recognition in your early years. Perhaps you are an over-zealous worker who stays late night after night, trying to please the boss and gain his recognition. In essence, you are reverting to the action-for-praise syndrome instilled by your parents. This tendency affects your well-being by restricting growth and reinforcing the feeling that you are not acting from your own center. Be careful what you do to gain love and acceptance. Evaluate the things you do out of a need to be loved and those you do out of joy. Do the same for the people in your life. Do you feel loved and accepted for who you are or for what you do?

What Are Your Most Blissful Moments?

Each of us has a different concept of bliss. Depending on the person, bliss may be walking in the woods, watching a sunset, or listening to rain on a roof. It's a feeling of perfect harmony that comes over us when we are in tune with nature. We do not feel threatened or imbalanced. List these moments and describe the role love played in them.

How Do You Deny Love?

What are the ways that you avoid love? Perhaps you make love trivial, escape from it, fail to communicate it or find fault with people so as not to accept their love. Look for the subtle avoidance mechanisms, such as overeating, displacing anger, or communicating dishonestly. Indeed, the most effective way to avoid love is to become involved in false and deceptive sharing.

What Do You Daydream and Fantasize About?

Make a list of your recurring fantasies, including those that do not appear to fit into your life. These daydreams reflect your inner needs and should become an integral part of your life. If you're excited by the idea of a trip to New Mexico to study Native American crafts, don't dismiss it simply because you don't have the money or it seems impractical. By doing so, you deny expression to an important part of yourself, the creative child.

The daydreams that occupy your mind need to be explored. They are essential parts of your nature. Keep notes about your fantasies and daydreams. Evaluate each one as a need in your life. They can be a new beginning.

Are You Filled with Love or Despair?

Love energizes us, while despair drains our energy. We must focus on love, not the negative force of despair, if we are to keep ourselves physically, mentally and emotionally charged. Both forces are potentially present at any given time. But we have choices about which emotion we will emphasize.

Are You Afraid to Express Love?

Many people do not express love for fear of being rejected, misunderstood or taken advantage of. They may pretend to be independent and aloof. They may act as if they don't need anyone to feel complete when, in fact, they are craving love. Or they may suffer quietly. You never know how these people truly feel because they act as if everything is okay. They have never been allowed to express their feelings.

List some of the ways in which you disguise your feelings, especially your need for love. Work to resolve these.

Can You Give and Receive Love if You Are Invulnerable?

You must be vulnerable to experience love. Like most people, however, you may try to be invulnerable because you expect the worst from people and fear getting hurt. As you age, you lose the ability to love others and feel their love in turn. Perhaps you can't even feel love toward your children. You're too busy to spend time with them, but they don't understand why. In the process, you hurt them, hurt your relationship and perpetuate the pattern by teaching them to become invulnerable. They, too, may one day be incapable of experiencing love.

Look at your patterns of behavior toward others. Then look at the patterns in the people around you. You may see in others what you cannot see in yourself.

What Limits Your Desire to Love?

Your ability and desire to love may be limited by anger, fear, envy, resentment or hostility. The more of these emotions you feel—and the more intense the conditioning from which they derive—the more frustrated you will feel in your ability to love. This conditioning must be addressed and changed. Write yourself a new contract on life. Examine the conditioning that causes you to believe and react in certain ways. Write down what you need and want from life, and then go after it. Work on replacing conditioned beliefs with the things you truly want.

Do You Suffer from Love Addiction?

Do you depend on someone else to make you feel good about yourself? Must others accept you before you can love yourself? If so, you may suffer from the love addiction that occurs in dysfunctional families and relationships. If you only feel good when someone gives you emotional strokes, you had better start concentrating on what's missing in your life. Think about the type of people to whom you are drawn. Note their positive qualities and develop these in yourself. By the same token, think about the negative attitudes that tend to attract you. See if you possess these attitudes toward yourself.

How Do Social Norms and Religious Morals Affect Your Ability to Share Love?

Organized religion has done more to suppress our natural desires and diminish true love than any other force in history. Religion has tremendous power to suppress love when it is separatist and laced with conditions and rules. Some religions tell us that we are not supposed to love people of other races, colors or religions. We learn to mistrust others and react negatively to them. They become the enemy.

On the positive side, religion can help you to understand your spiritual nature and the ethics and morals that should be common to all people. That makes religion a paradox; it may help you or suppress you, encourage you or deny you. Give some thought to your religion: What about it helps you to share love, and what causes you to suppress it?

Do You Blame Others for Not Being There for You?

Most children cannot express the anger they feel toward their parents for hurting or abandoning them. This is especially true of young children, who do not have the intellectual or physical capabilities to fend for themselves. Rather than speak up, they repress their feelings deep in their psyche. But these hurts will surface in distorted ways later in life. Often they are acted out in relationships, when you react to your partner as if he were a parent. You will blame others for the hurt caused by your parents, and others will blame you in the same way.

To have healthier, more constructive relationships, you need to address these issues as they arise. Learn to distinguish between the criticisms directed at you and those projected onto you. If you or your partner act as a substitute parent, then you must question whether the relationship is truly healthy.

Do You Allow Passion to Enter Your Communications and Experience?

You must be passionate about your life and dynamic in expressing your feelings. Passion gives you the momentum to go forward day after day, despite all the obstacles you encounter and the naysayers who want to limit your enjoyment and achievements. To actualize your passion—be it poetry, painting, dancing or medicine—you must be self-motivated.

Parents often encourage children to manifest an energy level that matches their own. They may express these restrictions openly with statements such as, "Calm down. There's nothing to get so excited about," or "Put on a happy face. You should be happy." Perhaps they are more subtle and simply do not respond when you express energies that are markedly different from theirs.

Compare your passions to the fears that have motivated and directed your life. What actions have you taken in life due to a fear of not being accepted, loved and secure? By removing those false security guides, you can manifest the passion that will take you the rest of the way.

What Are Your Innermost Expectations?

At every stage of your life, you must have certain expectations for yourself. If you don't, you will stop growing, and the dynamic forward motion of life will come to a halt. What's more, you should have the passion to implement these expectations.

List your expectations and then decide whether or not you can and will actualize them.

How Do You Validate Your Self-Esteem Inwardly and Outwardly?

When you feel good about who you are, no matter what you are doing, you validate your sense of self. And when you feel good about yourself, even in the face of failure, you raise your self-esteem. Many women suffer a damaged sense of self-esteem when their relationships stop working. They feel depressed, but may only display their emotions through anger or tears to someone with whom they feel comfortable.

Think of a goal or event in your life that did not work out. Did you feel good about yourself despite the failure, or did you consider yourself less worthy because of it? Most important, can you continue to pursue your dreams despite the risk of failure, or do you let it stop you?

Do You Try to Get Others to Validate Your Self-Worth?

Do you acknowledge people intellectually, or even try to please them, when you disagree with them or know they are wrong? While this tactic will gain you acceptance, it may very well cost you your self-respect. Making people feel good at your expense is not healthy. Only honest acknowledgement is.

In some cases, you may try to gain others' approval by allowing them to transgress your boundaries. You may allow them to enter any part of your life, at any time, for any reason. In the process, you will lose your sense of autonomy and subjugate yourself to the other person. This is especially true of women.

Note the things you do to please others even though these actions feel wrong to you. Evaluate your reasons for submitting to others. What would happen if you were to be yourself and honestly express how you feel? In what areas do you need to be more assertive? What steps can you take in that direction?

If You Told the Truth About Your Real Inner Needs, How Would the People in Your Life View You?

Don't be afraid to communicate your real feelings and needs. You'll never go forward unless you have the courage to express them. Indeed, many people go through life wondering "What would have happened if . . . ?" They are more concerned with how others will react and respond to hearing their needs than they are with having those needs met.

Think of what you would say to your boss or coworkers about your real needs. What would you say to your friends, family, lover? If a person cannot accept you because you communicate your needs, can you fulfill your needs within the relationship in spite of that?

How Do You Relate to Others, Positively and Negatively?

Pay attention to the effect you have on other people. How do they respond when you relate to them? You may discover that you are often too busy to listen to your children, or that you ignore certain people in the same way that others ignore you. Think about your reaction when other people do not know how to communicate with you. Do you try to find out more about them, or do you simply dismiss them as having nothing of interest to say because they are quiet? Some people have a difficult time communicating, but their silence does not mean they do not have feelings. Are you able to extend yourself to help another open up?

Do You Allow Yourself to Be Used by Others?

Sometimes we blame others for using us, when in reality we have set ourselves up to be used. This is a codependent pattern of behavior—the need to be needed. Then we feel anger, guilt, depression, the need to eat compulsively or some other displaced energy, all stemming from a negative situation we have created ourselves. Pay attention to your patterns of behavior, and analyze the circumstances when you feel you have been used.

Do You See the Larger Context of Smaller Actions?

Your viewpoint will become too narrow in scope if you do not recognize the bigger picture of your everyday actions. Suppose that you work in a munitions factory. Can you see that your work ultimately will be used for destruction, or do you consider yourself to be separate and removed from the product's purpose?

In Which Areas of Life Do You Feel Incompetent?

People commonly feel incompetent in the areas of life they have avoided. But you must pay attention to these areas and challenge yourself to become more proficient. Determine which areas are difficult for you now. How can you address them?

Do You Overreact?

Overreaction usually stems from insecurity. It is a defense mechanism that keeps you from going forward in an uncomfortable situation. By overreacting, you focus on the reaction itself rather than on a realistic plan to confront a problem and make constructive change. Consider this example: You know you need to eat better, but you sabotage yourself by saying, "Health food is too expensive. What's the point of eating healthy if I don't have the time or money to do it right?" Most of the time what you imagine is far worse than reality. You've overreacted.

Beyond that, you may overreact to minor things other people say or do. Instead of reasoning with them, you go into a rage and lash out at the person. If someone you are with wants to go to a particular restaurant, and you don't, you may become angry instead of talking rationally about the event. You believe that the only way for you to be heard is to scream. Needless to say, this can damage a relationship irreparably. It is far better to reason through a problem.

To make constructive changes in your life and maintain healthy relationships, it is important for your thoughts and behaviors to be appropriate. List the instances in your life when you have overreacted. Beware of these inappropriate thoughts as they arise and resolve to be more reasonable than reactive.

Do You Acquiesce to Authority?

Think back to your childhood. Did your parents or guardians only demonstrate affection when you were completely submissive to them? If so, you grew up believing that you must please those in positions of authority to gain their acceptance. Now, you might take the same approach to pleasing your boss or other authority figures. Perhaps you rush to get coffee for the boss, or you grin and bear it when you work late most every night. You think you must please people; they can't just like you for yourself.

Acquiescing to others does not make people like you more. To the contrary, it gives them the impression that you are weak, helpless and insecure. And it gives them more of an opportunity to take advantage of you. List the ways in which you acquiesce to authority to gain acceptance.

Do You Take Statements Out of Context to Justify Your Feelings?

People often hear only what they want to, not what is actually being said. They twist others' statements to justify their beliefs. If a friend tells you she was mugged by a black man and you conclude that all minority people are dangerous, you have used what she told you to justify your own beliefs. This way of thinking can keep you locked in your fears.

Do Your Belief Systems Limit You?

You can become stuck in ineffectual behavior patterns when you react out of habit. Rather than examine your life and initiate the process of change, you choose to recycle the same old doubts and fears. A homemaker who feels frustrated by this role, for example, may allow her belief system to prevent her from pursuing other avenues in life. She may feel that she is capable only of being a housekeeper, wife and mother.

If you follow the behavior patterns to which you are accustomed, you will continue to have the same doubts about your abilities and will remain frustrated that your needs are not being met. If, however, you expand your world and look toward other women who are overcoming similar obstacles, you will get the support and direction you need to change.

List the habitual types of behavior that keep you feeling trapped and frustrated. Think of new ways to deal with your problems. Look to role models and support systems outside of yourself for help in forming new paradigms.

Do You Respond to All Relationships in the Same Way?

You need to be adaptable in your relationships. Recognize that each relationship is unique. You may be able to share cultural interests with one friend, engage in sports with another and find a spiritual soulmate in a third. Note where you are rigid in your relations with others. Ask yourself, "What is unique about this person that can enhance my life?"

Do You Avoid Change Because of the Accompanying Pain and Anxiety?

Change is not a pain-free process, but that doesn't mean you should avoid it. If you want to correct a deformity in your back caused by poor posture, you will have to experience pain as you begin to straighten up. Sometimes the anxiety you feel when anticipating change is worse than the experience itself. If you fear the dentist, for instance, you may postpone taking care of your teeth. But once the dental work is done, you are happy you went.

You will feel anxiety and pain any time you let go of the predictable, such as an old job or a long-term relationship. A conflict arises because you are afraid to let go of what's familiar, even though you know that you must move on. To grow, you must work through the pain of relinquishing the attitudes, relationships and beliefs that no longer work for you.

Life is constant motion and change. To deny that reality and cling to the familiar is impossible; this approach will bring unhappiness and pain in the long run. Letting go, on the other hand, may be painful at first. But ultimately it will free you.

Do You Let Other People Define Who You Are?

Try not to see yourself through the eyes of others. You will give up your identity, autonomy and integrity by engaging in such codependent behavior. Another person can never know you as you know yourself and can never experience what you have experienced. Therefore, you may seriously shortchange yourself when you let another person define who you are.

Make a list of the qualities that define you. Look in the mirror and affirm who you are.

Are You Addicted to Your Relationship?

If you experience terrible anxiety and fear at the very thought of losing your relationship, you are addicted to it, and codependent. You may even believe that you cannot live without the relationship. As a result, you do everything possible to maintain your involvement, even if that means compromising your integrity, honesty, pleasure and growth. Your relationship becomes the antithesis of what it ought to be.

Now is the time to make a conscious effort to do things that are good for you. Focus on goals and experiences that add meaning to your life. Also, seek outside support to help you overcome your codependency.

Issues of Interest to Men

And the Masculine Side of Women

*Happy men have a passion for life; they
express themselves openly and with
vitality. They are content with their lives.*

Do You Hold Back Your Feelings?

In our culture, the typical male upbringing generally dictates
that we not show our emotions. For the most part, men are
encouraged to be active, achieve, and perform great feats. Any
feelings that distract from performance are to be suppressed.
Our society's undervaluation of the feeling function (if we let
them, feelings function as a form of intelligence) has paradox-
ically contributed to an underproductive, under-energized
workforce and to joyless relationships with others. We cut off
our feelings at a steep price.

People use various defense mechanisms to cut off their feelings. Addictive behavior is a common defense mechanism and
a potentially dangerous one. An addictive behavior can be anything that you do repetitively to avoid deeper pain. Do you run
from your feelings by overworking? Overeating? Buying things

you don't need? Spending hours in front of the television set? With any such addiction, you will feel that you do not have complete freedom of choice about performing the behavior. You will feel emotionally attached to it.

If this description rings true for you, now is the time to eliminate the addictive behavior from your life. By doing so, you will be able to grow and achieve real stability and peace. Any feelings that you avoid will always return until you deal with them. By running away from reality, you lose any opportunity to gain insight into yourself, and you do not treat yourself with respect. You may cause severe physical harm to yourself if your addiction involves the abuse of chemicals or foods, for example, and you may cause harm to those around you if negative emotions erupt explosively. You are not in control of your constructive energy.

To achieve balance, you must become familiar with your emotional life. Spending an hour each day writing in your journal will be of great help to you. Your writing will make you aware of what is working negatively in your life, and you will learn how to make changes that promote growth and happiness. You should set aside a specific time each day for this activity. Be sure to write in your journal when you feel yourself in the grip of a negative emotion. If your journal is not at hand, jot down a note to help you later recall what prompted the negative mood.

The very act of stopping to write about a feeling, rather than suppressing it, will help you break your usual negative patterns of coping. Never dismiss any thought, visual image or feeling that comes to mind when you are writing. To do so would only lead you to another defense mechanism—the tendency to minimize the importance of your feelings by saying they are stupid or of no consequence.

What Do You Want From Your Work?

If you're like most men, you tend to derive a large part of your identity and sense of self-worth from your work. Your job is a top priority, and it may take precedence over other aspects of your life. But have you considered what your motivations are in making work so important? And have you considered whether or not your current work truly fulfills your needs? For example, you may expect your job to meet your needs for the following:

- Identity
- Friendship
- Growth

Identity

Your performance at work affects the deeper meaning of your life. If you do well in your business or on the job, you feel good about yourself. There's a certain pride that comes from knowing you did a good job. You get positive feedback from others around you.

Friendship

The work environment promotes natural associations that can form into friendships. Some friendships stay in the workplace, while others carry over into your personal life. It's easy to see why such bonds are created at work. Not only do you have a lot in common with the people there, but you also see them on a daily basis.

Growth

Does your work honor your values? Or must you compromise your beliefs or feelings to conform to your workplace? For example, if your coworkers smoke and you are afraid it will affect your health, do you suffer in silence or are you willing to ask your boss to change the situation? If he won't, would you quit your job and look for a workplace that does not compromise your health?

If you must compromise your beliefs to maintain a job, eventually your whole life will be adversely affected. You'll stop caring about your work and yourself as well. Your work may become sloppy, or you may start to feel miserable and take it out on others. When you can't control your environment, you will feel out of control in all other areas of your life.

The lesson: You must evaluate your work honestly to determine if it respects your real needs. Ask yourself, does my job help me to grow intellectually, emotionally, socially and spiritually? If your work is personally meaningful, you will be much happier and healthier for it.

What Do You Want from Your Home Life?

Make a note of the things you have been taught to want from your home life and the things you really want. If you experience intense feelings that you do not understand, or cannot be flexible in certain respects, your conditioned (or learned) needs may be ruling your life. Some of these areas include:

- Dominance
- Hero identity
- Spiritual renewal

Dominance

Does your conditioning make you feel that you must be the dominant member of your family? Must the final decision always be yours? Are you afraid of competition from your wife and other family members? If so, you must recognize that these are conditioned responses. More important, they are far from conducive to a healthy family life. If you don't respect the abilities of others and allow everyone in your family an equal right of expression, you can expect deterioration in those relationships.

Hero Identity

Do you expect unconditional hero worship from your family members, or do you earn their respect and admiration? Give some thought to the actions you take, on a regular basis, to make your family look up to you.

Spiritual Renewal

Do you gain a sense of spiritual renewal from your home life? Does it revitalize you from the pressures of the outside world? You can use your home life to practice and reaffirm connection to others at a feeling and intuitive level.

You need to honor the peace and space of your home. It is unfair to you and your family to bring problems home from work. Be aware that you may be talking excessively and brooding about your job to avoid intimacy. So leave your problems at work, except for a short talk about the day's events that allows both you and your mate to put the day's problems behind you.

Is Your Life What You Really Want It to Be?

List the important areas of your life. These may include work, friendships, family, location, lifestyle and anything else that comes to mind. Note what works and what doesn't in each area. List your dreams and aspirations for each. Do you view your goals with pleasure, or do they reflect what you think you ought to want?

Begin to separate your real needs from those that are merely superficial. For example, if you enjoy wide open spaces, perhaps you shouldn't be living in the city. That doesn't mean you must move immediately, but this knowledge certainly can be factored into your long-term planning. You may have to consider practical matters such as job availability and school quality, but the time you spend researching the possibilities will stimulate your ability to transform your life.

You must learn to follow your heart. You may think of a long list of excuses to avoid making changes in your life—career responsibilities, family, lack of education—but these excuses ultimately prevent you from reaching your full potential. Allow yourself to trust your own perceptions.

What Are Your Heroic Qualities?

Everyone possesses certain heroic qualities or has certain heroic images to which they aspire. List yours. Perhaps you are capable of compassion, introspection, endurance, persistence, discipline, strength or courage. Do you manifest these qualities? If so, in what areas of your life?

Unless you examine your heroic qualities, you may overlook them. And this oversight could deny you a viable route to personal growth. Your heroic images help to motivate you. They serve as a catalyst for change that allows you to overcome your fears and move forward with your life.

Do You Define Your Own Life?

You must define your life by the needs and beliefs that are important to you, not by the standards of other people. Many people are a product of their upbringing, cultural heritage, peer pressures and other people's expectations.

The process of re-evaluating your needs and redefining your life is ongoing. If you don't like yourself, perhaps you are not acknowledging your true needs and living honestly. Instead, you are living out the stereotypes dictated by your earlier conditioning. If you do like yourself, then you will be comfortable enough to change the things that need to be changed. You must create an identity that fulfills your needs and desires and then make the dynamic changes necessary to live this life. Remember the heroic qualities you have just listed in establishing your identity.

What Are Your Successes and Failures?

Acknowledge your successes and learn from your failures. It's important not to berate yourself when you fail at a new endeavor. Instead, look at the ways in which you have grown from the experience. You've probably grown in ways you do not even appreciate. Recognize how your difficulties have strengthened you and acknowledge the new experiences you've allowed yourself to have. Don't dismiss these lessons in life.

Men tend to be too hard on themselves. They don't give themselves enough credit for the life experiences they have survived. Make a list of events in your life that have required you to confront major survival issues, such as the death of a parent, the loss of a job or the breakup of a relationship. Take an honest, careful look at the hardships you have been through. What lessons did you learn? Don't underevaluate yourself and your ability to respond to such crises.

Recognize your victories as well. You don't have to be a braggart and exaggerate the significance of your achievements, but you should enjoy your successes before letting them go. Too many people discount their accomplishments and thus deprive themselves of a well-deserved boost to their self-esteem.

Do You Follow Your Intuition?

Do you trust your own intuitive abilities, or do you feel you must be in control at all times to make your life work? It is often difficult to trust our intuitive function if we had early problems with bonding. Without a secure attachment to a protecting parent, the frightened child creates a false ego which may appear to others to be very strong. The child is pretending to himself and to the world. He reacts in whatever way he believes is necessary for survival. He may be compliant, aggressive, adorable—whatever will cause others to respond and attend to his needs. But the ego is not acting out of its own center; it is reacting rigidly out of fear. The frightened ego is threatened by the spontaneous feelings of our intuitive function (including spontaneous images, thoughts and body sensations). Spontaneity and feeling are frightening to the child who has learned to cut off his pain.

To recover our intuitive abilities, we must learn to recognize when we are being phony (that's our frightened false ego at work), and become more genuine little by little. We must look behind the front we have created and eventually allow ourselves to welcome all feelings, both positive and negative, because they will provide important guidance in life. They will allow you an understanding of yourself and others that cannot be achieved by rational thought alone. You will learn when to trust and when not to trust. You'll know when to say no. You will learn to set comfortable limits at work and at home.

Can you recall a time in your life when you did not follow your intuition? What did the experience teach you? Based on that experience and others, can you now allow your intuition to influence your thoughts?

If You Were to Die Today, What Legacy Would You Leave?

Make a list of the accomplishments and qualities for which you will be remembered. Is your legacy a positive or negative one? Are you leaving something for others or taking only for yourself? What have you created that's unique? Where have you taken a chance? If you take no risks in life, you can manifest no legacy.

Do You Associate with Negative People?

List the people with whom you associate. Are they a positive or negative influence? Some people manage to see the bad in everything. When you're around them, their negativity will rub off on you. As much as possible, dissociate yourself from the people who have a negative influence on your life. Instead, choose to associate with people who are positive and supportive of your ideas, your spontaneity and your honesty.

Are You Able to Say No?

Make a list of the times you said no—or wish you had—to acting in ways that betray your true self. How many times would you have prevented a problem had you done so? When you have the courage to say no, you take back the power to be who you are.

Are You Able to Make Commitments?
Do You Make Too Many?

Do you have a tendency to make more commitments than you can uphold? Analyze a typical month of your life to determine your patterns of making and keeping commitments. Be alert to the possibility that you leave no time for yourself.

Are You a Workaholic?

Work should not be all-important in your life, to the exclusion of all other interests. In our society, however, some men work so hard they forget how to relax. They even work around the house during their vacations. If you fit this workaholic pattern, you must begin to develop other aspects of your life. Let in other influences besides the work ethic. Otherwise, you may very well end up with ulcers, high blood pressure and other diseases as a result of the constant pressure.

Evaluate the time you spend working and the time you spend pursuing other interests. See if this division is in balance. If you work so hard that you haven't developed other parts of your life, you need to take time out for yourself. Only then can you do the things necessary for personal growth. Make a list of the non-work activities you might enjoy, and commit to doing one each week. If you are unsuccessful in taking time off, picture yourself enjoying a pleasurable activity. Note your thoughts and feelings about taking that time for yourself. Do you feel guilty? Out of control? Gratified? What else? Write down how you think others will react if you take time out for yourself. The reactions you imagine are probably your attitudes toward yourself. Try checking them out with people close to you.

Do You Communicate Honestly?

Make a list of your real needs. Do you let people know what these needs are, or do you mask them? Can you let another person know that he or she has hurt your feelings? One way you might do this is to say, "Right now I don't feel good about what you said." If you choose to say nothing, it will only build up as resentment. Think of how many times you have let an incident go by and then replayed the scenario over and over in your mind. All sorts of possible responses come to mind after the fact, but it's too late because you have not communicated honestly. Conversely, are you able to express positive feelings to others? You cannot control the past, but you certainly can learn from it. More importantly, you can resolve to express your feelings honestly when similar situations arise in the future.

How Attentive Are You to Your Personal Needs?

If you don't pay attention to your own needs, who will? No one else really knows you. They only know the aspects of yourself that you are willing to share. Meanwhile, part of what you share is your conditioned self, not the real you.

You need to get in touch with your real needs. These may include needs for nurturing, love, expression, compassion, humility, and openness. Define your needs and determine what you are willing to do to obtain them. How many of these nonworking parts of yourself are you willing to let go so that you can replace the old with the new?

Make lists of your real needs and your conditioned needs. Decide which ones you want to get rid of and which you would like to place more emphasis on.

Do You Take Time Out to Nurture Your Growth?

Personal growth comes from the learning process. But how many of us devote time each day to learning experiences? To check your progress in this area, make a list of the things you do to enhance your growth.

Like many people, you may believe there is a point at which learning stops. For example, you may think you have reached your full potential—and therefore can no longer grow—once you receive an education, master a career or have a family. But this is not the case, of course. We all need to learn and develop in certain areas throughout our lives. You may need to learn better communication skills, or more patience, for example. Or you may want to master a craft or to learn more about life. In any event, the things you want to know more about can enhance your life and make it more meaningful.

Are You Willing to Take a Chance?

Most men look for a secure outcome—a sure thing—before they venture into unknown areas. But this approach limits them from trying new things, since it is impossible to know the outcome of unfamiliar actions. As you approach the top of a hill, you never know what you will find on the other side. When you move or get a new job, you don't know what changes that action will put into motion. You need self-confidence to enjoy the process of change. Don't put limits on your life just because you can't control the outcome.

Are You Aware of Your Power and Control? How Do You Use Them?

No doubt you feel that you have control over some areas of your life, but not over others. You may have power at work and not at home, or vice versa. You must gain control of the parts of your life in which you wish to grow. The process of becoming self-aware will give you that control. Do not criticize yourself for feeling anxious or uncertain about this process. Instead, consider such feelings to be indicators that you have some work to do in that area. Never reject or avoid your feelings by engaging in substitute behaviors.

Finally, make a list of the areas in your life where you have control and the ways in which you use that power. Do you use it in a positive way to nurture relationships and aid other people? Or do you use it in a negative way to control others? Do you use control to make your life work in a more spontaneous way? Or do you use it to maintain the status quo?

There are two basic types of men: Those who are in control of their lives and those who are not. The first group uses their control in a constructive way. Being in control gives them a sense of power, but they do not abuse it. Rather, they use self-empowerment to create more and better options for living. They look at alternative solutions to their problems and choose the ones that are most feasible.

In the second group the men are angry about their lack of control. They emote a quiet suffering, a martyrdom. These people are likely candidates for illnesses such as ulcers, heart disease, constipation, obesity, and addictive behaviors.

Do You Compromise Your Beliefs in Order to Feel Secure?

List the ways in which you compromise your principles. Do you act meek on the job? Do you try to mask your insecurity by acting righteous at church or staunch and tough at home? If so, you must begin to face your fears and free your energy.

You may compromise your creativity for the security of a job you hate, for example, by reasoning that jobs are scarce and that you could never survive at the work you truly enjoy. That isn't true. Open your mind and change your values and beliefs so that you can pursue the interests that make you feel most comfortable. If your religious and educational upbringing has conditioned you to believe that your capabilities are limited, then you must overcome this conditioning before you can grow.

Look over your list of principles and decide which ones have true relevance and meaning for you. Start now to apply these principles in your daily life.

Do You Worship Strength? Do You Deify Leaders?

Most people overlook a hero's or leader's shortcomings because they want these models to have all the answers. They don't want their President to show vulnerability and say, "I don't have all the answers. They're too complex." They want him to be invincible. Similarly, their sports heroes can't do anything wrong. They would rather believe lies about such people than face and evaluate the truth.

Hero-worshiping becomes more prevalent during turbulent times. When the times seen uncertain, people like to fantasize about mythical heroes, such as Batman, Superman, Rambo and

Rocky. In fact, many men identified with Rocky, the underdog who overcame all obstacles to become a somebody.

You need to actualize your own potential, however, rather than project a fantasy. You need to become your own hero. Write down the qualities you admire in your heroes, and see how many of these you already possess. Then make an effort to develop the other ones. Everybody possesses these qualities, but some people simply have not found a way to manifest them.

When Do You Feel Vulnerable?

Imagine a spectrum with the macho-male image at one end and vulnerability at the other. Where do you generally fit into this spectrum? When you're vulnerable, you let your emotions and feelings show through, such as when you cry at a sad movie or express compassion for your fellow man. Most men are afraid to show such vulnerability because to do so connotes weakness and a lack of control.

But vulnerability is an essential part of the growing process. It allows you to transform by permitting a free flow of emotions that are not mitigated by the male defense mechanism. You become more dynamic, much like a reed in a storm that bends with the wind but does not break. Its vulnerability is what allows it to be flexible. When you're not vulnerable, by contrast, your shield goes up. You become stationary and rigid, and that's when you crack.

Some men, due to their own insecurity, are afraid of other men who show vulnerability. But being vulnerable does not mean that others can change your mind, alter your principles or take advantage of you. People who understand emotional and spiritual growth admire the trait of vulnerability in others.

Do you try to be vulnerable, open and sensitive? Or do you tend to follow the male model of being aloof and tough, with a "bear the pain" attitude? Write about the ways in which you could express your sensitivity. Picture yourself expressing your vulnerability to another person. What reaction do you expect from that person? This exercise will tell you a lot about your attitude toward yourself. If you imagine that the person berates your weakness, you are probably berating aspects of yourself that you have learned to call "weak." You may be drawn to people who berate you because you have been berated so many times.

Regardless of how you learned the original attitude, and regardless of what others think, you must know what you think about yourself. Don't get overly involved with projections about what others think. Follow your values.

How Do You Deal with Conflict?

You may deal with conflict in one of three ways: by being dynamic and meeting the situation head-on to resolve it immediately; by complying externally while denying your true feelings (saying yes when you mean no); or by glossing over the problem as if it did not exist.

Of these three, only the dynamic method allows you to get problems out of the way and move on to other things. Make a list of all the unresolved problems in your life. Try to think of a dynamic way to resolve each one.

How Has Your Childhood Conditioning of Right and Wrong Affected Your Life?

The training you receive as a child directly affects your concept of right and wrong and your self-concept as a man, including your notions about whether or not feelings may be expressed. This training will determine whether you feel disempowered or empowered in life, dominating or cooperative and spontaneous.

The rules from your childhood may cause you to react unrealistically to present situations. If your pet died when you were a child, for example, your parents may have told you that you had to be a big boy and not cry. In that case, you may not be able to cry as an adult. When we are rejected and do not deal with the rejection, it will continue to manifest later in our lives. The only difference now is that we will have chosen socially acceptable ways of displaying rejection.

Examine the following list of feelings and check the ones you might still be carrying from childhood. If you are unsure, try picturing yourself in a scene (at home, at work or during childhood) in which the feeling or attitude is being expressed:

helplessness	bravery
grief	calmness
domination	capability
defeat	inspiration
cheating	security
betrayal	helpfulness
abandonment	freedom
shame	gratification
fright	energy
being discounted	childishness
emptiness	contentment
envy	kindness
hate	mysticism
intimidation	poetry
loneliness	peace
persecution	relaxation
obsession	sexuality
rejection	tenderness
temptation	valor
vulnerability	wonderment
affection	heroism
bliss	selflessness

I have listed these categories because they are the ones that affect my life. You may have different emotions and feelings that need to be considered. The important point is that each one must be examined to determine if any remaining conflicts need to be resolved. Once a resolution is reached, you can free your personality to be who you really are. You will not be limited by your conditioning.

What Are Your Excesses and What Motivates Them?

When you feel discontented and angry—when things aren't going your way—you may tend to overindulge. You may overeat, overwork, chain smoke or overindulge in sex, drugs or alcohol. Some people try to resolve these symptoms without addressing the cause. If you overeat because you are not content, for example, you cannot resolve the problem by trying to lose weight. You must get to the root of the problem, your sense of discontent.

To begin this process, make a note each time you experience these negative emotions and each time you overindulge. Eventually, you may see a connection between the two. Everything has a cause and effect. Once you make the connection, it will be easier for you to resolve the underlying problems and eliminate any related excessive behavior.

When Do You Feel Content?

Learn to recognize the times in your life when you feel a sense of satisfaction—the times when everything feels right. Make a note of the events that transpired and caused this feeling, and then encourage yourself to linger in the moment. Too many men are almost afraid to feel good about their lives. If you always feel unappreciated by the people around you, it may be that you have lost the capacity to accept positive feelings from others. Perhaps you believe you don't deserve them. As a result, you may retreat to the comfort of the familiar—no matter how painful that reaction may be—and minimize the appreciation of others. You may not even hear their positive feedback.

Equally important, beware of the times when you feel good one moment and then terrible the next. That's withdrawal. It shows that you are not connected to your feelings. You don't accept yourself, and you're never satisfied with your accomplishments. This dissatisfaction forces you on to the next project and the same short-lived sense of accomplishment. You are acting out of a lack of self-esteem, rather than a genuine sense of achievement and the spirit of congratulation. Take the time and effort to recreate your good feelings whenever possible. Men tend to overlook these feelings. In the process, they miss out on one of the great joys of life.

What Things Do You Value in Life?

Do you value your family, friends and work? If so, how do you measure their value? Value is what you get from participating in the relationship, whether it be nurturing, love or friendship. If you do not have a sense of value, you will tend to take things for granted. You may have a wonderful person in your life, for example, but fail to fully appreciate the benefits received from the relationship.

Make a list of the people in your life and their value to you. Do you make them aware of their true value? By communicating their importance to you, you make it much easier for them to reciprocate. That means the relationship will be nurtured so that both of you may grow.

Do You Value Yourself?

List the things you like about yourself. Above all, you need to be happy with yourself. And you need to understand that nobody is perfect. If you tend to be your own worst critic, begin to allow yourself some room to be human.

Did You Gain Acceptance from Your Parents?

If you are like most men, you did not bond well with your father as a child. Our society dictates that a child's initial bonding will be with his mother, from the time of birth well into childhood. At some point, your father is expected to bond with you intellectually and nurture your abilities, while showing love and understanding when you fail.

But many fathers tend to be judgmental when showing their appreciation for a task well done. The reason is that a father wants his son to be a better man than he is. This approach will deliver the false message that your father is more interested in the results of your abilities than in a true loving relationship. You don't feel accepted for who you are, only for how you perform. You grow up with a feeling of resentment because you were never good enough to win your father's full approval. This sense of doubt can linger for years without resolution because you don't want to face rejection from your father at any age.

Some men feel that their mother's love also was contingent upon their successful performance. Our society promotes the so-called "masculine" values of rational thinking, specialization and the pursuit of perfection. Men are encouraged to seek perfection by isolating and exaggerating some aspects of their personality and excluding others. A more intuitive approach to living values the intelligence of our instincts and feelings as well as our thoughts. We often learn these functions through our mothers, as they teach us how to care for ourselves. When we honor our instincts and feelings, we know when we are tired, comfortable, truly receiving love, and so forth. Due to their own upbringing, some mothers did not bond with people who valued their feeling, intuitive function. These mothers will be unable to support that function in their sons and daughters. If your parents did not learn to balance their energies, you will probably have to develop this sense in yourself as part of learning to nurture yourself.

You may compensate for a lack of love in different ways. Some people mistrust love and become excessively aloof, while others strive to be overachievers to gain acceptance. You may try to please others all the time as a form of compensation. All of these are misconceptions about the true nature of love.

You need to acknowledge your need for love before you can receive it. First, you must be loving to yourself. Accept yourself unconditionally for who you are. Then learn to share love. And finally, forgive your parents, especially your father, for not showing you the love he felt. One way to do this is by writing a letter to your father. The letter will serve its purpose whether or not he accepts it, because you are the one who needs the healing. By forgiving your father, you free yourself.

What Are You Willing to Sacrifice to Be Who You Really Are?

A real man must stand up for his beliefs. In many cases, it will require sacrifice to do so. You must live out your beliefs, not simply exist in silence. Otherwise, by your silence, you will condone things in which you do not believe. You know that your neighbor is abusing his children, for example, but you choose to remain quiet. By not speaking out against his abuse, you have compromised your basic principles. Men don't like to live at less than their potential. There's no pride in that, no self-respect or self-esteem.

You don't have to accept that your conditioning was right or normal. You don't have to do things just to appease other people. You need to stand up for your ideals, even in the face of adversity. Otherwise, the conflict between your inner and outer selves will begin to wear you down. It can eventually lead to physical and mental illness.

Courage is all it takes to be who you are. Better to be honest about your beliefs—even if they differ from the socially accepted standards—than to suffer in silence and wreak havoc on your mind and body. If you live by your honest feelings and show true love, you will be respected and admired by other men, even if they don't express their admiration openly. You will make them wonder what it is that gives you inner peace and happiness—and what it is that they don't have themselves.

List both your good and bad qualities. Life doesn't work if you express only your good qualities and have a dark side that you do not acknowledge even to yourself. Until you face your total being, both good and bad, you can never grow. You will not be able to move forward with your life if you have any unresolved conflicts of principle because you are not a well-defined person. You will get caught up in the world of make-believe rather than in the reality of your life.

What Is a Balanced Relationship?

A balanced relationship meets the essential needs of both people. That doesn't mean, however, that each party must give to the relationship in equal proportions. Rather, it means that you give of yourself to the best of your ability. If you give more than you can reasonably offer, or if you withhold a part of yourself, the relationship becomes imbalanced.

Take an honest look at what you need from your relationship. Do you express these needs to your partner? If you do not understand your own needs and share them with your partner, you cannot expect to have a good relationship. It's unreasonable to expect someone to recognize your needs automatically, without your saying anything. Your partner can't read your mind, after all, and you will end up feeling frustrated and angry. Honest communication is essential to a balanced relationship.

How Do You Know When a Change Comes from Your Real Self Versus Your Ego?

When contemplating changes in your life, remember that the ego always looks to gain advantage, while the real self simply seeks to explore and grow. What's more, your ego generally externalizes things and blames other people for your problems. It takes the responsibility away from you. The ego would rather try to change everyone around you than change who you are. Your real self, on the other hand, will explore your inner nature and lead you to positive changes.

Do You Fear Death?

If you feel out of control in your life, you may develop a fear of death. This connection often occurs when people look at the past and determine that they haven't accomplished anything worthwhile. They have yet to fulfill their dreams or aspirations.

When you get up each morning, tell yourself that the day belongs to you. Say to yourself, I'm taking control. What I do today will affect my life. I'm going to use positive thoughts, deeds and actions. I'm going to actualize my higher self. I'm going to give joy, be open, and listen carefully before I react to anything. I'm going to discard any negativity.

Throughout the day, be aware of the positive things that result from this approach. Good things will be returned to you, and this positive feedback will reaffirm your sense of control and enhance your self-esteem. Remember, too, that you need to re-establish who you really are as you take charge of each day. Don't be afraid to show your vulnerability as well as your strength. When you live fully as yourself every day, you will lose your fear of death. Death holds no power over you when you have control over your life.

Are You Easily Provoked to Anger and Other Negative Emotions?

Certain situations may cause you to experience negative emotions, such as anger and depression. When this occurs, you need to evaluate your response to the situation. You may be reacting according to your conditioning. Suppose, for example, that someone cuts in front of you in his car and you feel like running into him. You are the one who will suffer from the internal frustration this type of anger generates. You could just as easily recognize that the other driver's actions do not affect you.

You have the freedom to take any approach you choose to the situation. But you lose this freedom if you respond according to your conditioning. Therefore, you must overcome your conditioned responses to take a more reasoned approach. Ask yourself if there are alternative explanations for another's behavior. Imagine yourself in that person's situation. If your anger is justified, is it very important that you express it? Before you react in anger, evaluate the situation and see if the anger will make any difference or whether it is just a learned reaction.

How Do You Resolve Pent-Up Emotions from Childhood?

Our childhood emotions can be the underlying cause of many present-day problems. We may react adversely to people who say or do something that subconsciously reminds us of our past. For example, you may be in a relationship with a woman who reminds you of your mother. And you may end up admonishing her for your mother's shortcomings. Until you resolve your latent desire for fulfillment, you will continue to blame her for the things your mother did not provide.

Make a list of the needs, events or experiences that were overlooked or denied during your childhood. Also, list the things you missed because you had to shoulder responsibilities that your parents didn't or couldn't. These situations caused you deep-seated pain and anger that carry over to this day. You may need to evaluate the items on this list one by one to identify those things that are influencing your life, both positively and negatively. Only after you resolve the negative issues will you be able to forgive and forget so that you can live your life free of the influences of the past.

How Do You Handle Deception and Betrayal?

Everyone knows what it feels like to be deceived. And once you have been betrayed a few times, you will begin to recognize the signs of deceit early on. The person may fail to make eye contact, or he or she may assume a certain body language. Your intuition will tell you what is about to happen. This intuition can help you to avoid the same pitfalls.

Naturally, you will feel hurt when you are betrayed. However, you need to forgive the person and let the negative emotions go. Then you can get on with your life and the things that really matter.

When Should You Challenge Authority?

You don't have to accept authority when it is self-serving and abusive. Indeed, you should challenge it. If you find yourself thinking of excuses not to act, you are allowing your insecurity and fearful, negative feelings to undermine your resolve to live by your principles.

Be wary of anyone who professes to have all the answers for you. This precaution is essential. A goal in life is to develop your own inner guide. We allow others to have an undue influence on us because we do not know ourselves or our values. When we make contact with our own higher self, we will discover that we created the illusion that other individuals, and society at large, have power over us.

Do You Have Trouble Ending Relationships?

If you feel trapped in a relationship that is not nurturing, and your partner appears to want to continue the relationship, then you need to examine your past. Maybe you were not allowed to say no or were not encouraged to assert yourself. Dig into your past to find the origin of these feelings. Undoubtedly, you will find that there were many such incidents in your childhood.

How Do You End Relationships?

When you want to end a relationship, accept responsibility for its breakdown and explain that you are not the person he or she needs you to be. Don't blame or intimidate the other person. By accepting responsibility yourself, you allow the other to save face. In some cases, this approach will leave you open to ridicule. But if the relationship ends successfully, you have accomplished your goal.

You should be in a relationship because you like being there, not because you are codependent. All relationships need to be based on mutual respect and positive reinforcement. That's the real reason that you should be with someone.

Do You Seek Help When You Need It?

Men are conditioned to be loners. As a result, they have a difficult time expressing their need to be accepted and bonding with other people. To do so, they believe, would make them appear needy. Meanwhile, they grow up admiring role models who were always alone. These heroes of the past, like the cowboys, would ride off alone into the sunset. Some men will confide in one close friend, but most are reluctant to seek professional help or group support.

In the 1990s, men are finally beginning to open up and get in touch with their feelings. They are learning to express themselves with the help of professional counseling or support groups. This is a first step toward growth. See whether you get in touch with your inner feelings.

What Behavior Characteristics Do You Want to Change?

Some common negative behaviors include the following (you may experience these as gut reactions or have a vague sense that they apply): You need to control all conversations; you have trouble expressing your feelings; you selectively choose what you want to hear; you hold rigidly to a point of view because you are afraid to change; you reject anything that does not fit your perspective; you maintain an image and reject whatever does not fit your self-concept; you have over-committed yourself and feel burdened by responsibilities; you're unsure of how to do things.

Make a list of five characteristics that you would like to begin to change.

What Repetitive, Negative Patterns Do You Participate In?

People who do not have control of their lives will recreate patterns of disharmony that have proven to work for them. If yelling or threatening always helps you to win an argument, then you will continue that behavior pattern. Even though the other person has become quiet out of fear, you will not attempt a more reasonable approach to handling a disagreement.

You need to find reasonable and healthy ways to communicate and live your life. That means you must respect other people. Always consider what it would be like to be on the other end of one of your conversations. Look at the long-term consequences of your actions and ask yourself, "Would this make me feel good?"

Make a list of your repetitive negative behaviors. Try to understand why other people react to you as they do. Change these behaviors into more positive ones.

Are You Who You Want to Be?

The professional community often divides people into type A (high stress) and type B (passive) personalities, but this is an overly simplistic paradigm. Many people thrive under stress; they work day and night and socialize night and day. These people manage to commingle their personal and work lives. They create balance by doing the things they love to do.

Creative people, by their very nature, often are volatile and expressive because they allow the energy of the unconscious (the emotional, the unexpected) to disrupt the dominance of the ego. An overly strict ego or an overly structured external environment can discourage creativity. What would happen if you were to tell an artist such as Picasso or Dali that he must work from nine to five, or that he must not be so highly excitable? You would destroy the basis of their creativity. Painters and other artists need to express their internal zeal to give us their gifts of poetry, dance, music and writing.

By our willingness to adhere unquestioningly to meaningless conventions, we have dehumanized and depersonalized the society in which we live. We must not look to others to tell us who we are, what we should value, how to look, what to eat, how to feel. When Mao Tse-tung's cultural revolution sought to set universal norms for China's population, creative and artistic expression was suppressed. This most powerful and important source of social and personal renewal was denied, and China ended up with a sterile society.

Creative expression is the energy of life. People who have not found the courage to express themselves can easily become depressed. Long-term depression is the leading emotional disease in our society today. It is also the impetus of many physical diseases, since psychological depression decreases the body's immunity. Expressive people are seldom depressed. That is not to say that they never feel transient negative moods. People who are open to creativity and personal growth will allow all feelings into their consciousness in order to learn from them.

Begin to act on your insights. Perhaps you will find the courage to give up a nine-to-five job and start a business you really love. You may even look forward to working 12-hour days because you enjoy what you are doing. As long as you express your real feelings and maintain balance in your life, you will thrive.

When you change, you challenge the reality of people around you. People close to you may feel unsettled by your new energy level, or they may feel that your relationship with them is threatened by your freedom and self-expression. They may envy your ability to tap your creativity. But you should not let the negative reactions of others hinder your growth. Your courage may ultimately prompt those around you to make positive changes as well.

Men are beginning to realize that they have been complacent for too long. They would go to the ballpark and scream and yell, but, for fear of losing their jobs, they suffered in silence if their work conditions were unhealthy. They would go to church and sit by passively, never questioning or challenging anything as they muttered an occasional "amen" and "pass the till."

Finally, men are accepting responsibility for what they must say and share with others in order to express their creativity and add meaning to their lives. As this trend continues, there will be less anxiety, less abuse, less alcoholism and drug addiction, and more family harmony.

Make a list of the times you suppressed your creativity or were unresponsive to situations that really required your attention. Then make a list of the times you expressed your real feelings in a meaningful and caring way for your own benefit or that of your fellow man.

Do You Struggle for Power?

Are you out there struggling to accumulate power, or do you recognize the natural power that each of us possesses? You need power so that you can live your life, but if you assume you don't have it you will let someone else have power over you.

To use your inherent power, all you really need to do is make a decision about what you are willing to do for yourself and the ideals in which you believe. People often try to make you feel that you are not empowered in life. If you believe that, you won't make decisions on your own. You will be conditioned by society. You'll eat the four basic food groups, for example, which has been a major contributor to disease for the past 50 years. Even as you're eating yourself to death, you will believe that you're doing the right thing by following these food guidelines. A more rational—and empowered—approach is to make your own decisions about the right and wrong foods to eat.

You need to follow your intuition. When you feel that something is right but the structured power around you says it's not, follow your instincts and go by your own experience. It's only when you stand up for yourself that you can use your power in a constructive way. Otherwise, someone else will use power against you.

Are You Egotistical?

Do you believe it's important to satisfy your ego? Many people seem to think so. Consider all the executives who do not hobnob with the general society. Instead, they display the trappings of success by frequenting exclusive clubs, elite restaurants and exotic resorts. They drive expensive cars and own extravagant homes with many more rooms than they need. They pay high prices for these homes so that they can live in exclusive neighborhoods and display their social status. In short, they do anything to get the merit badges of life.

Most men seem to have a great need to be acknowledged. They're always looking for recognition, either through their business life, where they become high-powered executives, or through their recreational activities, where they become the head of the bowling league or the softball team. They want to have something that you don't have.

Occasionally you will find a man who simply hangs out with life and enjoys it to its fullest, with no need to impress anybody. This takes a mature, balanced, whole person. In the past, our nation had many such men. But with the advent of the Doctor Spock baby-boomers came the philosophy that everybody had to be a winner. Men adopted compulsive behavior and put the pedal to the metal to get as far ahead as they could, as fast as they could.

The baby-boomer generation raised and spent three trillion dollars with very little to show for it except a lot of debt, pain and destroyed lives. The greatest amount of cocaine addiction in history occurred within this upwardly mobile group, which used the drug for a supposed energy boost. The baby-boomer's destructive dependence on drugs and alcohol was no accident; it was concurrent with their need to achieve.

In today's society, people are under a tremendous amount of stress. We have become a nation of emotionally stunted people because we have believed in things that we do not need. We overconsume to prove to others that we have significance, all because of the fact that we're really very insecure. A man who is comfortable being a man doesn't have to overextend himself. He doesn't have to prove anything. People intent on proving that they're acceptable often try so hard that, ultimately, they never achieve that goal and never feel content with life.

Do You Have the Time and Patience to Be Who You Really Are?

American men have become very impatient. They want material possessions now—and more of them than they can possibly use. They're willing to get themselves into debt to show that they deserve these things. Once they assume this debt, however, they don't handle the pressure well and start breaking down. They resent having things they don't really need, and they generally punish themselves and others for this state of affairs.

Americans have become gluttonous. They're out of shape, lazy, unfocused, undisciplined and unhappy. This is the most addicted society in history—one that has spawned tremendous anger. Hostility is manifest all around you through exhibitions of violence, particularly in sports such as football, the roller derby, gladiators and wrestling.

This cycle of gluttony and anger doesn't occur as much in cultures where men are happy about being men. They're content with their lives. We can take a lesson in patience from other cultures. Maybe what many American men need to do is take a trip to Europe. If you were travel to Milan, Florence or Venice, you would see that men there are physically fit. These men have a passion for life; they express themselves openly and with vitality. They are never in a hurry. At noon, they close down their businesses to join their family for a meal, a short siesta and a relaxing conversation, and afterwards they return to their work rejuvenated. They usually work until about seven at night, have a light dinner, and then enjoy their family and social life for the rest of the evening. You won't find them vegetating in front of the television set because these people have a zest for life. They're eternally romantic and express passion in everything they say and do.

Further into the countryside, you will find villagers in their 80s and 90s who still tend their flocks, their gardens, or their grandchildren every day. They live in small communities of four to ten homes that are separated by farmland from the next hamlet. Thousands of these small communities dot the countryside. This is where the population at large lives.

These people have a reason for living. When you ask them what that reason is, they say that they really enjoy life. They certainly don't have fancy cars and all the latest gadgets. They're not rich and they don't have money in the bank, but none of this worries them because they know they have a reason for living when they rise each day. They've learned to master what they do. Craftsmanship takes time, patience, understanding and apprenticeship. You see men in the countryside weeding their gardens with the precision of a Zen gardener. They don't try to rush nature. They live within a natural time frame. You can't pull on a rose to make it grow at an unnatural pace. Everything will happen when it needs to happen.

List all of the things you do on a daily basis. Are you an expert in any of them? Maybe you should identify the ones that are important to you, and then devote more time and attention to perfecting them. Eliminate some of the others that have little meaning in your life.

Are You Cluttering Up Your Life with Material Things?

Look at all the material possessions in your life. Identify those you really don't want, need and use, and then get rid of them. Give things away. Let other people enjoy what you've long lost the ability to appreciate.

Once you give something away, don't bring in a substitute right away to take its place. Rather, learn to scale down. It's better to have less debt and more freedom than to be enslaved to new things you do not need. Use this newfound freedom to take care of your real needs, to create real priorities for yourself and to make better use of your precious time.

When you start letting go of the things that no longer serve you, you begin to lighten your load in life. There's an old saying that those who want to travel far in life must travel light. When compiling your list of things that you no longer use or need, include the clothes you haven't worn in years, the TV set you haven't turned on for months, and the old tires in the garage that do not fit your car. Think of people who could make use of these items.

Are You Living in the Present?

It's fine to have long-term objectives, but if all your goals are in the distant future, you may never get around to enjoying them. Why put your life on hold? Instead, begin to view each day as special—one that you won't have next week or next year. Life is short and you never know when it will end. That doesn't mean you should live irresponsibly, but it does mean that you must recognize that today counts.

Make a commitment to put your energies into today. By living your life one day at a time, you reaffirm your choices and live life to the fullest. No matter what comes, you will make each day a constructive one in your life. Every morning when you get up, look at life and see what positive thoughts and actions you can take to confirm your legacy. Can I do something for others? Can I be patient? Can I be compassionate? Can I take care of my own mind and body? Can I allow myself to grow? Can I be intimate and open with others? Can I live with what's in my heart? You can do all of these things.

Once you set these ideas in motion, they will become a pattern of behavior that works for you. You will start to feel more relaxed, light, confident, honest and flexible. You will have a much greater range of intellectual and emotional happiness.

Make a list of the things that matter in your life. Are you doing these things now and living a positive, dynamic life, or are you always planning for some time that may never come in the far-distant future?

Intrinsic love is the energy that allows life to thrive. Ultimately, you must choose what type of a life you want and how you want to live it. It's a choice you make by deciding to be consistent and positive. All the right situations in the world will not grow if they are not nurtured by love.

How Do You View Life?

Some people believe they are a victim of circumstances. Good and bad things just happen to them, no matter what they do. Other people believe that their active participation in life helps to shape their circumstances. With the second philosophy, you take an entirely different approach to living. You are more likely to wake up each day and affirm your needs, knowing that your conscious effort makes a real difference in each day's events.

You might face the mirror each morning and say, "Thank you, God, for this day. I'm glad to be alive because this moment is the only one that I can really change." This attitude allows you to focus on an immediate concern, such as the need to change the way you eat, the way you live, the people you live with, the way you communicate, the way you spend time and so forth.

This approach to life will give you a different mindset. It is an important prerequisite for changing your life because it emphasizes the things that are important to you. There will always be some things that you cannot control, of course. But you will feel greater harmony in any situation if you believe that your life is in control. Suppose that you get stuck in a traffic jam. If you change your perception of the experience, you will feel less impatient and more relaxed. You have not changed the reality, but you have changed your experience of it. Make a list of the aspects of your life you need to change.

Do You Exaggerate Your Problems?

Many people think their problems are insurmountable, when, in reality, they are just blown out of proportion. Perhaps these people have become spoiled by too many gifts and options. American welfare recipients, for example, eat more food than some of the wealthiest families in impoverished nations. Imagine that you live in a war-torn nation like Somalia, where people must fight just to survive. Owning nothing but the rags on your back, you hunt for food in the bushes at night surrounded by hyenas and lions. You don't have a home and must spend your time traveling from one battlefield to another, watching your children die from starvation. What wouldn't you do then to have your basic needs met with things you forgot were important.

If you feel resentful because you have hardships in life, you are expressing an inflated opinion of yourself. You've forgotten what real suffering is. All human beings have problems. If you find meaning in your limitations and don't make mountains out of molehills, you will gain an awareness of your strength.

Do You Project Your Shortcomings onto Others?

It is often the case that we cannot acknowledge our own shortcomings, but react strongly to the shortcomings of others. When you are feeling hypercritical, judgmental, bitter, cynical or sarcastic toward someone, stop. Take your intensely negative feelings as a signal that the very attribute that so enrages you in others may be an aspect of yourself as well.

It does not matter whether or not the other person possesses the negative attribute. What matters is that you have something to learn about yourself in this area. You probably feel as intensely intolerant toward yourself, albeit unconsciously, as you do toward the offender you have targeted. If you make an honest effort to recognize and change the conflicts in your own life—and are willing to acknowledge that you can grow beyond them—you can do so.

In addition, become conscious of any tendency you have to idealize others. In this case, you project everything positive onto others and expect them to embody the positive qualities you possess in an undeveloped state. Focus on developing your own positive qualities instead.

Do You Use Your Time Properly?

The only thing in life you can really call your own is your time. Why waste it? Use your time wisely by paying attention to your real needs, not the superficial ones that can rob you of time and energy. Take time to nurture yourself. Allow the child in you to come out and help guide you in the nurturing process.

Are You Looking for Love?

The idea that you must look for love is the wrong way to view this aspect of life. You are love. Love is inside of you; it's not something outside of yourself. If you open up and share your vulnerability and intimacy, you will draw people to your inner light. They will feel the love you represent. And when you meet people who are willing to do the same, you will automatically bond with these people.

Are You Conditioned to React Rather Than Reason?

Insecure people are hypersensitive, and they retaliate easily. Others must be careful not to step on their egos or trigger their emotional minefields. These people react rather than reason, a pattern of behavior that usually starts in childhood when their parents teach them words and gestures to be used as defense mechanisms. Before long, they have been inundated with rules that cause them to react in ways that are excessive and counterproductive.

You must learn to trust your sense of reasoning. Otherwise, your exaggerated attitude toward people may generate excessive responses. Make a list of your common reactions and try to identify proper responses to be used in their place.

Do You Retaliate?

Retaliation, in and of itself, is an infantile behavior. It's an inhumane way to respond to other people. When you strike back at someone, you show your need to be right at any cost. If you catch yourself thinking about retaliation, stop to consider both the reasons why and the consequences of doing so. What am I angry about? Why do I want to retaliate? What will happen if I do? How would it feel to be on the other end of what I am about to do or say? If it doesn't feel good, then you shouldn't act on this negative impulse.

Are You Both Competitive and Cooperative?

Both of these qualities are important, and each has its place in life. In the best of circumstances, they can complement each other in a highly effective way. In long-distance races, for example, athletes often do best when they run together at first and help each other to maintain the pace. Then, at the end of the race, they run competitively.

I'll never forget a race I entered in Washington. About 15 athletes participated, all of us trying to make the national qualifying time. During the competition, a highly skilled athlete—one of the best of all times—noticed that one of the less-experienced runners was starting to pull back from the group. He gave up his lead position to help this runner.

The less-experienced racer, who was having cramps, told the other athlete that he didn't have the energy to continue. The experienced athlete helped him through that difficult stage with some guided visualization. He paced with the runner until the man was able to get back into the race. As a result, the racer who almost dropped out made the qualification time by one second. The spirit of camaraderie during a competition distinguishes a real athlete from an insecure one.

Cooperation is an important quality in all areas of life, but some men have difficulty showing it. They equate it with weakness because they fear others will take advantage of them. These men believe they must win at any cost and that any means will justify the end. They are feared by others, but at the same time they artificially isolate themselves.

Today, men are beginning to understand the need to cooperate. Being cooperative makes them more likable as human beings. When they need help themselves, people will be more patient, tolerant and accepting of them. In the end, they get the same amount of work done and everyone involved feels they have won. They can create win-win situations.

Cooperation is especially vital to relationships. Being overly competitive is unhealthy because it promotes fear. If you always need to have the first and last word, for example, normal interactions become impossible. No matter what anyone says, you deny its value and, in effect, disempower that person. You use words defensively to control others and make them feel subservient.

When you work as a team, on the other hand, you talk openly. You realize that both people must contribute to a relationship to make it work. In any relationship, you must discuss what you feel comfortable doing, what decisions you feel comfortable making and to what degree you feel comfortable making them. This keeps the relationship balanced.

Too much competition creates a gross imbalance that affects the relationship on every level. One partner takes on too much responsibility while the other becomes overly dependent. The person who is in control makes even the most mundane decisions, like where to eat. He assumes that his decisions are always right and that his partner must enjoy the relationship because there are no complaints. But compliant people seldom complain, at least directly. They may complain to their friends over the phone or sublimate their feelings by watching soap operas, but they are afraid to speak to you face-to-face about what's bothering them. If you are overly competitive, the first step to changing your behavior is to recognize what you are doing. Can you see where you are exercising unnecessary control?

Do You Go Along with the Group?

If you are compliant by nature, you accept the status quo without question. Your identity derives from the groups to which you give your support. Belonging to these groups makes you feel accepted. You may be the type of man who works at the post office for 40 years and never complains about the system of which he is a part. Instead of looking for things to reform, you adapt to given conditions as long as your basic needs are met. You never think of starting your own business, even if you have the financial ability to do so. You feel much more comfortable being a part of someone else's business.

People who are dynamic by nature tend to challenge the establishment and take certain risks rather than play it safe. If you are a politician, you are the maverick who takes on controversial causes, not the cautious politician looking for a guaranteed career path. If you are a doctor, you question standard medical practices and use the techniques that work for your patients even if they are not sanctioned by the medical associations.

This type of person can't comprehend working for someone else. One hour's work in a post office would be too much. You'd rather be on the street. You have a disdain for the ordinary, especially when it means sacrificing your freedom and your identity. You are a constant seeker.

These two basic types of men (or women) can be classified as supportive and dynamic. Society needs both in order to function. Without innovative men and women, we would have no one to lead the way. We would have no Frank Lloyd Wright, Robert Moses, Voltaire, Buddha, nor Christ. Without supportive people, we would have no one to execute ideas. Society needs cooperation between these two groups, the dynamic and the supportive.

Do You Follow Your Intuition?

People who do not develop their insights will pay an enormous price. Those who obey authority blindly allow totalitarian rule and fascist ideologies to exist. In Japanese culture, where the individual is subordinate to the group, people are not motivated to become autonomous because they receive all the support they need at home and at work. This support results from dedication to the work principle, which goes unquestioned and unchallenged.

American society tends to be more flexible. Here you can gain the insights you need to be both autonomous and to work with a group when necessary. But it takes some effort to do so. In the 1940s and 1950s, when people did not acknowledge their own insights, men believed that real men would only eat huge steaks and fries and other high-fat foods.

The basic-four-food-group diet was a major contributor to coronary heart disease and cancer, but the average man would consider it unacceptable to be a vegetarian. Men would rather weigh 250 pounds and be headed toward sickness than be a 165-pound vegetarian with normal biochemistry and health. Vegetarians were regarded as being gay or communists.

Many people are still very primitive when it comes to developing insight. But some men have indeed identified their real and honest needs. They see what they really want to be, really want to do and who they really want to do it with. They no longer feel constrained by their religious and social positions.

Do You Work Within Your Physical Limitations?

You must accept your limitations before you can overcome them. When you ignore these limitations, you do yourself more harm than good. Perhaps you want to start an exercise program, but you're overweight because you have not exercised for some time. Your blood pressure is too high and your cholesterol and triglycerides are elevated. If you do not acknowledge these limitations and exercise in a reasonable way, you run the risk of dying from a heart attack or stroke.

You must honor your body's condition and realize that you cannot improve your health instantaneously. Take your time and perform the actions necessary to compensate for your limitations. You may need to have a cardiovascular stress test, an EKG test and even a musculoskeletal examination to determine what types of exercise you can perform safely.

Do You Prepare for Change in Your Life?

Positive change requires preparation and work. The results don't simply fall into your lap. If you're not happy at work, for example, you must prepare for the job you really want. The transition may require that you train yourself, familiarize yourself with the new job and possibly advance your education so that you're the best qualified candidate for the job.

If you do not make this effort, in all likelihood, you will go nowhere. You'll complain all the time that you feel trapped in a job you do not like. You will be a perpetual victim. This is true of many men who work in the coal, steel and auto industries. A good percentage of them complain about working the same old boring job day after day at a fixed wage. But when their factory finally lets them go, they feel betrayed. They take their anger out on the union for not having negotiated a better deal.

While outside factors may contribute to your problems, you must recognize that you are ultimately responsible for your own happiness. You can't rely on your union, corporation or boss to change the things that bother you. Think of what you must do to make your life work in a meaningful way. Think of ways to overcome any limiting circumstances. If you don't, you make yourself a victim and allow others to exploit you. But once you take control of your situation and initiate the process of change, you will find that others support your efforts.

It's your choice. You can either sit around and moan at home when you get laid off or you can take positive action. Instead of drowning in self-pity and longing for your old job, use the time to rebuild your confidence. Perhaps you could get some training in another profession, one that is more to your liking and that offers a better guarantee of work.

Another option is to create a home-based business. I know one family that turned their garage into a bakery when the husband lost his job. They didn't cry in their beer and let their lives go down the drain, which would have compounded an already negative situation. Instead, they read up on baking, watched videos, took workshops, went to auctions and bankruptcy sales and put together their own small business.

They reasoned that they could supply higher-quality and better-priced goods than the processed junk food found in supermarkets. Starting the business gave them a sense of confidence, and over time the little bakery expanded. They began to advertise and even had their children make home deliveries. Today it's a thriving business.

People operate all sorts of successful home-based businesses now. Some homemakers sell crafts, others teach remedial reading to children. There are a thousand paths you can take if you choose not to be a helpless victim. Reject the status-quo mentality that says you must wait to be called back to your old job or find a similar job that offers you nothing more than a dead end. You don't have to follow standards that do not work for you.

What False Assumptions Do You Have?

Most people live with many false assumptions. See if any of these sound familiar to you: You assume you're going to marry the right person and live happily ever after; you assume that the way you were raised is the way you should raise your children; you assume that the way you've been taught to eat in the past is the way you should eat now; you assume that your job will be there forever.

People accept such ideas as fundamental truths because of their conditioning. According to a concept known as cognitive dissonance, our early training stays with us the rest of our lives. This training, no matter how unreasonable or impractical, becomes a person's standard throughout life.

You need to examine the source of your beliefs. Ask yourself, am I really happy with the things I was taught to accept as a child? If not, what beliefs made you feel uncomfortable and unhappy? Are you passing on these very beliefs to your own children? Perhaps your mother gave you food every time you complained as a child, and to this day you eat whenever you feel upset. Becoming aware of the roots of your problems is an important first step to overcoming them. The key is to allow yourself to start over again.

What Male Stereotypes Do You Adopt?

Most American men respect an all-purpose list of "male" attributes—authority, control, power, strength, dominance and invincibility. They're terrified to show compassion, uncertainty or any sign of weakness. Thus they will quickly resort to violence to settle an issue.

Where do these images come from? Many were fabricated in Hollywood, where actors such as Marlon Brando and James Dean personified the American male hero of the 1950s—the tough, defiant loners who chose to play by their own rules. There was also John Wayne, who portrayed the all-American leader protecting society's standards. His character exemplifies the typical male ego, which says that we are a first-rate power that must maintain our control at any cost.

Unfortunately, this belief has bankrupted our national economy. It has justified an overtaxation of the population, the production of arms when we have no one to fight and the production of unnecessary weapons at a time when the stockpile in our nuclear arsenal could kill every man, woman and child 47,000 times over. This system exists solely to perpetuate the male ego's concepts of strength and invincibility. To fuel the myth that such weapons are needed, people are made to feel paranoid and fearful. They believe that only their leaders can be trusted, that their very lives depend upon their government's ability to guard and protect them.

But governments, much to their shame, fabricate enemies and build them into real threats for the public consumption. The United States government has made Cuba's Fidel Castro seem like a legitimate threat. The truth is that he couldn't fire off a banana peel, let alone a rocket. We could have annihilated him in about a week had we chosen to, but we needed him to perpetuate the Cold War in the Western hemisphere.

We played the same game in Nicaragua and several other Central and South American countries. But the height of this folly was in trying to make Saddam Hussein's third-class army appear to be invincible. They were such poor soldiers that they couldn't win a war with Iran in eight years despite their collection of high-tech gear. In the weeks before Desert Storm, we made them into a Goliath, as if they were a major threat to American security.

As in the past, this technique did the trick of confirming that we are powerful and in control. But in the process, we devastated a country, caused the death of about 300,000 people, spent about $100 billion and caused several hundred Americans to die from our own friendly fire. After some 200,000 bombings, we left pretty much as we came and Hussein remained in power.

The male image also associates power with money; hence our fascination with men who become millionaires and billionaires, such as Donald Trump, Michael Milken and Ivan Boesky. We admire their big homes, beautiful women, fancy clothes and sports cars, and we dream of attaining these things ourselves.

We never question how these men get their money or power. We never wonder about the types of deals they make. An objective look at many of the people we admire would reveal that the takeover artists of the 1980s caused the displacement and loss of five million blue-collar jobs. Not until they were caught and convicted for overt illegal actions did we realize that they are not the great white knights we thought they were. In reality, many such men are megalomaniacs who don't care about anyone but themselves.

We males have a warped concept of success, power and control. It's based upon winning at all costs and doing everything possible to get ahead. How many hugely successful American men and their families earned their fortunes honestly or ethically? Perhaps none of them.

Do You Look to Others to Support Your Ego?

Men tend to surround themselves with people who strengthen their identity and do not threaten to expose the qualities about them that they fear most. In a male-female relationship, for example, a man who is insecure about his masculinity will look for a woman who does not require him to be masculine. If you base your identity on your physical appearance, you will choose a woman who always comments on your manly appearance and flatters your ego. You won't have someone in your life who challenges you with comments such as, "Shape up, I don't like your infantile attitude. You're sexist and inconsiderate." Your partner will be an extension of your ego, whether or not your self-image is a healthy one.

A healthier relationship is one in which the partners respect each other's differences but continue to support the relationship. You help each other to recognize faults and make improvements. You may say, for instance, "Come on, now. You're exaggerating, and it's making you look foolish to other people."

Granted, it is difficult to hear the truth at times. I know someone, for example, who always embellished his conversations to make him seem a little bit better than everyone else. One time he left the room and I saw one man turn to another and say, "Isn't that unfortunate? He keeps exaggerating all the time just to get some attention."

I knew this person very well, so I asked him privately if he knew he looked foolish every time he made up a story. He became livid and did not talk to me for a year. Then one day he told me that he had finally come to terms with his compulsion to exaggerate. When I first spoke to him, he had denied his feelings because he was so fearful of them. Our relationship became stronger and healthier for this experience.

It's important to have people in your life who are honest, who will speak to you candidly without humiliating you in the process.

What Motivates You to Change?

Like most people, you may attempt to make changes in your life when you feel that your self-esteem is at stake. For instance, you may make a New Year's resolution to lose weight because you don't like what you see in the mirror. You feel depressed and unsettled by your appearance, so you compensate for your feelings by going on a crash diet or a faddish exercise program.

The problem is, changes based on what you do not like generally cannot be maintained. You'll adopt new behavior for a while, and then go right back to your old habits and your old appearance. A better approach is to conduct an objective evaluation of the adjustments you need to make at any given time, and then develop a realistic program for change. Consider the way you are now and the way you want to be. Then adjust your lifestyle, your perceptions and your reality accordingly to achieve those changes. With this approach to change, the effects will be longer-lasting.

Do You Undermine Yourself?

Anything you do that has a negative effect on someone else ultimately will come back to affect you as well. You become a part of everything that you share with other people, good or bad. Think of this before you gossip about other people or attempt to undermine them. In the process, you will undermine yourself.

What's more, you will demonstrate a lack of character. I never trust anyone who gossips about others because I know they wouldn't think twice about doing the same to me. If I find out that someone has cheated or stolen from others, no matter how insignificant the incident, I keep my distance because sooner or later that person will cheat or steal from me.

Don't overlook these types of behavior in yourself and in others. They are barometers of what lies beneath the surface. You become what you express to others. If you express hate, you become that hate and disrupt your life. Conversely, when you project love, kindness, openness, sensitivity, understanding, care and compassion, you allow these qualities to come back into your life.

Do You Feel Threatened By Love?

If you feel threatened and cut off from love, you will lead a sad and lonely existence. You won't know how to be intimate with people who enter your life. You won't know how to express your real needs and desires and to be your real self. And you will be afraid to share this undeveloped part of yourself for fear that others will perceive you as immature. It's like being afraid to open your mouth in the dentist's office when he just wants to take a look. You're terrified. You have resistance to it.

Perhaps you mistrust love because you were hurt at some point in your life. For example, you may have felt love for someone who only betrayed and abused you. At that point, you decided not to be open to love again because the consequences were so painful. Now you don't trust anyone who comes into your life. You've closed yourself off to the possibilities.

By reacting in this way, you limit your potential for future happiness. If a woman breaks your heart, and you mistrust all women from that day forward because you assume they will hurt you, you are seeing only the negative possibilities. If you drink one glass of spoiled milk, does that mean you should never drink a glass of milk again?

You may even seek out women with the same qualities as the first to confirm your worst expectations. If a woman leaves you for another man, you may decide that all women are prostitutes as a defense mechanism. You start to look for other women on 42nd Street in Times Square, where you are likely to find prostitutes. In this way you confirm your low image of all women.

A more positive response to this experience would be to look for women in healthier environments. Then you will find women who are willing to share romance, love, openness and joy. You must actively seek out the experiences you want to have in life.

Do You Deny Yourself the Pleasure of New Experiences?

Many people deny themselves new experiences because they do not want to relinquish their well-entrenched habits and old ways of thinking. Suppose that a friend invites you to the opera. You turn down the invitation at once, rationalizing that you don't need to see male dancers jumping around in tights. Besides, you think, Monday night football is on (even though you've seen it a hundred times before). In the same vein, you are likely to turn down the chance to see a folk festival, a rodeo, a poetry reading, or anything out of the ordinary.

By living such a routine existence, you will deny yourself the joy and the growth that new experiences offer. You will be afraid to allow such experiences into your life because you would have to alter your perceptions. Many men fall into this pattern, allowing their lives to become stagnant after high school or college. But if you are open to new experiences, it doesn't have to be that way.

Do You Have Attitudes and Behaviors That Sabotage Your Health, Happiness and Growth?

Some of your attitudes and behaviors can prevent you from doing things that are in your own best interest. If you are somewhat lazy, for example, you might like to sit around and watch television on Saturday mornings. Then, when a friend suggests going for a jog, power walk or bicycle ride, you find it difficult to break your routine. You might get defensive and deny the benefits of exercising, and you might even overreact and make your friend feel bad for having suggested it. Since you work hard all week, you argue, you need Saturday mornings to do what you want to do. You feel upset that someone is infringing on your time and wants you to do something else.

That sort of thinking can undermine you. Why not look instead at the benefits that come from a change of pace? Ask yourself, is this something that will make me feel healthier, live longer, be happier, have more energy and be a better person? Poor attitudes and unhealthy behaviors also can sabotage your relationships at work. Let's say you feel threatened because a female coworker is getting a promotion and you are not. To retaliate, you make sexual remarks about the woman in an attempt to dehumanize and dismiss her as nothing more than a sex object. You're trying to make her seem incompetent and incapable to others. And you're trying to show that your male insight, knowledge and intellect are superior. Of course, nothing productive will ever come from this approach.

Why Do You Please Others?

In a relationship, doing something to please the other can be either constructive or destructive. It depends on why you do it. If your intent is to show respect and appreciation of the other person—for example, you surprise your wife by preparing dinner for the family one night—then the action is constructive because it shows your unconditional love for her. You don't expect anything in return for your efforts.

In a codependent relationship, on the other hand, you will try to please your partner out of a need for acknowledgement. In that case, you are not acting from your own inner strength, direction and purpose. You are living in the shadow of someone else's life. You may fear punishment for not doing what is expected of you, or you may expect to be rewarded for your efforts. Neither reason is good.

Make a list of the things you've done to please other people and the reasons why you did them.

How Do You Respond When Others Attack Your Dignity?

When someone attacks your dignity—or makes you feel uncomfortable in any way—you must decide whether or not you will allow that person to control the way you feel about yourself. If you do, you are relinquishing control of your feelings to that person.

Understand that other people are entitled to like or dislike you. You have no control over that. But you can control how you regard yourself. Self-respect and acceptance of yourself come from within, not from what other people think of you.

Make a list of the feelings you have about yourself. How do

you feel about the way you dress and act? Do these feelings come from you or from other people?

What Are Your Weak Points?

It seems to be human nature to focus all of our attention on our strengths. This allows us to perpetuate the false image that we are totally successful. Donald Trump, for instance, appeared to be enormously successful—and initially was—in his business dealings. But how successful was he in his marital life? He betrayed his wife by associating with another woman. That isn't success; it's failure. If he had ended his marriage and then pursued someone else, his actions would have been more acceptable.

Make a list of your weak points. You must be willing to deal with these qualities in order to have a whole relationship. Only by addressing them can you ultimately grow and thrive.

Dealing with Negative Emotions

*By mastering the powerful energy of
anger and putting it to work for you,
you can create almost anything you want
in life.*

Do You Get Angry?

Everyone experiences negative emotions, such as anger, hurt, and feelings of betrayal. But most people have a difficult time expressing negative feelings, particularly anger, to others. Learning to manage this emotion can be rewarding. In some cases, anger is our primary response to a negative situation; in others, it may mask other feelings that you find even more difficult to tolerate, such as shame. In the latter case, learning to express your anger constructively will help to uncover other important emotions as well. Freeing your anger will allow you to feel more energized.

You may have trouble showing anger in appropriate ways because our society does not encourage such expressions. Early on, in fact, we are conditioned to contain our anger. We learn to rationalize our silence by saying we deserve whatever is making us angry, and we believe we are powerless to change the situation. In reality, the opposite is true. Anger is a tremendous motivator when it is channeled constructively.

By joining together with other angry people, you can become a great force for social change. When women boycotted meat in 1978 because the price was too high, the cost came down within two weeks. When people protested the use of MSG and sugar in baby food, the manufacturers took it out. When concerned citizens said that dolphins should not be caught along with yellow fin tuna, the practice was stopped.

Enormous change occurs when a few people focus their anger constructively. For this reason, those who have an investment in the status quo discourage anger. They don't want to jeopardize what they have attained. Middle and upper-middle class whites and blacks often do not speak out for fear of losing their symbols of success. But the irony is that once you are afraid to speak out, you become disempowered. When you lose your voice you become invisible. Suppressing angry feelings is ultimately destructive to your well-being. It can even make you physically sick. One way or another, you must learn to validate your anger and express it properly.

Think of something that angers you. Write it down. Does this anger motivate you to change the situation in a constructive way? If you are suppressing your anger, think of an appropriate way to express it instead. What first step can you take?

Why Do You Get Angry?

You may experience anger for a variety of reasons. Some of these include:

- Feeling powerless
- Being victimized
- Failing to communicate

- Getting defensive
- Feeling betrayed
- Feeling hurt
- Feeling attachment and loss
- Feeling guilty
- Having unresolved conflicts
- Feeling insecure
- Having your beliefs violated

Feeling Powerless

In this case, you feel angry when you cannot control your circumstances. An example: You are being audited by the IRS. A stranger is sitting across from you who in all likelihood will impose a penalty against you for something you have not done. You feel frustrated, fearful, powerless and, ultimately, angry in the face of this bureaucracy.

Write about a situation in which you feel powerless. It could be something that happened to you as a child or something occurring in the present. Get in touch with your anger. Express these feelings on paper.

Being Victimized

Victimization causes a deep and persistent anger. Children who are victims develop especially strong feelings of anger that may surface in unhealthy ways later in life. It may take a lot of work to resolve such feelings. People who were sexually abused as children, for example, may have difficulty having healthy sexual relationships as adults. Each sexual encounter reminds them of their victimization, sometimes subconsciously. They need to do much work, alone or in groups, to let go of their past. Otherwise their anger will continue to manifest in unhealthy ways.

Think of a situation in which you felt victimized. It can be a major life trauma or something small. Get in touch with the anger this event stirs in you. How did you react to the event? How did you use your anger? Did you resolve the situation constructively? If not, what steps can you take to do so now?

Failing to Communicate

When someone does not communicate with you, or vice versa, the indifference will create anger. Conversely, you show others that you care by communicating openly. This approach to a relationship is healing. Recently a newspaper article told of a domestic fight between the head of a ballet company and his wife. The husband was arrested for becoming violent with his wife when she refused to talk about their failing relationship. How much violence in the world would be avoided if we communicated openly and honestly?

Think of a person in your life with whom you have trouble communicating. How does that obstacle anger you? Write down what you would like to say to that person.

Getting Defensive

People in powerful positions who must protect their image will become defensive and angered if challenged. I see this all the time with doctors. Recently, for example, I stated on a radio show in New York City that the HIV virus alone could not cause AIDS, since many people with the disease do not have HIV. A doctor on the show insisted this was impossible, but a short time later my findings were confirmed. It was made publicly known that HIV was not a necessary component of AIDS. But the doctor never admitted he was wrong because his ego was hurt. An empowered person would have been more open.

Write about a situation that made you angry. Was your ego involved, or were you expressing your true beliefs and facing someone else's ego? In what way did either of you become defensive? Try to make an honest assessment of the situation.

Feeling Betrayed

No one likes to be betrayed, especially by someone they trust. You feel hurt and angered by the experience and lose all faith in that person. You wonder when they will lie to you next. It's important at such times to express your anger to the person. Don't hide your feelings, be honest.

Feeling Hurt

I was on a television show once when a man launched a vicious verbal assault against me. I had never been attacked in that way before and I didn't know how to react. Afterward, he laughed to someone that he had made mincemeat out of me on the air. I walked up to him and said, "You denigrated me because I wasn't willing to engage in a verbal attack. I wanted to deal with issues. Why did you insult me in that way?" He answered, "That's how you win."

I came away feeling very hurt. I felt as if my intellectual and spiritual sanctity had been violated, and I felt a lot of anger. But I soon realized an important lesson. I didn't have to be like that person. In fact, in his folly he showed me the tools I needed to gain strength. I learned that strength comes from humility, not from arrogance. I learned that people who attack others just to look strong are really very weak.

Recall a time when someone hurt you. Did you turn the anger in on yourself or did you express your feelings openly? Were you able to separate yourself from the person attacking you and not absorb it? How have you become wiser from the experience?

Feeling Attachment and Loss

The more attachment you feel toward a person or thing, the more its loss will provoke anger. Think of the times in your life when you experienced the loss of a job, a friend or a loved one. If the loss angered you, then you were measuring your success by the things you had accumulated. You felt these people and things made your life more secure.

You need to examine all the losses in your life. Did you feel angered by loss or were you able to let go and move on? In times of loss, it may help you to make this affirmation, "When one door closes, a bigger and better one opens."

Feeling Guilt

In today's society, we feel a lot of pressure to conform to narrow, specialized roles. Societal attitudes often are reinforced within the family unit, and people are encouraged from all sides to feel guilty about being different or expressing what is unique to them. Guilt makes us feel controlled or manipulated; hence, it is a primary source of anger. It makes you afraid to take risks, to challenge yourself and grow. It keeps you in line with thoughts such as, "Good boys don't do this, and good girls don't do that." It negates anything on the other side of the accepted paradigm, including joy, happiness and new horizons. How has guilt kept you under control? Can you get in touch with the anger fueling that guilt?

Having Unresolved Conflicts

When someone says or does something that you believe is wrong, you may internalize the conflict and start an argument in your head. The many things you should and should not have said will run through your mind, and you may berate yourself for not having had the courage to stand up to the other person.

You're angry with that person but you're equally angry with yourself. You feel like a coward.

The problem with this response to conflicts, however, is that you are listening to the wrong voice. The negative voice inside you has been allowed to supersede its positive counterpart. That negative voice has enormous power to mute the positive voice and prevent it from having an equal say.

In this way, you can carry multiple unresolved conflicts with you through life. And when you finally do express yourself from this passive position, the response is generally out of context. You may express such rage that you end up hurting yourself and others. Needless to say, you can never solve your problems constructively in this manner.

Think of an unresolved conflict in your life. Meditate on the situation. What does your higher self say to you about it? If any negative voices or feelings appear, ignore them. Can you accept that you did the best you could at the time?

Feeling Insecure

Insecurity breeds anger. By definition, codependent people are insecure and, therefore angry. But they suppress their anger to maintain a stable relationship. Their anger then manifests in unhealthy ways. What are you insecure about? What makes you angry? How do you manifest your anger? What steps can you take toward feeling more secure?

Having Your Beliefs Violated

Your beliefs provide you with a sense of security. Thus, you feel threatened the moment someone challenges them, no matter how gently. You become defensive and angry. The more you have invested in your ego, the greater your need to be right. Being right becomes more important than doing right. Much conflict in the world today stems from this source.

What types of challenges to your belief systems upset you? Why do they make you feel uncomfortable? Picture yourself in your challenger's shoes. Can you see his perspective on the issue? Why or why not?

How Does Your Anger Manifest Itself?

When you are angry inside, the emotion may express itself in many ways, some more healthy than others. The more common manifestations of anger include:

- Rage and aggression
- Repression, suppression and sublimation
- Disease
- Passive-aggressive behavior

Rage and Aggression

Rage is a destructive expression of anger. When you express rage, you can become very imbalanced. Rage can escalate into violence, as often happens with street gangs.

Repression, Suppression and Sublimation

Rather than express rage outwardly, most people turn the feeling inward. This type of suppression can be devastating because it allows the rage to eat away at you. It can cause you to become sick and dysfunctional.

People usually cope with anger in dysfunctional ways. You may try to feel something other than anger by throwing yourself into unproductive activities, such as compulsive sex, eating, drinking or drug addiction. Perhaps you become a workaholic, complying with an inner voice that says you can make the anger go away by doing your work perfectly. At the same time, though, you will feel even more angry at the inner tyrant who will not allow you to rest. You may sublimate your anger by committing your life to a cause that is likely to be related in some way to the primary source of your anger. Or you may spend too much time watching television, listening to the radio, or talking to people. You keep busy so you don't have to feel your anger.

Many people displace feelings of rage by watching violent contact sports, such as boxing, football and hockey, or by watching violent movies. By supporting the aggressive actions of others, you sublimate your own rage. Why do you think most people supported the Gulf War? Do you think they really cared about Saddam Hussein or the political issues involved?

Do you identify with any of these forms of expressing, repressing, suppressing or sublimating rage? If so, write down some ideas for more constructive ways of dealing with your anger. Recognize that these dysfunctional behaviors will disempower you and prevent you from getting to the root of the problem. Instead, you must get in touch with who and what makes you angry. Write down what you are truly angry about. You can even write a letter to your parents or another important person in your life expressing this anger. Delivering the letter is not important; what counts is to actively recognize your anger.

Disease

Due to the connection between mind and body, disease and anger go hand in hand. Truly happy people have far fewer diseases than unhappy people. Therefore, you need to think about the ways in which your anger affects you physically. Try to resolve the problems and issues that create mental pressure before they can affect your health.

Passive-Aggressive Behavior

Many people withdraw from their anger and deny its existence. This often happens as you age, especially if you have not had a fulfilling life. But the denial of anger can lead to passive-aggressive behavior. You smile on the outside but feel angry on the inside. Your negativity expresses itself in behaviors for which you cannot be clearly blamed but that cause distress for others. For example, do you overcommit yourself and then drag your feet about doing what you said you would do? Do you make nasty comments and then tell the other person that you were only joking?

Think of ways that you deny your anger and withdraw into yourself. Can you get in touch with what you are denying? Can you identify any passive-aggressive behaviors you exhibit? What first steps can you take to changing a negative life situation into a more positive one?

How Have You Dealt with Anger in Different Stages of Your Life?

As a child, teenager, young adult, adult and mature adult, how have you processed anger? Note the different behavioral patterns in which you have engaged. For each stage of life, determine when your anger caused you to react to situations and when it motivated you to take action and make positive changes.

What Does and Does Not Work in Your Life?

Make a list of the things that work in your life. This exercise will help you to see that control empowers you. It makes you feel positive about yourself and allows you to deal with issues in a constructive way. Then make a list of the areas of your life that do not work. You should be able to respect what works and focus your attention on what does not.

What Fears Do You Have?

Some of your fears are realistic, others are not. Unrealistic fears are conditioned, such as the fear of trying something new. A woman with grown children who stops herself from going back to school to further her education has a fear of trying something new and different. She is allowing her growth to be limited by unrealistic fear.

Don't give all of your fears legitimacy. Learn to distinguish between fears that are reasonable and those that are not. Once you expose your fears for what they are, you will be taking a first step toward eliminating them.

Why Do You Suppress Anger?

The thought of rejection may cause us to suppress our anger because we want to be liked and accepted by others. We may silence our anger because we do not want to be punished for expressing our true feelings. When I oppose policies of the Food and Drug Administration, for example, I run the risk of making them act more aggressively and maliciously toward me. Most people do not want to deal with such hostility. You may feel exactly as I do on certain issues, but you suppress your anger because you fear the consequences.

Perhaps you are afraid that anger will cause you to lose control and hurt someone. But this will only happen if you are full of rage and destructive anger. When your anger is justified and focused, it can only be healing to express it. Our society uses control to keep you from speaking out in your best interests. Losing control is healthy if it turns a negative situation into a positive one. Consider the environmental movement of recent years. Anger directed in a beneficial way has led to many constructive changes in our environment.

Notice the ways in which you suppress anger. What types of situations cause you to suppress your feelings? What are your reasons for keeping it in? Write down actions you can take to express that anger in a constructive way.

Have You Found Healthy Ways to Express Hurt and Anger?

From this point on, resolve to deal with your anger in healthy ways that will lead to positive changes. By mastering the powerful energy of anger and putting it to work for you, you can create almost anything you want in life. Here's how you can start this process of self-expression:

- Be honest with yourself
- Seek support
- Focus on the problem
- Direct your anger
- Think first
- Be active, not passive
- Act, don't react
- Don't hurt anyone
- Let go of pain and fear
- Stop compulsive behavior
- Give up perfectionism
- Learn new responses
- Organize your life
- Act in your best interests
- Make your word your bond

- Set attainable goals
- Take charge of your life

Be Honest with Yourself

Have an honest dialogue with yourself each morning about what is bothering you. Give yourself the time to reflect on these issues in a place where you will not be distracted.

Seek Support

Share your feelings with someone who will understand your needs and your reason for being angry without criticizing or judging you.

Focus on the Problem

Evaluate one problem at a time. Keep your energy focused on finding and promoting solutions until the problem is resolved.

Direct Your Anger

Your ability to channel anger can make all the difference in whether your feelings are positive or negative. Properly directed, anger can be a driving force in your life. But if channeled incorrectly, it can become mentally and physically destructive.

There are many avenues for expressing anger constructively. An artist, for example, can use his or her work to express anger and frustration toward society. Think of what a protest would be like without artists' posters, folk singers' songs and poets' verses. Its perspective would be limited without these constructive expressions of anger.

Think First

The old adage that tells us to count to ten when we feel angry has a great deal of merit. Reflection allows you to think before you react. You can consider what you want to say, why you want to say it and what will happen when you do. You can think through your options and react in a rational way. In the process, you free yourself from conditioned responses and focus on those that will improve the situation.

Much of your pain emanates from your conditioning. Think about the origins of this conditioning. How can you change your perceptions? If certain words or gestures upset you more than they do other people, this is due to your conditioning. The key to resolving such conflicts is introspection. It allows you to determine the sources of these conflicts and the purpose they actually serve. It gives you an opportunity to become aware of old patterns of behavior that are destructive to you and to replace them with more positive ones. Through introspection we become more acutely aware of the inner workings of our minds and emotions.

Be Active, Not Passive

If you are passive in a situation that calls for action, your submissiveness will allow other people to take advantage of you. And this experience, in turn, will breed even more anger. Take action to resolve such situations. Seek support if necessary.

Act, Don't React

Every time something angers you, ask yourself whether you will act or react to it. Being active allows you to maintain a sense of focus; being reactive does not.

Don't Hurt Anyone

Uncontrolled anger can lead to violence on many levels. Domestic violence results from unmitigated anger, while war results from the egotism of leaders. Conflicts should be resolved before anyone suffers. As the saying goes, "First, do no harm." When something angers you, try to remove yourself from the situation. Think of yourself as a referee in the altercation. Call time out. What would you ask these people to do before they engage in conflict? By taking a few seconds to remove yourself from direct conflict, you will be able to evaluate the situation more fairly.

Let Go of Pain and Fear

When your pain and fear no longer serve you, learn to let go of them. By doing so, you will be free to express yourself constructively. Remember that you cannot feel freedom until the pain is removed; these opposing feelings cannot exist at the same time.

Look at the causes of your pain and fear. Examine these feelings and say, "You've been with me for a long time, but I no longer need you. I'm going to try something else." Let it go, knowing that something better will take its place. Continue to reaffirm this goal and you will find a way to accomplish it.

Stop Compulsive Behavior

You know when you are about to act compulsively. It doesn't just happen on its own. You don't just open the refrigerator and eat a three-pound cake without knowing it, for example. You know exactly what you plan to do, and then you do it. Therefore, you should be able to stop compulsive impulses the moment they start. Have a constructive dialogue with yourself. Say, "Hold on. This is the wrong voice. There is no way I'm going to listen to you. You have no power or control over me. I'm in control of my life now. Good-bye." When you refrain from compulsive actions, they will eventually begin to go away. And you will create new, positive habits to replace these compulsions.

Give Up Perfectionism

You may pursue perfection to justify living in an imperfect world. But this urge will make you angry with yourself and the rest of the world. Stop looking for perfection and look instead at the realities of life. You must be honest about who you are because that's your starting point. Evolve from there and don't be impatient. You can't force a rose to grow on schedule. It grows when it is ready to do so, according to the laws of nature.

Learn New Responses

If you always react according to the same old formulas, learn to respond to life in new ways. You can write your own script in life and make active choices. How will this script be different from the one you were given? This is your chance to eliminate the things that do not work for you, such as the dictates of your upbringing, your education and the way you relate to others. Of course, you can't alter events that have already occurred. But you can redirect your life from this point on.

Organize Your Life

Get rid of the junk that clutters up your life. It feels good to eliminate things you don't need. Pack it up, give it away, throw it away—whatever it takes to start fresh. Clean up your desk, your closet, your car, and your body. The physical world reflects the mind. To respect your environment is to respect yourself. By clearing your surroundings and getting organized, you will rid yourself of the clutter and some built-up anger as well.

We're foolish not to organize our lives. We need certain systems to make things work. If a person's desk is cluttered, it may indicate that he or she does not feel comfortable with order. Order, after all, means you're getting something done. You have a beginning, middle and end. You plan to follow through on what you start, not leave calls unanswered and projects sidetracked. You're going to start something, create a blueprint for finishing it, stay focused and get it done.

Some people have trouble getting started because they know from experience that an inner voice will criticize their every imperfect effort. You must change this scenario. Get started, no matter what. Ignore your negative voice. If necessary, it can speak to you later. You're not going to be compulsive or obsessive. You're not going to push yourself beyond normal limits and judge yourself and others harshly by how something gets done. What makes a difference is that it gets done. But it doesn't happen unless we are organized.

Ask yourself where you are lacking in organization. Is it discipline? Do you feel uncomfortable when you know that you will not follow through on a specific task? A lot of writers never finish books or articles. They sit down, they get fidgety, they go to the refrigerator. They look for the phone to ring or they turn on the television to distract themselves. Many people spend too much time distracting themselves. Those who accomplish things are the ones who get organized and then focus in until the task gets done.

Act in Your Best Interests

Make a list of the things you do that do not serve your interests. Why do you take these actions, and who benefits from them? Don't be afraid to break the old patterns you created when you were acting out of guilt or fear. Concentrate on doing things that will benefit you.

Make Your Word Your Bond

People become disenchanted when they cannot trust what you say. Then you have nothing on which to establish or maintain relationships. Frightened or insecure people are particularly prone to lying about who they are. They feel their true selves are not acceptable, so they lie about what they feel and do. A related maneuver, typical of teenagers, is to lie to feel independent and in control. While knowing that she must become autonomous, the child may fear that autonomy will alienate her parents. She does what she wants, but hides any behavior of which her parents may disapprove.

This pattern can repeat itself in adulthood. People may lie because they fear that being an individual will lead to negative feelings in a relationship. They may lie to feel the power of being the only one to know the whole story. Or they may feel so disempowered in life that they lie whenever the opportunity presents itself. They believe they have no resources within themselves to bring good things into their lives. There are no good reasons for lying. All spiritual traditions warn against it because lying impedes the development of the self and true relationships with others.

Unfortunately, lying has become the norm in today's society. Many people use words as a means to an end, with little regard for the commitment that goes with them. A prime example of this schism is a political campaign and its ultimate results. You must stand by your word, even if it is based on a bad decision. It forms the basis of your integrity and serves as a foundation on which to build your self-worth and self-esteem.

Your word reflects your values to others; it shows that you are trustworthy. Suppose that you misprice something you plan to sell based upon an incomplete analysis of the relevant factors. Someone takes you up on the offer and you accept. It is your responsibility to stand by that price, even if it costs you time or money to do so. As you go through life, you must leave a legacy of being true to your word. People will respect you for it. While others cannot expect miracles from you, they can surely ask that you keep your word.

Set Attainable Goals

Don't overwhelm yourself by attempting to change too much at once. You will only revert to your old habits. Instead, take one bad habit at a time and replace it with a good one. If you maintain a schedule, you have a much better chance of turning your life around. You may decide to eliminate one bad habit a week. If you are trying to improve your diet, you could eliminate sugar the first week, meat the second, caffeine the third, and so forth. Or you might work at a slower pace, eliminating one item every two or three weeks. The point is to make your goals attainable and the results evident.

Take Charge of Your Life

There comes a time when you must redirect your spirit and intellect to develop the persona you will project the rest of your life. That means you will have to be responsible for all of your actions all the time. You will have to stop living like a warthog, take chances and choose the options that move your life in a more powerful and positive direction. Now is the time to get going and do it.

Beating Self-Defeating Habits

*The person who can let go of the past
and move forward is the one who will
find life most rewarding and exciting.*

Are You Carrying Other People's Burdens?

Are you always trying to second-guess someone who has not given you clear instructions? Are you frustrated because you can never please the other person? Do you feel you are inadequate at work because no matter how hard you try you're chastised for doing something that's not quite right? Is your motivation undermined because your successes are never acknowledged? Do you have to beg for acceptance on a daily basis?

If you grew up under such conditions—or now work within them—you no doubt feel insecure. But you are far from alone. American businesspeople tend to be severely critical of those they supervise. Your work isn't good enough, right enough or consistent enough to please them. It's one thing to meet attainable goals; another thing to strive to attain artificial values set by people who feel inadequate themselves and are trying to put their shortcomings off on others.

Always be on the lookout for people who continually berate you and never show any appreciation of your accomplishments. Beware the person who wants you to be more than you can reasonably be.

Do You Have Problems Helping Someone?

Have you ever tried to teach others a simple task and found that they never quite get it, even after repetitive trials? The problem does not stem from their intellect, but rather from their belief system. They simply do not accept what you are saying. In such cases, we must have honest two-way communication and allow others to be who they are. Otherwise we may develop a codependent relationship. They will not change their beliefs for the long term, but merely adapt to us.

When you interact with someone like this, always watch to see how they respond. No matter what they say, you have to watch what they do. If they don't respond to your direction, it's best not to chastise them. Recognize that their beliefs may be hard to identify, confront and relinquish. They may truly want to learn from you, but at the same time they are frightened by a new belief system. If a person says he wants to be healthy but continues to eat a terrible diet, he probably believes that what he eats cannot really hurt him. You can see that his words and actions do not coincide, but the contradiction is not evident from his point of view.

To bring about change, you must develop a two-way dialogue. It never helps to force your will on others. It may take time and effort on your part, but you must help them to modify their belief system and integrate it with your own. If this happens, the changes that occur will be valid within their belief systems. If this does not occur, accept that their beliefs, for whatever reason, differ from your own. Respect this difference and allow them to maintain their autonomy. There is never only one right way to do anything. One religion or system of wellness will not suit everyone, and each human being is entitled to have his beliefs without being ridiculed for them.

List any problems you have had in this area and write down your observations. See if a lack of two-way communication has contributed to the problem. Can you see a way that the other's beliefs can be integrated with your own?

Do You Have Disparities in Your Own Beliefs?

Do you think or say one thing and do another? If so, you need to watch yourself to determine where you are imbalanced. Your belief systems derive from your intellect, intuition and conditioning. If your feelings and intelligence tell you that a situation is wrong for you, but you do nothing physically to change it, then you have an imbalance.

The more extreme the imbalance, the worse its manifestation will be. If you stay in a bad relationship or work situation, you will feel uncomfortable even though you have rationalized that it is the right thing to do. You may even become physically sick if the discomfort continues for a long period of time. Some people, however, are totally unaware that their lives must be in balance. They feel safer adapting to a bad situation than identifying their real needs. They never ask themselves if their actions and choices fit with their personal ideologies.

Consider the creative person who needs time and space to pursue his craft. Since it's tough to pay the bills in our society on pure art, the artist may have to compromise his principles by taking a job on Madison Avenue. There, he must produce artificial, self-deprecating artwork to sell harmful products, such as cigarettes, and work under extremely stressful conditions. It's no wonder that Madison Avenue has such a high rate of turnover.

This person may rationalize that the job is not forever. But every day that he must compromise his integrity, he becomes more and more angry. Eventually, he will begin to attack his personal values with the artificial values he has been made to accept. He will start to make excuses for himself, such as, "I don't have enough money to support myself on my own" or "I'm not a good enough artist yet, so I'll do this just for a little while." Little by little, he gives up a part of his life.

To have true health, you must be balanced on all levels. You must be in tune with your real needs and react to them in a positive way. And you must look for creative solutions to your needs instead of giving in to your fears. Make a list of your genuine beliefs and refocus your agenda on them.

Do You Examine the Systems in Which You Believe?

You may be placing the blame for problems on a variety of potential culprits when the fault really lies with the system you have accepted. For example, many people in the 1980s wanted to build up home equity, generally because they were insecure. When real estate prices fell in the early 1990s, they were wiped out financially because they had bought into a system of beliefs that created artificially high prices.

The real value of property was no longer critical; it only mattered what people thought it was worth. The same belief prevailed before the Great Depression, which was caused not by economic collapse but a lack of confidence. The economy of 1929 and 1930 was booming, but everybody wanted to get rich without having to work for it. They bought stock with only ten percent down and expected to make millions of dollars.

Speculators would buy up companies with small profit margins and boost their value 40 or 50 times. When the average man saw this taking place, he bought in while the values were going up. Soon enough, however, the speculators would pull out. The little man was left to think the prices were still on the rise when in fact they were heading south. Eventually, values dropped to their true level and the game collapsed. This started a widespread panic over all the artificially inflated values.

The same thing happens again and again. For instance, ten years ago in New Jersey an acre of land worth $2,000 suddenly was valued at $50,000 or $60,000. People snatched it up, convinced that its value would double each year. They financed most of it and then waited for a million-dollar payoff. But history repeated itself and the property finally dropped to its real value.

Any belief system with artificial values will eventually have its day of reckoning. Make a list of your values. In your belief system, what has real value and what has inflated value? Challenge the ones that have inflated value.

Do You Feel Threatened by Change?

Perhaps, like most people, you find ways to justify your resistance to change. You may deny that you need to change at all when you feel threatened. But think about what precipitates the feeling of threat. Many people don't like to acknowledge their mistakes and therefore have a fear of failure. If they were to try something new and fail, they would focus on the failure rather than give themselves credit for having tried.

Take the person who wants to stop smoking but avoids this positive but difficult task because she believes she will only start smoking again. She justifies her fear of failure by believing she will not get cancer. In fact, she may believe that cigarettes do not cause cancer. Only after she is diagnosed with the disease will she give up the habit. Unfortunately, people in our society do not learn by prevention. Most wait until the worst occurs before they respond.

Don't feel threatened by the process of change. List the areas in which you need to make life-enhancing changes, such as giving up drinking, smoking or other bad habits. Evaluate each one to see if you can improve your health by taking certain actions today.

Do Your Relationships Overshadow Your Beliefs?

In codependent relationships, the partners have unrealistic expectations of each other. The relationship becomes all-important and you forget what is personally meaningful to you. You don't know what your genuine needs are because you allow the demands of the relationship to supersede your own beliefs.

In any relationship, it's essential to maintain a degree of independence. Recognize the importance of your own beliefs and distinguish your values from your partner's. To have a healthy relationship, you must first have a relationship with yourself so that you know and understand your real needs. Then you can select the qualities that you best appreciate in yourself and share them with another human being.

There's a lot to be gained when you enter a relationship knowing who you are. You know what you can and cannot give to the relationship. You can negotiate your needs and expectations in a realistic way, rather than assume your needs will be met and give your power to the other person. You can maintain your autonomy and avoid the formation of a co-dependent relationship.

Make a list of the important relationships in your life. Identify those in which you cannot be your real self. These are the ones you need to work on.

Do You Deny That Problems Exist?

Throughout history people have had a tendency to ignore their problems. In my family, nobody ever acknowledged openly that anything was wrong. If a relative were to walk around naked in someone else's backyard, they would deny that he was senile. They were completely unwilling to accept that a problem existed. Problems can only be resolved when we get to the root of them. In the 1950s and 60s, our society remained silent about alcoholism, drug addiction and child abuse in dysfunctional families. We did not encourage people to bring these issues to light. Although we have become more open today, many problems remain hidden. Occupational hazards in the workplace may not be discussed, for example, because management does not want to acknowledge their existence. Rather than risk your livelihood by speaking up, you also deny that the problem exists. It's easier to live with the lies than to fight for change.

Make a list of problems in your professional and personal lives that you have not brought to light. You must resolve as many of these as possible to grow. If your problems appear to be insurmountable, then you may need the help of a support group.

Do Your Associates Betray Your Confidence?

It's painful to learn that someone you confided in has betrayed your trust. Suppose you tell a coworker or friend that you are looking for a new job, and on your next review the supervisor says, "I understand you're looking for a new job." This breach of trust will make you wary of extending your confidence to anyone. But you shouldn't chastise yourself for having trusted that person. As you become more connected to your intuition, you will be less likely to reveal yourself to untrustworthy people.

Think of an incident when you were betrayed by someone you believed was a friend. Did this experience teach you to pay attention to your intuition?

Are You Afraid of Reaching Your Potential?

Sometimes we have great potential but stop just short of realizing it. I have seen people with the makings of great athletes pull back and drop out the moment they started to reach that potential. They realize that once they start on the path to success their lives may never be the same. They're afraid to let go of the familiar, even if it is not right for them, and to face the uncertainty on the road ahead. They anticipate the negative possibilities of change instead of positive ones, such as joy, happiness and new experiences.

The person who can let go of the past and move forward is the one who will find life most rewarding and exciting. Each day can bring something new to life if only you go after it. List the mental and physical roadblocks that prevent your self-expression. What are you afraid to give up? How would your life be more fulfilled if you were to express those things? Make a positive step in that direction, even if it is a small one.

Do You Resolve Your Conflicts?

When you run away from difficulties your whole life is impaired. Consider the person who never devotes the time needed to bring a project to completion. When the inevitable obstacles arise, he becomes distracted and discouraged and may even quit. By jumping from project to project, and not completing any of them, he is never able to take command of his life.

Your early conditioning may have taught you to avoid difficulties. Perhaps your family tolerated frustrations when things didn't go as anticipated. Can you remain open to new ideas when they don't go as planned, or are you afraid of the unexpected? Are you still trying to please someone else? If your family did not give you unconditional time and attention, if they did not acknowledge your efforts, you may carry a grudge today that stops you from resolving conflicts.

Learning to solve problems and see projects through to completion is a skill that you can still acquire. Make a list of any continuing conflicts in your life and try to resolve them.

Two major factors prevent people from resolving conflicts and moving forward with their lives:

- Believing you're not enough
- Fear

Believing You're Not Enough

You will limit your growth if you always chastise yourself for not achieving enough. You must learn to be reasonable in your expectations and acknowledge your efforts. Recently I participated in an indoor race at West Point. The man who removed my number after the race said, "It didn't look like you put much effort into that." I ignored him because I had satisfied my criteria for success by completing the race. Even if I had raced slower, in fact, I would have accepted that my effort was complete. Ironically, I later learned that I had broken a national record.

It's important to accept all attempts at growth even if the results are less than perfect. If you only acknowledge the best job possible, you will become stagnant and angered by your own imperfections. Recognize that you cannot improve every single time you try. Life has various plateaus that serve as balancing stages. These plateaus give us time to think about the direction of our lives and get things together. If you reprimand yourself for not advancing, then you will negate much of what you have learned up to that point.

Write about the times that you have chastised yourself for not achieving big results. Think of something positive you have gained from the experience.

Fear

We live in a time of gross uncertainty; nonspecific fears are universal. Since people do not know how to resolve these fears, they blame them on other people or situations around them. They stop themselves from engaging in new activities by rationalizing that they will not like it anyway or that something is bound to go wrong.

Fear and uncertainty can make you feel out of control. An inability to cope is counterproductive to the process of resolving conflicts because it makes you feel depressed and helpless. Then you wait for someone to rescue you. You may form a codependent relationship with the first likely candidate to come along. Millions of baby boomers joined cult groups in the 1970s and 80s because they believed their lives were out of control. They looked to gurus for the answers. They wanted someone else to resolve their conflicts because they did not feel capable of taking on the responsibility themselves.

The same situation can manifest itself in personal relationships. You act as if you want to fulfill another person's needs but really have a hidden agenda to take care of your own. You might think, "If I use praise or submissiveness as bait to develop a relationship, that person will take care of me." Your neediness compels you to form codependent relationships when you fear the challenges of life. You barter away parts of yourself to keep unhealthy relationships alive.

Make a list of the things you feel fearful about. Then make a list of your positive attributes, such as persistence, flexibility, and understanding. How can these virtues help you to resolve the conflicts you have listed? Learn to tolerate some uncertainty. You will never be able to control everything, and trying to do so will only make you feel more helpless.

Do You Have Self-Defeating Behavior in Relationships?

How do you know if you or a potential partner has a tendency toward self-defeating codependent behavior? Look for the following signs:

- Having obsessive feelings
- Overreacting
- Dredging up old issues
- Overlooking uniqueness
- Violating boundaries
- Not growing
- Buying into negativity

Having Obsessive Feelings

You constantly need positive reinforcement because you crave love and attention. When you are excessive you express feelings inappropriately. But no one deserves to be the sole focus of all your psychic energy. It is overwhelming to them and unproductive for you. You must determine what it is that you feel you need so desperately and then begin to understand that need in light of your own psyche. Learn to develop the good and to reject what is not helpful within you.

Overreacting

If you overreact to insignificant events, think about whether your response is unreasonable. You may be resorting to childish emotions to have your demands met. For example, you are so insecure in your relationships that each incident and each statement by the other seems to have enormous significance for your well-being. You must scrutinize everything they say and interrogate them about every nuance of a statement. You cast events in the worst possible light out of a fear that something that might affect your safety will slip by you.

Your overreactions create an environment that feeds rage, anger, frustration and anxiety, and leaves no space for genuine positive feelings. If people do not deal with you in an appropriate way, express honest reactions. But consider the possibility that you have not communicated correctly before you react with inappropriate anger or rage.

Dredging Up Old Issues

You keep dredging up old arguments because you never resolved the issues through honest communications. You're not being honest about the real nature of the problem. You are blaming others for their insensitivity to your needs because you hold them responsible for your nurturing.

Overlooking Uniqueness

A person who is not growing generally treats all relationships in the same way. You do not recognize what is unique in a relationship. To understand how dysfunctional this approach is, consider a coach who demands that every athlete train and perform in exactly the same way. He refuses to account for differences in body type, age, bone structure and so forth. It's a terrible way to deal with things. You must learn to respect the individuality of people and relationships.

Violating Boundaries

You have no right to invade other people's personal beliefs. But if you are codependent, that's the first way in which you will try to influence them.

Not Growing

If you focus on immediate problems but overlook their spiritual, emotional and intellectual elements, it's a sure sign that your growth has stagnated. This stagnation indicates that you are out of balance and overly focused on your problems. In fact, the only way that you can resolve problems is to consider them from higher levels.

Buying into Negativity

If someone you know always bitches and moans, and you accept what he says or does, then you are supporting codependency by participating in the negative behavior. Try not to make excuses for this situation. Just see it for what it is. You don't have to be critical, just honest.

What Do You Do When Things Get Tough?

When you are under extreme stress—the IRS audits you, you lose your job or you have an interpersonal crisis—you are likely to experience despair and helplessness. You feel out of control, perhaps even nauseous, and try to abandon the situation by seeking the quickest way out. Unfortunately this approach never works because you cannot run away from your problems. What you need to do instead is look for ways to get through crises.

In times such as these, one technique that may prove useful is positive visualization. When I face a conflict, I visualize a long road with a beautiful, beaming, healing light at the end. This image reminds me that the crisis is a part of my spiritual journey. As I travel this path, I notice the dragons and demons of my existence all around me. But rather than focus on them and be consumed by hopelessness and despair, I concentrate on the heroic qualities that will give me the strength to overcome my problems. I think about the virtues that have aided me in the past and present and that will support me in the future.

When you pay attention to your best qualities, you will find answers to your problems. When you concentrate on the problem alone, you will remain in crisis. Here are some of the good qualities you need to look for in yourself:

- Love
- Creativity
- Honesty
- Openness
- Trust
- Purpose
- Self-respect
- Sensitivity
- Life-affirming attitude
- Patience and caring
- Self-control
- Spirituality

Love

One of the most positive virtues you can have is an unconditional love of life and self. When you need to resolve a crisis or break negative patterns, look at your situation lovingly. Hate will only reinforce the negativity.

Creativity

Creative people have options. You have the ability to express yourself in deeper, more meaningful ways. And you can deal with your problems in new, original ways.

Honesty

Be honest with yourself about the nature of your problem so that you can approach it in a more realistic way.

Openness

You must be open to change, new values and new beliefs. Sometimes a problem signifies that you are holding onto something you need to let go of, such as a relationship that no longer contributes to your growth or your partner's. If you can let go, you may find the answer to your problem.

Trust

Trust that the process of change will be beneficial. Nobody is born a champion, and we all have problems to overcome in life. To get us on the road to change, however, we must trust the process of growth and our own definition of what is important and meaningful.

Purpose

When you have purpose in your life, you will be healthier and better equipped to overcome crises.

Self-Respect

Self-respect allows you to react from your needs and intuition, not from a sense of obedience.

Sensitivity

When you are sensitive to yourself, other people and the world around you, your real nature will manifest. Being cruel is the opposite of being sensitive.

Life-Affirming Attitude

People who take a positive position are inspirations to the world. I think we're all tired of hearing words such as but, can't, won't, shouldn't and couldn't from people who deny life.

Patience and Caring

A patient person realizes that the effort needed to accomplish something is worthwhile and that nothing comes all at once. Being caring allows you to empathize with others. People who possess the opposite qualities are restless and uninvolved.

Self-Control

You are able to control your own life without trying to manipulate others.

Spirituality

People who recognize a higher power know they are not alone in solving their problems. People who lack a spiritual connection try to resolve their problems in worldly ways with fraud and deception.

To this list of virtues, you could add many others that will help you to break your negative patterns. The more you focus on your assets, the stronger you will become. Becoming strong will make it easier for you to resolve conflicts.

If It's My Life, Then Let Me Live It

When you are in balance, you will be resolving your fears, acting on your intuitions and desires and feeling satisfied with your life.

What Do You Want to Make Important in Your Life?

Examine the different areas of your life and determine the elements that are important about each. Make a list of those you feel are critical to your well-being. Until you identify these areas and write them down, they may appear to be insignificant. If physical health has meaning to you, write it down. Otherwise, you may miss the connection between wellness and diet and continue to eat too many fatty foods such as hamburgers, pizza or french fries.

Once you decide what is meaningful in each area of life, determine what you must do to act in a way consistent with your priorities. What follows are some areas you might want to consider:

- Relationships
- Financial security
- Spiritual growth
- Sexual fulfillment
- Career growth
- Personal time
- Play time

Relationships

Define the qualities that you want from your relationships. Are your needs different from those you were led to believe are important? Perhaps you associate with businesspeople rather than the artists you really like because you are expected to mingle with the former. Think about what elements would comprise an ideal relationship for you. You must define what you want from a relationship before you can make it a reality.

Financial Security

What does financial security mean to you? To what degree does money—or the lack of it—dictate how you live your life? Some people use a lack of money as an excuse not to live their lives more fully. They may never travel and rarely socialize. And some people who have a lot of money live an equally limited existence. They become overly responsible and never find time for their friends and families. Others with limited incomes lead wonderful, happy lives.

The point is that wealth, in and of itself, is not a determinant of happiness. Why, then, do most people center their lives around money? In large part, they are seeking security. But they may become prisoners to money in the process. For example, many people work at jobs they hate "just for the money." Other people center their lives around money to gain acceptance. Newlyweds, for instance, often rush to buy a home and have a family they cannot afford because their families expect them to. As a result, they go into debt and need to work two jobs.

To avoid the pitfalls of money, you must reassess your material needs. When you want to buy something of significant value, ask what you must sacrifice to own that possession. Is it worth it to you? Can you give it up if you choose to, or will you become too attached to it? Is this something you really want or is it a status symbol that others expect you to own?

Spiritual Growth

Is spiritual growth important to you? Are you guided by your conscience or do you live by your animal nature? Do you have real concerns about the world, your fellow man and the quality of life in the world? If your generation and those of the future do not live with and address these concerns, you will suffer for it.

There are people on the streets who have all but eliminated conscience from their daily lives. They lie, steal, cheat, rape, and kill without remorse. This sociopathic attitude has become commonplace in all levels of society. Some bankers, corporate raiders and executives do basically the same thing. They are motivated strictly by gratification and are not at all concerned with the consequences of their actions.

Are you complacent about the world, or do you live your life according to a set of principles? Do you address things that you feel are inherently wrong, or do you simply allow them to happen? Are you aware of the quality of energy you put out every time you say, do or think something? Do you contemplate the positive or negative consequences of your actions? To become more fully empowered, you must be the one small voice that speaks out for yourself, your world, and the things of value in it.

Sexual Fulfillment

Is sexual fulfillment important in your life? Think about the role it plays and the ways in which you can fulfill your needs in a healthy way. If you have a spouse or lover, when was the last time you talked about your real needs in an open, honest way? When was the last time you considered their needs as part of your sexual fulfillment?

Career Growth

What are your career aspirations? This time next year, where would you like to be in your career? Have you planned for your professional growth and developed a plan to implement it? Recognize that you will never go anywhere if you do not have a plan and the desire to get there. You won't be able to break through the frustrations and limitations of your present position or profession.

Of course, you can find a million and one excuses to avoid taking the actions that will expand or change the direction of your career. But you could just as easily find a million and one reasons to alter your career. It's all in how you approach it. Excuses such as, "I don't have the time, money and support" are cop-outs that can be turned around and used in your favor. If you lack the proper education for a given career, for example, consider it an opportunity to devise imaginative approaches to the profession. Formal training may give you a set path to follow, but a lack of training will give you original insight into the situation.

Once you achieve the first success, you will identify the next goal you must accomplish. As you climb further up your ladder of success, you will recognize additional goals that are easier to achieve and more rewarding each time you attain one. If you have internal desire, you can do anything. There's nothing you can't do if you start with "I will" rather than "I can't."

Don't be discouraged by the time it takes to see results. All things happen in good time if they are worth waiting for, and you shouldn't defer, limit or ignore your goals simply because they take longer to achieve than expected. By focusing your attention on them, you will be able to nurture them to completion with favorable results.

Personal Time

Be sure to devote some time solely to your interests. My personal time is important to me because I am continually in the public eye and need time to rebalance. If someone shows up when I need to be alone, I don't hesitate to politely let them know that I will get back to them as soon as I can provide them with my time and attention. I would rather spend a shorter amount of quality time with someone than a longer period during which my attention is diverted by some other need.

Setting aside personal time each day can help to foster your creative, intellectual and spiritual growth. But to do so, you must create boundaries that cannot be crossed. Allowing others to transgress your intellectual and creative boundaries is not without consequences. For example, has anyone ever said to you, "Do you really think that way?" or "You don't really believe that, do you?" That person is showing no respect for your thoughts and feelings. In effect, he or she is saying that you are incapable of making an intellectual judgment on your own.

Most people are never encouraged to develop their own thoughts and beliefs. Early on, parents try to mold their children into who they want them to be instead of allowing them to develop into who they naturally are. In school, students are not supposed to have opinions that differ from their teachers'. Like parrots, they learn to say and do what is acceptable. At the same time, they lose sight of their real thoughts and feelings. This carries over into all phases of adult life. You only do what your doctor says, for example, and dismiss all forms of alternative medicine as quackery.

Unfortunately, children cannot fight back when adults transgress their boundaries or they will be rejected by their families. But you can learn to assert yourself as an adult. When someone asks for your opinion, give it to them in an honest and straightforward manner. This approach affirms what is legitimate for you.

You also need personal time to be creative. It doesn't matter what you create, so long as you receive pleasure from the creation. Many people prevent themselves from creating because they cannot justify the time involved. If it isn't marketable, they say, why devote time to it? As a result, they shut down their creativity. They have been programmed to believe that doing something for the fun of it is a waste of time. But if painting relaxes you and allows you to express yourself, don't let others tell you that it's only worthwhile if you create artwork that can be displayed.

Stop thinking that you must justify your actions and your mode of expression to anyone. Nobody's judgment should deter you from your creative outlets. The value of engaging in any particular activity comes from your inner perspective.

Play Time

Like most people, you probably do not give play time much credence. You take life too seriously. You get into heavy relationships and serious situations. You think play is something children do and grown-ups have no time for. In reality, life can be fun at any age. By allowing yourself time to play you lighten your load and keep your life in balance. Associate with people who understand that play is an important part of relationships. Lighten up. Have some fun with life.

What Do You Plan to Do to Change Your Life?

You've decided what is important to you and where you need to modify your life. Now you need a system to implement the necessary changes. Otherwise, change is simply not going to happen. You will see glimpses of what you want to change rolling through in your mind but you will never do anything about it.

Using all the lists you have developed here as a guide, make a schedule that allows time to concentrate on all the important areas of your life. Focus on the actions that will turn your life around in a positive direction. How can you use these times to your best advantage? What are the first steps you need to take to refocus your life? Don't feel that the first schedule you make is the one you must live with for the rest of your life. You can modify it as your life patterns change and continue to concentrate on the areas that will empower you.

What Beliefs Limit Your Growth?

As difficult as it may be, you may need to modify your beliefs to create positive change in your life. Take an honest look at your current beliefs. Which ones limit you, and what defense mechanisms do you use to hold on to them? Are you willing to do what it takes to let go of these beliefs? This is a difficult exercise because everyone tends to surround themselves with people and things that reinforce their beliefs—their parents, religion, school, job, and friends.

Sometimes you need to get away from familiar surroundings to gain a new perspective on your beliefs. One person who joined my detoxification program told me that being with our group helped him modify his beliefs and eliminate negative people from his life. Previously, he had always made excuses for their behaviors and attitudes. Now he can relate to more positive people. But he had to get out of his environment to see the situation objectively.

Your environment and the people in it may be healthy, positive and nurturing, or they may not. Be honest in your assessment and see your surroundings for what they are. Don't condemn or try to change what you cannot. You must respect others' rights to live as they see fit. To change your own life and belief systems, however, you must carefully examine them to see what works and what does not.

Do You Express Your Autonomy?

Autonomy is crucial to growth, and yet many people fear it. They don't want to stand out from the crowd, and believe they must live their lives in an average way to be acceptable to others. Living to please others is pointless. No matter what you do, some people will support your efforts and some will not. People see things from different perspectives because they come from dissimilar backgrounds. Therefore, their attitudes and beliefs might be right for them but wrong for you.

Granted, it is difficult to be autonomous in a society that values homogeny. Children are taught to think and behave in the same way. Those who think and feel differently from the group run the risk of being ridiculed. This also happens to people in the health movement. One day when I talked about my book, *Good Food, Good Mood*, on my radio show, a man called in and said, "I'm not one of those 'health food nuts' but I'm getting more fiber in my diet." He couldn't just admit that he felt good about the changes he was making. Instead, he had to show his friends that he was still a part of their group.

People distance themselves from anything that appears to be extreme. And in our society, doing something that announces to the world that you are an independent person is extreme. Living in a nontoxic environment is extreme. Detoxifying the pollutants from your body is extreme. But that doesn't mean you should not pursue these goals by being an autonomous individual.

Make a list of the ways in which you would like to express your autonomy. What would you like to do that is meaningful to you but appears extreme to others?

Do You Accept Responsibility for Too Many Things?

Make a list of all your responsibilities and then prioritize them so that the most important ones will receive the most time and attention. Accept that you have certain responsibilities that you cannot change. But also look to see if you have taken on responsibilities that are not necessary or beneficial to you. If you spend time agonizing over things that you do not need to be responsible for, you will not have time to make beneficial and meaningful changes in your life. You should be responsible, but you should choose what you will be responsible for.

Do You Do the Things That Give Your Life meaning?

Make a list of the things you do for the simple joy of doing them. If you jog each morning, for example, you may feel tired and achy but you've also accomplished your goal of enhancing your health. If at the end of the day you haven't put any garbage food into your body, you've made a positive step toward better health. If you do things for others but expect nothing in return, you've helped society and also rewarded yourself. When I jog in the park and find a rock or a stick in my path, for example, I always remove it so that other people won't have to contend with the hazard. It's not important to be acknowledged for such acts; the satisfaction of helping others is reward enough.

You must respect yourself before you can respect others. Respect for yourself, others and the world around you is what makes life meaningful. Don't procrastinate about doing the things that are meaningful to you. Don't put off a vacation because you don't have the time or money, and don't put off a relationship because you are too busy working. You will limit your existence if you play these games with yourself. You need to live your life every day in a meaningful way. Life is much too precious not to live it to the fullest.

Are Unreasonable Fears Holding You Back?

The following fears often are used to justify a lack of progress in life: taking a chance, competition, autonomy, intimacy, letting go, being open, being criticized, being unaccepted, losing control. Make a list of your fears and work to eliminate the ones that are holding you back.

When you make a change that you originally feared, you typically find that your fear was an illusion and that the dreaded results never materialized. Perhaps you need to change some aspect of your job, such as working new hours or taking a longer lunch, but you're afraid to approach your boss. Really, the worst thing that can happen is that he will say no. But if you prepare yourself well, you can show the boss that the change will not affect your work or productivity. You'll be happier and he will benefit from your continued productivity.

As this example shows, you must concentrate on the good that can result from change, not from the fears that deter you. When I lecture on natural health to a group of medical students, I fully realize that many people in the room will not accept the things that I am telling them. In fact, many will be angry with me. But the benefits of having even one person respond favorably to my lecture eliminates any apprehension I may feel. When you act on the things you fear, you become more empowered with each success, and your unreasonable fears will begin to dissipate.

What Other Things Are Holding You Back?

In addition to unreasonable fears, consider what other attitudes, behavioral patterns and physical constraints are holding you back from making positive change. These may include the following:

- Home
- Food
- Addictions
- Blocked communication
- Burdensome priorities
- Isolation
- Overresponsibility
- Too much restraint
- Lack of curiosity
- No sense of adventure
- Overlooking opportunities
- Unhealthy competition
- No relaxation
- Insecurity
- Avoidance of conflict
- Unrealistic goals
- Barriers
- Limits
- Materialistic values
- Irrelevant rules
- Lack of support
- Failure
- Holding back

Home

Does most of your time, money and attention go toward owning and maintaining a home? Has it become the driving force in your life, causing you to sacrifice other important goals? If so, step back and see if your home has become an obsession. If it's taking most of your time and energy, perhaps you would be better off renting.

Food

What role does food play in your life? Do you live to eat or eat to live? Your food should be dedicated to making you healthier. It should be enjoyable to eat but not a pastime or an obsession. What modifications do you need to make to eat better and obtain a healthier lifestyle?

Addictions

What addictions do you need to clear out of your life? Typical ones include cigarettes, coffee, food, alcohol, relationships, sex, and work.

Blocked Communication

Are you willing to communicate openly? Can you be honest about your needs? Can you allow people to see the real you instead of the one they have grown accustomed to? You'll have to prepare others for the fact that you're changing. Tell them that you are committed to making changes in your life and that you would like them to recognize the true you instead of the imitation. Let them know what the real you will be, without being intimidating or apologetic.

As you make changes, notice whether or not they accept you

for who you are. You will want to maintain a relationship with the ones who do; the others may need to go by the wayside. Remember, too, that communication is the most important aspect of any relationship, and the changes you make may very well alter the nature of your communication. If you have been dominant, you may begin to listen more. If you have been submissive, you may become more dominant and speak up for yourself.

Burdensome Priorities

Priorities are the parts of your life to which you devote specific blocks of time and attention. Make a list of your current priorities. Do you do these things by choice or because you are expected to? Are you willing to establish healthy priorities and rid yourself of unhealthy ones? The most difficult priorities to release are those that stroke your self-esteem, such as sending your child to an expensive school you cannot afford or working two jobs to finance your materialistic success. But some priorities are burdens that you must lift to live more fully. Other people may say you are being irresponsible, but your first responsibility is to yourself. Any priorities driven by guilt need to be eliminated from your life.

Isolation

Do you isolate yourself from the events around you, or do stay abreast of what's happening in the world? As social creatures, we don't live in a vacuum. We are a product of our environment, and everybody has a subtle influence on the world. Life will not go on as usual because you are complacent; rather, your complacency will allow others to gain a controlling influence that may not be in your best interests.

How can you become more aware of and involved in critical issues, such as the environment, human rights and animal rights? Choose the ones that are important to you and resolve to make a difference. Even if you don't join a formal organization to express your interest in an issue, you can influence others through the sincerity of your conversations on the issues that have meaning for you.

Overresponsibility

Do you express your independence, or are you tied to your relationships and responsibilities? I once went on a trip with a friend who felt he had to call home every few hours. It was obvious to me that he was more involved in the events of his home life than in enjoying himself on the trip. Sometimes you just need to let go and get away.

Can you get away from your everyday life? Can you enjoy an occasional retreat from your familiar surroundings?

Too Much Restraint

What do you do to show spontaneity? Do you ever do anything on the spur of the moment? Do you climb a mountain just because it's there? Do you take a day off from work and drive to the country?

Make a list of the things you do that are uniquely yours. What sets you apart from other people? Do you dress in an original way or have original ideas? Do you do anything that is absolutely different?

Lack of Curiosity

Are you curious about life and nature? Do you enjoy learning new things just for the sake of learning? As children we have a natural curiosity that is unblemished by ulterior motives. But as adults we allow our curiosity to be overshadowed by the mundane aspects of life. Before we know it, we have lost sight of our learning abilities and become stagnant and complacent. Eventually, we channel all of our efforts into making money and doing what's expected of us. We no longer take the time to explore life.

Average adults allow their curiosity to be satisfied by short, canned experiences, such as watching television or going to the movies. Or perhaps we accumulate knowledge for the purpose of display. Few adults take the time to satisfy their curiosity with a nature walk, a trip to a museum or even a good book. What do you do every day to express your curiosity?

No Sense of Adventure

How often do you head out into the unknown, without a clear idea of what will happen? Without some adventure in your life, you will become a boring person. Many people go on Freedom Bound Journeys, where they rough it for a week and forego their creature comforts. Despite the lack of any modern conveniences, they return from the adventure feeling exhilarated. Do you have any adventure in your life?

Overlooking Opportunities

Do you seize opportunities when they present themselves? Or do you sit around and wait for opportunity to knock? If you let new adventures in life pass you by without responding, you will no doubt regret it. Most people don't take the time and energy to create their own opportunities. They want the opportunities to come to them. But if you don't work to create opportunities, then you normally don't have the motivation to take advantage of them when they do arise. You miss out on a lot of life's excitement.

Unhealthy Competition

Unhealthy competition stunts personal growth; healthy competition enhances it. Competition is healthy when you relate to your own past accomplishments, rather than go head to head with someone else. When I race I don't compete against anyone else on the track. I compete with myself to try to do better each time. Sometimes I enter races knowing that I don't have a chance to win because I will be racing with Olympic champions. I enter for my own satisfaction. Racing with such people—and having my time logged in an official record—motivates me to beat my previous time.

No Relaxation

People who must occupy their minds at all times do not know how to relax. It's important to take the time to mellow out each day and eliminate the tensions of life. You can't do this by watching television, reading a book or otherwise occupying your mind. You need to let your mind relax after a hard day, just as you let your body relax after physical exercise.

Insecurity

Be secure in and of yourself. Don't rely on unnatural, man-made security to make you feel good about who you are. In today's workplace, which is rife with cutbacks and layoffs, people have learned that they can no longer rely on the outside sense of security that provided workers before them with a sense of protection.

Clearly, true security comes from within. When you live out your values and feel satisfied with your relationships, you will be secure. Recently I talked to a woman working at a health-food store in a small artists' community in New Mexico. When I asked her what she did prior to moving there, she said she had been a corporate lawyer. She had become disenchanted with the rules and regulations laid down by authority and went to New Mexico to do what she wanted and be who she was. For her, financial security, job security and relationship security were not as important as being with herself. The way in which you view security determines what you will do with your life.

Avoidance of Conflict

How do you handle conflict? Do you view it as an opportunity to grow, or do you run away and hope that the conflict will resolve itself? If you're intimidated by conflict, you will not grow. The same conflict will simply reappear in your life. Think about whether you are resolving your conflicts.

Unrealistic Goals

Have you always set goals for yourself? If so, evaluate them to see if they are healthy, positive and realistic.

Barriers

How do you view things that seem to stand in your way? Do you give up immediately and use the barrier as an excuse not to continue, or do you view it as a challenge and resolve to meet it head-on?

Limits

Do you recognize that many of the things limiting your growth are artificial and can be overcome? You can motivate yourself to transcend any situation.

Materialistic Values

Examine your values to determine if they are superfluous. Do you impose artificial limits on your social life by associating only with people of a certain social status, economic level or education? Do you value material existence more than nature? Look at all the people and experiences you are missing out on in life by subscribing to these values.

Irrelevant Rules

Is your life controlled by rules and regulations? Take a hard look at your sense of independence. Is it limited by all the things you are expected to do?

Lack of Support

If you do not get real support from your friends and family, it may be time to devote more energy to people who will support your efforts to grow and change. Real support is unconditional, while the support we get from most people is shallow and self-interested. Most people don't want to see you change because they are not ready to change themselves. A drinking buddy will not want you to quit drinking, for example, because then you will not have anything in common. You must give up certain relationships and look for more supportive ones.

Failure

Your failures should serve as learning experiences, not measures of inadequacy. No experience is a true failure if you learn from it in ways you did not anticipate. These beneficial lessons ultimately aid the process of growth. When you try something and fail, you may learn that you are not really cut out for that area and need to channel your energies into other endeavors. Equally important, failure can be a time of reassessment. Perhaps your presentation or audience was wrong in a new business venture, and you can now approach the goal in a different manner. As long as you are afraid of failure, you will never take chances and you will never grow.

Holding Back

When you have an idea, do you actualize it or ignore it? Do you have the confidence to share your ideas with a support group? Better yet, do you have a support group that allows you to share your ideas without ridicule? You need to share your ideas with people who help you make them happen. If the people who support you cannot help you directly, they may lead you to the right people to make your ideas materialize. When you have faith in your ideas, you will find creative ways to overcome the obstacles that limit most people.

Do You Try to Reduce Your Negativity?

Negative attitudes can make you feel disempowered, helpless, and controlled by others. Make a list of things you were negative about today. Think of ways you could have turned these events or feelings into positive situations. Try to visualize the end results.

Do You Have a Purpose in Your Life?

Having a purpose in life gives you direction and allows you to focus your time and talents on your goals. Without a purpose, you will wander aimlessly through life, dissipating your energies without accomplishing meaningful goals. Be aware that you may need to change your purpose as you grow. The important point is to maintain a clear view of what you want to accomplish so that your efforts will be concentrated.

If your purpose in life is unclear, make a list of things that are important to you and things that you like to do. Use these as a guide to help you find your purpose.

How Can You Modify Your Behavior?

Once you identify behaviors you want to change, you must trace the roots of these behavior patterns. Otherwise, you will continue to perpetuate the same old behaviors over and over and nothing will change. When you trace a behavior to its roots, it becomes easier to let it go. And, of course, any behavior that adversely affects your mental or physical health should be at the top of the list of those you want to modify, such as smoking, drugs, alcohol, eating habits, anger, violence, and stress.

Are You Overlooking Certain Realities?

Most of us only examine the beliefs presented to us by our religion, school, parents, friends and work. But some of these beliefs limit your ability to find solutions to problems. It's important to examine other beliefs with an open mind. In the 1960s, for example, many people went outside the Western culture to examine Eastern religion. This willingness to explore other ideas gave them new insight into the meaning of life.

When you have an open mind and a spirit of adventure, you may discover hidden ideas, beliefs, values and solutions in places you otherwise would not have looked.

What Things Do You Purposely Avoid?

No doubt you have certain goals in life that you always find an excuse not to pursue. Make a list of these, since identifying them is the first step to facing them. Be sure to include everything you avoid in the major areas of your life, such as your career, your relationships and your family. This exercise allows you to focus on the ones that are important to your growth and fulfillment. It also helps you to clarify any concepts in your life that are ill-defined and therefore difficult to modify.

What Parts of Your Life Are Out of Balance?

Put the various elements of your life into proportion, according to the real value they have for you. Your work and your pleasure each must have its own time and place. When your life is in balance, you will be satisfied with the way everything is going. You will be happy with your work, for example, rather than doing a job you dislike or wanting to make a transition to a new job.

For practical purposes, balance can be defined as a state in which everything that can be dealt with has been dealt with. There are no festering problems nor unresolved questions lingering in your mind. There are no inner conflicts that gnaw away at you. In essence, your life is in order: You are eating the right foods, doing the right exercises on a routine basis, talking out your problems, resolving your fears, and acting on your intuitions and desires.

When you concentrate on one area of your life, the others do not interfere with the tasks or pleasures at hand.

Conversely, an imbalance in any area of your life will carry over into everything else you do. When unresolved problems cannot be set aside, your mind will not be on the task at hand.

Thus, you cannot forget about your work problems when you are at home with your family, or your work suffers because of unresolved problems at home.

For this reason, you need to deal with unresolved conflicts as they arise. At the very least, get them out in the open so that you can acknowledge they exist and need to be resolved. This approach will allow you to focus your time and attention on one area, without dissipating your energies in other parts of your life. Maintaining this essential balance is one of the keys to a better life.

Rediscovering Your Real Self

*To be a healthier person, value your
uniqueness and look for the people in the
world who will accept you just the way
you are.*

Do Your Parents Expect You to
Live Out Their Dreams?

How do your parents respond when you pursue your ideals?
Do they support your efforts to express these ideals, or do they
burst your bubble and dictate how you should live? Suppose
your father expects you to be a football star because he never
reached the big time himself and sees you as his proxy ego. But
you would like to be a pianist because music expresses your
artistic nature. If your father verbalizes his disapproval of this
"unmasculine" choice, he denies your real needs.

The question is, do you need your father's opinion to reaffirm that you are okay? If so, you will deny yourself the satisfaction of doing something meaningful and try to live for him
instead. You may even be successful at it, but you will never

be fulfilled, because it is his dream, not yours. The same is true of women, of course, who often make choices to gain their parents' approval. Men and women alike must curb the tendency to live through their parents' egos.

Be honest in looking at all areas of your life. Have the courage to see what is before your eyes. You will destroy your instinctual and intuitive self if you do not let yourself know what you know. Anything you do not want to see is the very thing you need to see. You will become curious about many things when you stop narrowing your reality through denial of what is painful to you. When you question your conditioning, you will free yourself. When you eliminate negativity from your life, you will find your creativity.

Are Your Relationships Dysfunctional?

Tell other people the truth about yourself; otherwise, you will encourage dysfunctional relationships. You must be able to define your real needs and express them to others. Your relationships should acknowledge and honor those needs. Why choose to stay in any relationship—be it with a lover, family member, friend or job—if your needs are not addressed? If the relationship only allows you to recognize artificial or socially contrived needs, you will be completely unfulfilled.

The longer you display false happiness, the more you feed a dysfunctional relationship. If someone tells you repeatedly that your thoughts are wrong or stupid, he is transgressing your intellectual and emotional boundaries. And if you allow yourself to be invalidated this way, you will only have merit when someone of importance agrees with you. This process fuels insecurity, which will cause you to look and listen very carefully to see how other people view reality. With no reality of your own, you will try to match your actions to their reality so that they will continue to accept you. But the moment you go against anyone else's views or beliefs, you are discounted.

Are You Conditioned to Condone Injustice?

Government, industry, religion and other institutions exert an enormous amount of control over people. In all walks of life, we see examples of what happens to those who voice a challenge to authority. Consider the Amish woman who quietly challenged the subservient role of women in the Amish religion. She said that women should have the right to join in the governing process. What did she get for her efforts? She was reprimanded by the church and then excommunicated when she persisted. Her husband divorced her and her children were brainwashed to abandon her. The church's influence was so strong that every single friend and family member turned against her. But what had she really done to deserve such harsh treatment?

For another example of the injustices spawned by institutions, one need only look at organized medicine. Patients who choose a non-traditional approach to treatment, such as nutrition or vitamin therapy, are considered to be irrational by society at large. And the doctors who offer these treatments are branded as quacks. The controlling boards of the medical establishment do not hesitate to punish doctors who do not abide by their standards.

No matter that the doctor is healing patients. He or she will pay for traveling an alternative path. One doctor in California, for example, offered nutritional therapy to cancer patients who had not been helped by radiation or chemotherapy, the mainstays of conventional medicine. He helped more than 260 patients strengthen their immune system and overall health without the side effects of conventional therapy.

What did he get for his efforts? Marshals broke into his

house and arrested him and his wife. Later he was convicted of a felony, but not because his patients were dying or his method was scientifically unacceptable. In fact medical literature supports the efficacy of nutritional therapy. And it was not because his colleagues did not support him. Many people came forward to testify that his treatment made sense.

He was convicted and sentenced to hard labor for one reason alone: He went against the institutional grain and chose something different. He rejected the prescribed treatment of chemotherapy, surgery and radiation, none of which truly help heal cancer patients. The laws of California favor the medical monopoly so overwhelmingly that anyone who steps over the line, no matter how well they succeed, will be destroyed. Any doctor who has deviated since has also been destroyed.

Isn't it strange that no one from the church, the media or the political and educational communities came forth to intervene on this doctor's behalf? They did not say, "This doctor is treating people and they're getting well. We're crucifying him for it. That doesn't make sense." Here again, the established system we have been conditioned to accept simply does not face any challenge.

In fact, our conditioning teaches us to accept the many contradictions, inconsistencies and failures within our belief systems. We resign ourselves to living within the system and silence the objections raised by our mind and spirit. We fail to recognize that our social systems are based on pure economics, and we don't question whether industry has the people's interests at heart, which it clearly does not. If society tells us to live and eat in ways that produce disease, we become prisoners of disease. If the meat industry tells us to eat cancer-causing meat, we deny this cause-and-effect relationship because we have been brainwashed to believe that meat is healthy.

The paradigms set forth by society are powerful forces indeed. Trying to change them can be like trying to move a mountain. Even so, you can take small steps that will eventually change an unjust system. First and foremost, you must redirect your energies from unjust systems to those that support your beliefs. You can buy household products that do not use animals in their testing and invest in companies that do not violate human rights. You can encourage healthier farming practices by buying organic food. As more and more people take such actions, small change becomes a trend, which, in turn, becomes the norm. New paradigms are created through the process of enlightenment.

Make a list of the things you truly believe in. Are you supporting these beliefs with your time and money?

Do You Waste Time in Relationships That Prevent You from Growing?

In all likelihood, the patterns of healthy and unhealthy behavior that you learned in childhood are with you today. But remember the first rule of empowerment: You don't have to justify anything to anyone at any time when you are on your own. You don't have to consult with, share with, or get approval from your family. It's your life. You can live it as you wish.

Our families condition us to be obedient for so long that we continue to seek their approval throughout life. You probably know the routine: You take a boyfriend or girlfriend home to get the family's approval. Who's marrying the person anyway, you or your family? When you want to change jobs, move or start a new career, you consult with your family to make sure the change will be accepted. Why? It's your life, not theirs. This is not to say, of course, that you shouldn't share growth and happiness with your family, provided they are supportive of your ideas. In that case, they will see that you are taking positive steps toward personal growth. They will help you in your decision-making process and you will benefit from that support.

But if the love you received was conditional, a sense of fear will haunt you for the rest of your life. You will fear abandonment, which makes us feel that we are alone, unlovable and unworthy. You'll spend your whole life trying to make someone else love you. You may overwork and overstrive. Spontaneity will fade from your life because you cannot release the child in you, whom you believe to be unacceptable. In the end, everything you do will be aimed at making others feel comfortable with you. You will act like a compliant child no matter how old you get. It's just a game, but a vicious one indeed.

To be a healthier person, you must stop the game. You don't have to be obedient to anyone, nor must you alter your nature to gain the acceptance of others. There are people in the world who will accept you just as you are. Look for them.

Make a list of all your important relationships and evaluate whether or not they are healthy. Are others supportive of your beliefs or do they try to influence you with their own?

How Do You Deal with Stress?

There's no denying that today's society produces enormous stress. The sad part, however, is that we have very few healthy mechanisms for alleviating that stress. The average American, with too many unpaid bills, may try to release stress by watching *American Gladiators* on Saturday afternoon. The announcer gets them worked up at the prospect of watching a tractor roll over other cars. What does that say about our coping mechanisms? Does it really resolve stress to watch someone crush the top of six cars in eight seconds?

The strange methods of relaxation adopted by our culture show no appreciation of the higher values in life, such as spirituality, intellect, and creativity. Instead, society encourages us to form addictive habits, supposedly to alleviate tension, when in fact they compound the stress. For decades, movies and television commercials influenced people to smoke, drink and take prescription drugs to relieve daily stress. To this day, good health habits and whole, healthy meals are not depicted. If all you ever see are people who drink coffee on the run, you will revert to this image when trying to subdue stress. I'd much rather watch an 80-year-old woman skate at Laguna Beach or see a 90-year-old man run a marathon. That, to me, is normal. The hippies of the 1960s also showed us how to have fun with life and to express ourselves with bright colors, dance, and music. For the most part, their attitude about life was a healthy reaction to their parents' disapproval of fun. Their nonsmiling, serious parents never let them forget the sacrifices they had made for them. They expected their children to become just as obedient, contrived, controlled and powerless as they were—the perfect prescription for passing on stress-related diseases to the next generation.

America's addictions manifest themselves in our powerless attitudes, our lack of bonding and honesty and our inability to actualize life. We tend to overlook real values and instead seek a false utopia. We want to escape the everyday monotony and boring routines of our lives. Therefore we look for something to distract us from the seemingly unchangeable nature of our lives. Coffee, alcohol, cigarettes, cocaine, marijuana and crack—all of these appear to give us the high that will take away the pain for a moment.

We turn to drugs when we don't feel good about who we are and when we are not encouraged to engage in life. The kid on the street taking crack, the adult on Wall Street taking cocaine and the politician sidling up to the bar have one thing in common. They're all in pain. But rather than be honest about the cause of the pain, we blame others for our addictions—the South American coke dealers, the cigarette manufacturers, the bars that serve alcoholics. The truth is that if we put every cocaine dealer in the world in jail, coke would be back on the streets in six months.

A crisis cannot be resolved by addressing the symptoms alone; you have to dig deeper to get to the cause. But that would mean acknowledging that your guiding paradigm is flawed. As a nation, we don't want to admit that our biases, prejudices, and lazy thinking are erroneous. It's too painful. Instead we choose to blame others for our problems, pointing the finger at anyone who is not a part of us. This hostility leads us to create artificial, unnecessary conflicts in the world.

Ultimately we end up with misdirected, stressful lives. We try to relate to other people through soap operas, trashy novels and magazines, movies, and even the evening news. Why would you be interested in someone else's sex life? Perhaps you don't have one of your own. Why would you be interested in someone else's success? Perhaps you don't feel successful in life. What do you gain from soap operas, which are filled with treachery, adultery, murder, deceit and lies? That's not real life. Participating in someone else's pain and discomfort may allow you to escape from your own feelings, but it's a negative way to deal with stress. People who are living their own lives don't have the time or inclination to worry about how other people live.

And what about the news? Every evening, we see that people have been murdered, burned in car wrecks and so on. Will this make you feel good and enhance your life? We should be reading books or watching shows that provide insight and information and contribute to our growth. No wonder so many people are dysfunctional, since we receive so little input on being functional.

What Causes Stress in Your Life?

To deal with stress effectively, you must identify stress-generators in your life. Some of the common ones include:

- Family
- Personal environment
- Career
- Relationship
- Self

Family

Families can create stress by transgressing the boundaries of their members, assuming that they have a right to do or say anything they want to another family member without respect for his or her feelings. Stress also is created when a family member is inflexible, impatient and unwilling to listen and learn. You must deal with such stress as soon as it arises.

What's more, you may not spend enough quality time with your family because you don't make the time, or you devote too much time to matters of less importance. Ideally, much of your time should be spent with family, friends and yourself. If you're spending it elsewhere, you are allowing superficial needs to overshadow essential ones.

Make a list of the stresses in your family life. These are the ones you need to change.

Personal Environment

Your environment may be stressful if it's too small, too large, too noisy, too hard to maintain or too costly. Have you ever said to yourself, "I could enjoy life more if I didn't have the stress of maintaining this expensive house or lifestyle?" You may fool yourself into believing you will enjoy yourself once the house is paid off or the kids are gone. But that day never seems to come.

Sometimes the only solution is to let go. If your house is a true burden, consider getting rid of it. This can be a real challenge if you have a large emotional investment in the house. To ease the transition, visualize the advantages of living in a place you can afford. In other cases, you may need to get away from your immediate surroundings to determine whether or not they are healthy for you. You may discover that your present environment is satisfactory after all or that it needs to be changed.

I once met a man in a small New England town who had

returned to the town following a stint in the Midwest. He had moved away to work as a computer scientist, but eventually realized that his 15-hour workdays did not allow room for him to have a life. With that awareness, he made the decision to return to his roots and live a more balanced life. The desire to return had been in the back of his mind for some time, but it was his time away that made him appreciate what he originally had.

When he came home, he bought an old house and spent much of his time fixing it up. He was able to relax because he could easily afford the house and didn't have to devote so much time to work. And he was able to spend more time with his family, his friends and himself. He earned only one-tenth of his former salary, he said, but his life was a hundred times better.

That's going home in the right way. Your essential needs really have nothing to do with the things you are conditioned to want. All across America, people are returning home with this attitude, but not necessarily to the home they came from. They are going to environments that feel like home and make them comfortable. If you don't feel that you belong in your environment, you will feel out of place in everything you do.

I meet many people in my travels who tell me they can never commit themselves to anything because they don't feel comfortable with their situation. As a result, they always have one foot out the door in their relationships, their work and every phase of their lives. These people are always confused, always in crisis. They can never give their full energy to anything or anyone.

List the things you cannot afford in terms of time and money. Assess their importance to determine which you might be better off without. Then list the aspects of your environment that make you feel comfortable or uncomfortable. Do you have a burning desire to live in a different sort of environment, or are you happy where you are? To perform this analysis, learn more about other parts of the country that interest you.

Career

Is your career too limiting, competitive or demanding? Does it just not feel right? If your career is in crisis, whatever the reason, you must address the cause of that stress. Identify the conditions behind these feelings; then, either change the conditions or change your career.

To get to the root of your problem, listen to your inner guides. They are in touch with your intuitive feelings and thus will give you good guidance. All you need then is the courage to follow through on your decision. I meet men and women across America who are starting over in their careers—and feeling much better for it. They undergo some tremendous changes, but the process allows them to live in a more enjoyable, stress-free way.

Make a list of the aspects of your career that concern you. Can you change these things, or do you need to change your career entirely?

Relationships

If you accept the traditional paradigm, which teaches us to feel threatened by anyone who is different, then your relationships will be stressful. How many people have you rejected in your life without knowing why? Do you look for excuses or minor flaws in others to justify your inclination not to socialize with them?

It's not an unusual tactic. Take a look around. You never see the rich with the poor, the educated with the uneducated, the beautiful with the ugly, the healthy with the sick. That's because people feel threatened outside of their narrowly defined categories. If they have difficulty listening to their instincts, they also may have trouble determining who is safe. To broaden your life, you must accept different realities and respect people for who they are. If you show your respect in a noncompetitive way, you will have the opportunity to learn from people of all types.

The imbalances in relationships can create stress as well. You may be too dominant or overly submissive. Your relationship may be too sexual or not sexual enough. You may be giving too much time to the relationship or taking it for granted. You may feel jealous or you may provoke jealousy in your mate.

Whatever the imbalance, you can only solve such problems by identifying the issues at hand and getting them out in the open. If you cannot be honest about your real needs and feelings, nothing will change. Don't worry if you are initially afraid to talk about the problems. Once you start, you may find that the process enhances the relationship. When you bring your feelings to light, you may even find that the other person thinks and feels the same way. If you cannot talk your problems out, it may be time to let the relationship go.

Make a list of the relationships you have now and the ones you would like to have. Evaluate the ones that could be most beneficial to you and nurture these relationships.

Self

With a balanced life, you have time for your body, mind, spirit and emotions. Those who lack this balance may throw all their energy in one direction, to the exclusion of all else, or they may scatter their energy among too many areas.

If you are not careful, you can easily overcommit yourself. Learn to say yes when you mean yes and no when you mean no. Have the self-assurance to know that you can give an honest response. You may find that the only time you are truly honest is when you yell in anger; otherwise you conceal the truth behind hidden agendas. Wouldn't it be better to be happy and honest?

To eliminate stress, you must be consistent in your life. It doesn't pay to go overboard in one direction or the other. Many people experience too many swings in their lives: They become too lonely or too excited, they need someone or they become aloof, they can't express themselves at all or they over-react. To end these gyrations, establish balance and focus on healthy endeavors. Allow yourself to heal by taking the time to play every day, not just on weekends or holidays.

What First Step Are You Willing to Take to Initiate Change?

Decide today to change something in your life, and then take a first step toward making that change. What first step do you feel comfortable taking? Don't worry if it is not the best or most appropriate step. Don't let an imperfect step stop you from taking any action at all. Just begin. Take the first step.

Consider this example: A person with a kind nature, who tends to be taken advantage of by certain people, decides to become more assertive and confront these people. He has identified the change he wants to make, but he may not be certain what to do when the situation next arises. The important part is that he has resolved to assert himself. As a first step, he may read a book on the topic or join a support group to help him overcome his doubts and fears.

In time, your small successes will build your confidence in making important changes. You will be using a challenging situation to change, grow and express your true nature. List the areas in which you need to change, and commit to taking a first step, whether alone or with the help of a support group.

What Do You Do That Is Boring, Meaningless and Unfulfilling?

These activities will disempower you and rob your life of excitement and spontaneity. Human beings are social by nature, but that does not mean you must lose your uniqueness to exist in a larger society. You are free to be original and spontaneous as long as you show respect for other people's values.

Write about the areas of your life that you find boring, meaningless and unfulfilling. Which would you like to eliminate? What would you like to do instead? Think about how you can express your uniqueness and, in the process, give your life more essential meaning.

What Types of People Do You Look Up to?

Frequently the very qualities you admire in others are the ones you yearn to express yourself. In people you look up to, you see an essential part of yourself that you were never encouraged to develop. Suppose that you were once excited by the idea of a spiritual journey and you meet a man who has been on a spiritual path for some time. You admire him for having persevered and attained great peace and insight. In your own life, you had done more "practical" things by taking a job, marrying and having children. As the years passed, you felt more and more bound by your responsibilities. Now your encounter with this man reminds you of a part of yourself that you had almost forgotten. You wonder if pursuing a spiritual path would bring greater happiness to your life.

Pay attention to the qualities you admire in others. Identify the people you look up to and the characteristics in them that you respect. Ask yourself, do I need to express these qualities in myself? No one else can complete your development for you, and an awareness of the qualities you admire in others can be key to understanding your own needs.

What Purpose Do Your Work and Relationships Serve?

Ask yourself what you are truly striving for in your work and relationships. Is the work you do essential to your life, or do you work for financial rewards only? Are you in an ideal relationship, but somehow you and your partner do not work toward personal ideals? Re-evaluate the essence and purpose of your work and relationships. Perhaps they have gotten off track.

Beyond that, define the roles of the important people in your life. What do these people mean to you? This process may enlighten you about the reasons behind your relationships. And it will help you to evaluate whether these people should or should not remain a part of your life.

How Do You Express Love, Intimacy, Vulnerability, Anger, Pain, Hope and Other Emotions? With Whom Do You Share Your Feelings?

The emotions you feel comfortable expressing may depend on who you are with. For example, you may be able to express love and intimacy, but not negative emotions, with your partner. Instead you feel more comfortable sharing any fear and insecurity about the relationship with a close friend. Consequently your friends know more about how you feel toward your partner than he or she does. That makes for incomplete communication within the relationship.

Identify any feelings that go unexpressed in your relationships and address these incomplete emotions. Perhaps you and your partner could write a poem to each other expressing your feelings in a constructive way. You can express more through verse and rhyme than through talking because you must break down your thoughts and feelings to write a poem. In conversation, by contrast, you may rationalize your feelings away and generalize your thoughts and spoken words.

This is a particularly good exercise for men because they tend to hide their feelings. Women, on the other hand, are usually more connected to their emotions.

Write a Poem or Story About the Unlearned Lessons of Your Childhood, Young Adulthood or Adulthood

By writing about the unfinished lessons of your childhood, you can help put your past behind you. This exercise may take months, but it is well worth the effort. To start, sit down quietly and recall the past. As you look at your life, see the lessons that you never had a chance to complete. If you are like most people, past circumstances have limited your potential for growth. And the older you get, the more difficult change may be. If you can find out what is missing in your life, you can open yourself up to greater fulfillment.

Imagine how your life would be different had you completed these unlearned lessons. Let's say that you were musically inclined as a child but never given the opportunity to take music lessons. As an adult you have lost touch with that creative part of yourself. By rekindling this desire through visualization, you may be able to incorporate the talent into your life once more. You may not be the professional musician you once could have been, but you can make music a creative outlet for your personal enjoyment.

Repeat this exercise for the young adult and mature adult stages of your life. If you were to learn new lessons today, what would they contain that your previous lessons did not allow? In performing this analysis, look at the following areas of life: family, sexuality, denial, service, friends, money, religion, self-esteem, career, men/women, armed forces, food, school, rituals, sacrifice, death.

Let Your Spiritual Guide Help You Complete Your Development

Dysfunctional qualities usually result from incomplete development of some aspect of your life. To address this problem, imagine that you have a spiritual guide who is taking you back in time to explore your unlearned lessons. Remember in *A Christmas Carol*, when three spirits take Scrooge on a tour of his life? In a similar way, your spiritual guide will present him- or herself to you. Take a moment to close your eyes and visualize your spirit guide now.

Next, ask your parent(s) or other people who were essential to your development to appear. Imagine that you are all going back to times in the past when your development was hindered. You may see yourself playing alone as a child, for example. You feel lonely because no one is paying attention to you. Communicate these feelings, which you were unable to verbalize then (and are still carrying), to your spirit guide and your parent. You might say, "Look at little Timothy over there. He is playing with imaginary friends because you didn't give him any time. He's running into his room now because he's terrified by your screaming. And when the lights go out he's going to talk to his little friends about you." Repeat this process for each painful memory to heal the spirit of your parents, teachers or others who contributed to your lack of development.

Then look at yourself as a teenager and identify painful experiences that have not been communicated and resolved. If a girl was date-raped as a teenager, for example, she may not have told her parents for fear they would hold her responsible and view her with shame. As a result, she has suffered silently for many years and may even be physically sick. Now she can ask her spirit guide to show her parents the emotional pain she endured due to a lack of love and support. By explaining such feelings to your parents, you can forgive them and let go of the past. You will resolve the pain and complete another important lesson.

Remember, the guide is teaching your parents about the pain by showing them what the child is feeling. In effect, you're working on a spiritual level to get to the core of the incomplete parts of your development. You're seeing how your past affected you, and you're allowing yourself to forgive your parents and others who played an important role in your development.

What Areas of Your Life Need Attention? Are You Addressing Your Essential Needs?

Are you ignoring important areas of your life because they appear to be out of your control? You may be afraid that you will feel bad about yourself if you fail at a new endeavor, or you may worry that others will judge you by such failures. Don't simply deny that needs exist in order to avoid dealing with them. If your relationships are unhealthy, for example, you must engage in healthy relationships to grow. Start by learning some lessons from your past relationships. Examine the constructive and destructive aspects of each and ask yourself which essential needs were being met and which were not.

Look at other areas of your life as well, and strive to fulfill your essential needs. Let go of everything else. Once you identify your true needs, it will be easy to walk away from the nonessentials. I've built some beautiful things in my life, including a restaurant, a ranch and a farm, but I let them go the moment they were no longer essential to me. The change came easily because I could break my connection to them when they no longer served my needs.

Clearly our essential needs can change as we progress through life. A 40-year-old spends his day differently than does a 20-year-old because his feelings about mortality change. Few 20-year-olds run in the park, while thousands of 40-year-olds do so because exercise has become more essential to them. It helps them feel younger and healthier and slows down the aging process.

What is essential to your well-being today? What things do you hold onto out of habit, even though they no longer serve an essential function in your life? Focus on attending to your essential needs, and let go of the nonessentials.

How Do Your Perceptions Distort Reality?

Your perception of the world may prevent you from enjoying life. When your perceptions distort reality, they can affect you more than the event itself. If you are in a beautiful meadow, do you perceive the grandeur of nature or unseen hazards such as snakes and lizards? The danger in letting perceptions overshadow reality is that you lose sight of what is real and important.

What things in your life could be viewed as misdirected perceptions? Which perceptions bother or intimidate you? List the perceptions that limit your happiness and well-being. Try to reassess the situation in a more positive light.

Begin to Reconstruct Your "Real Self"

Where does this process begin? First you must accept your imperfections as a part of your being. Then you can identify ways to transform each imperfection and eliminate it from your life. Although few of us like to acknowledge the parts of our lives that do not work, you can only grow by recognizing the weakest part of yourself. One liability can negate many assets. Just as you cannot build the Taj Mahal on a foundation of quicksand and expect it to stand, you cannot expect to change without an honest assessment of your flaws.

Work on one shortcoming at a time. Ask yourself, "How can I convert this imperfection from a weakness to a strength?" Stay with the imperfection until you have resolved it. Don't deny the problem; deal with it. If necessary, get feedback from another person or a support group to help you with the process.

Are You Living a Role That Masks Your True Self in Order to Cope?

Many people get caught up in archetypal or culturally prescribed behavior patterns. Some of these include: 1) the predator/aggressor/dominator; 2) the prey/victim/submissive/blamed; 3) the savior/warrior/hero; 4) the magician/illusionist/escape artist. See where these or other roles appear in your life.

The predator needs to conquer, dominate and control, while the prey is a submissive victim who takes the blame for everything. The magician seeks to escape reality. Many people, particularly artists, can identify with a need for fantasy and illusion. And saviors, for their part, generally have been hurt in some way. To compensate for the pain, they strive to win favor and praise from others and thereby raise their self-esteem.

They want someone else to validate their life when, in fact, this validation must come from within.

You may exhibit various combinations of these behaviors at different times. But these roles can mask your inner self, so be alert to the ways in which they show up in your life.

How Do You Use Control and Guilt?

Control itself is neither constructive or destructive. What matters are the reasons behind your use of control. For example, do you try to induce guilt in others when they begin to make positive changes? Suppose your husband makes noticeable improvements in his physical and mental health by joining a health club. If you feel threatened by these changes, you may retaliate by making him feel guilty for spending time away from the family. Similarly you may use guilt as a defense mechanism to avoid making much-needed changes in yourself.

List the control and guilt mechanisms you use, and then examine your reasons for using them. Are your reasons for controlling a situation constructive or destructive? Do you try to improve the situation or do you become vindictive? Do you make someone else feel guilty because you are afraid of change?

Can You Separate Real Needs from Conditioned Needs?

Learn to distinguish between the things you are conditioned to want and those you truly need. Our conditioned wants are not necessarily bad; in some cases, they may reflect our true needs. But you must separate the fact from the fiction so that you can abandon the conditioned needs that do not represent your true self. For example, you may have been conditioned to believe that living in a luxury apartment is a symbol of success and a key to happiness. When it comes right down to it, though, you would be much happier in a little country home.

Define the Boundaries of Your Inner Self

Be wary of people who try to attack your thoughts and make you think as they do. No one has that right. Your inner self is a place where you can be comfortable. If people try to invade this space, let them know that it's off limits to them.

Make a list of the thoughts you have that are exclusively yours. Then write down the ones that are influenced by others.

If You Expressed Your Real Self, What Type of Confrontation Would Occur? What Would Change?

When you begin to identify and express your real needs, sooner or later you will come into conflict with someone. Here is where you must take control by standing up for yourself and continuing to express your inner truth. Consider such confrontations as opportunities for growth. Initially other people may resist the changes you have made, but you must persevere to establish your newfound sense of self.

Just Do It

*Take control, discover what you want and
then let people know that you are ready
to share your positive energies.*

How Would You Fare if You Put Your Life on Trial?

Make a list of people in your life—family members, friends, coworkers, supervisors, religious leaders, teachers—and then describe their opinions of you (based on your perceptions). Assume that your character is on trial. These people will be weighing the good and bad. How do you fare? Where do your weaknesses lie? Is there a consistent misperception? Perhaps they all perceive you as stingy when you see yourself as giving. As your own attorney, how do you defend yourself? If their perceptions are correct and the fault lies within, what can you do to change their perception of you?

What Types of Circumstances Make You Feel Good or Bad?

Look at a typical period of time in your life. Identify the elements that make you feel good and those that make you feel bad. Some of these may include:

- Acceptance
- Security
- Calmness
- Freedom
- Happiness
- Relief
- Relaxation
- Balance
- Words
- Sound
- Taste
- Smell
- Touch
- Other people's behavior

Acceptance

Acceptance creates positive feelings. When people accept you unconditionally, you emote good feelings.

Security

Security also generates a positive response. List the things that make you feel secure, such as self-esteem, love, appreciation, or feeling comfortable.

Calmness

Nature creates serenity because it doesn't require anything of you. There's a natural rhythm to listening to the rain on the roof, watching a sunset or sunrise, or watching the moonlight on a quiet lake.

Freedom

You will feel free when your life is in control, but you do not have to control others.

Happiness

What makes you feel happy and carefree? Can you get in touch with the inner child? When the child within comes out to play, you forget your troubles and do things just for the sake of doing them. You don't worry about making mistakes. You lighten up and enjoy the moment.

Relief

This feeling usually follows a crisis, when you no longer have to deal with the tension and anxiety created by the situation. The stark contrast of these times makes you appreciate everyday life all the more.

Relaxation

You feel relaxed when you can be yourself and don't have to do anything special, such as when you sleep in on a Sunday morning. The opposite feeling occurs when you try to please others because you are engrossed in projecting an image that you want them to see. You should be able to relax a good part of the time, not just in rare moments.

Balance

Any action or behavior taken to an extreme will adversely affect your sense of well-being. If you exercise excessively or not at all, you are unbalanced. If you eat too much or too little, you're unbalanced. If you cannot express love or you show love to the point of obsession, you're unbalanced.

To achieve balance, then, you must be at peace with who you are. This process requires focus, attention and time spent on self-development. When you identify your excesses and balance them, you will find the time to be a whole and happy person.

Words

Words have the power to offend, control and demean when they are purposely used that way. You may have been conditioned to respond to certain words with submission or anger. It's no accident that the term "boy" was used to address black men. It was meant to dehumanize and disempower them, just as the word "girl" kept women in their place before the advent of the women's liberation movement. People didn't have to treat you like a man if they called you boy, and they didn't have to respect you as an intelligent woman if they called you girl.

Make a list of the words to which you react. You'll be able to view them differently—and maintain control of the situation—if you can hear these words without getting emotionally involved. Try to accept them as just words. Equally important, make a conscious effort to use words that encourage other people. Why not make people feel good about who they are? Think about what it feels like to be on the other end of what you are sharing.

Never gossip. If you have something to say to someone, talk to him or her about it privately. Don't threaten or intimidate, just say what you feel. If someone does something that concerns or displeases you, don't automatically assume that he or she is wrong. Give others an opportunity to explain their side, and you just might see the situation from a different perspective.

Sound

Think of the sounds that make you feel good. Try to surround yourself with these sounds as much as possible.

Taste

Take time to savor the foods that taste good to you. Even if you're having a quick snack or lunch, chew your food slowly and really experience the flavor.

Smell

Pleasant smells provide a great psychological boost. In fact, many hospitals are now trying to facilitate the healing process by replacing medicinal odors with pleasant aromas.

Touch

The sense of touch is a healthy stimulus. We demonstrate true love when we hold hands or hug. Unfortunately, our society discourages hugging because we characterize it as sexual. In the process, we overlook one of the greatest therapeutic actions available to us in life.

Other People's Behavior

Modern society breeds paranoia in many people. But as long as you fear others, you will never be in control of your life. You will feel helpless, rejected, insecure, anxious, controlled, sad, apprehensive, tense and weak. Believe in yourself and know that you can handle any situation.

What Causes Your Life to Stagnate?

Have you ever noticed that you tend to rely on the same old excuses—and recycle the same old doubts—when you want to avoid making changes in your life? Suppose that you make excuses not to go out with your friends time after time. By doing so you are purposely sabotaging your chances of meeting new people, even though you later complain that you never meet anyone.

Make a list of your standard excuses and examine them for this type of interference.

How Do You Compromise Your Principles to Gain Acceptance?

Like many people, you may substantially compromise your true needs to gain acceptance from others. In doing so, you make your own needs secondary to those accepted by the person or group from which you want to gain favor. As long as you allow this scenario to continue, you will have to circumvent your needs.

Examine your relationships and the social and professional groups to which you belong. Determine if these relationships interfere with your true needs.

Do You Share Your Best Qualities?

What qualities do you have that make your life exciting? These might include the gifts of joy, creativity, spontaneity, openness, fellowship or benevolence. Learn to recognize these qualities in yourself and to share them with others. Allow yourself to experience the benefits and deep appreciation that can come from giving a small part of your life to somebody else.

List your best qualities and describe the ways in which you benefit from sharing these characteristics.

Do You Focus on the Negative?

Many people dwell on what does not work in their lives. They forget that their daily life, for the most part, does indeed work; otherwise they wouldn't be here. They tend to forget the events in life that have fostered their growth and happiness and the moments of true passion. Some people believe they had a terrible childhood, for example, because they allow the bad memories to overshadow the good. As victims of the past, they limit their growth to retaliate against their parents for the things they did not do or the encouragement they did not provide.

List the good things you remember about your childhood. Recall the times your friends and family encouraged, helped and directed you. You will discover a lot more positive instances than you thought. Perhaps your father spent a lot of quality time with you on fishing trips or at ball games while your mother taught you to cook or sew. There's a lot to feel happy and satisfied about when you reflect on positive experiences. By acknowledging these beneficial times, you will appreciate life more than if you allow yourself to be overwhelmed by the negative.

Do You Accept Other People as They Are?

One of the most difficult challenges in life is to allow people to be themselves. Usually we try to make others conform to our perception of what they should be, rather than accept them for who they are and go forward with the relationship. Much time and energy are wasted in relationships due to these minor differences. You must recognize that it's impossible for two people to agree about everything, and then choose your friends according to their overall qualities, not the small details. If you are compatible in the most essential areas—trust, honesty, integrity—this will be the basis of your relationship.

Make a list of your relationships and consider whether or not they meet your fundamental requirements. Can you accept another person for his or her overall characteristics, or are you bogged down in the petty differences?

Do You Respect Other People's Feelings?

Remember that all of your communications should support or enhance your relationships. The way in which you communicate is an active choice. Before you say anything, always ask yourself what it would be like to be on the receiving end of the comment.

It's important to remain aware of this issue in your day-to-day dealings with people. Keep a list of anything you say that's abusive and anything you say to others that you wouldn't like to hear yourself. Then make a commitment to becoming more positive in your communications. You receive the benefits many times over when you give positive input to others.

Do You Have Trouble Making Decisions?

Decision-making becomes extremely difficult when you haven't taken the time to define your needs. Perhaps you walk past a discotheque and feel drawn to go in and dance. But another part of you feels uncomfortable about visiting such places alone. You feel conflicted between an inner desire and your conditioning.

When you're in control, on the other hand, decisions become intuitive. There are no contradictions between your inner nature and your outer actions. You have the confidence to be straightforward in fulfilling your needs.

Do You Have Someone with Whom to Share Your Intimate Self?

True intimacy means that you share your most private and inner thoughts in the most vulnerable and honest way. It is an unfolding of the heart, mind and spirit. It's important to have such a relationship in your life, where you allow someone to see every aspect of your being. There are no inner secrets or hidden agendas; you can be your true self without fear of being judged, corrected or manipulated in the process.

How Can You Recover the Missing Parts of Your Life?

You need to know what's missing in your life before you can go out and find it. If you have not received unconditional love, for example, then you must find someone who has unconditional love to share. Many people like to think that problems and negative situations will correct themselves, but the fact is they never do. You are the driving force behind change in your life; you are the one who must actively seek to fulfill your needs.

Have faith in yourself and the confidence to know that you can form fulfilling relationships and direct your energies toward fulfillment. Identify what's missing in your life by examining the things that bother you. Forget about blaming others for your problems. It's a wasted effort. Take control, find what you want, and then let people know that you exist and are ready to share your positive energies.